IMMUNOLOGY AND IMMUNE SYSTEM DISORDERS

Additional books in this series can be found on Nova's website under the Series tab.

Additional E-books in this series can be found on Nova's website under the E-book tab.

IMMUNOLOGY AND IMMUNE SYSTEM DISORDERS

MAJOR HISTOCOMPATIBILIT[Y] COMPLEX

BIOLOGY, FUNCTIONS AND ROLES IN DISEASE

IMMUNOLOGY AND IMMUNE SYSTEM DISORDERS

MAJOR HISTOCOMPATIBILITY COMPLEX

BIOLOGY, FUNCTIONS AND ROLES IN DISEASE

NATALYA V. SEMILETOVA
EDITOR

Nova Science Publishers, Inc.
New York

For permission to use material from this book please contact us:
Telephone 631-231-7269; Fax 631-231-8175
Web Site: http://www.novapublishers.com

LIBRARY OF CONGRESS CATALOGING-IN-PUBLICATION DATA

ISBN: 978-1-61942-999-4

Library of Congress Control Number: 2012931080

Published by Nova Science Publishers, Inc. † New York

CONTENTS

Preface		**vii**
Chapter 1	Prophylactic and Therapeutic Approach for Adult T-cell Leukemia Based on Targeting Anti-tumor Immunity *Tomohiro Kozako, Shinya Hirata, Makoto Yoshimitsu and Naomichi Arima*	**1**
Chapter 2	MHC Class I Antigens and Tumor Immune Escape *Ping Yu and Chi Lu*	**17**
Chapter 3	MHC Exchange between Cells and its Functional Consequences *Kathryn Brown and Wilson Wong*	**25**
Chapter 4	MHC Diversity and Wildlife Health: Lessons from Tasmanian Devil Facial Tumor Disease *Yuanyuan Cheng and Katherine Belov*	**43**
Chapter 5	TNF Block Haplotypes Reveal Diverse Pathways between TNF and Disease: Implications for Understanding Neuropathy in HIV Patients *Constance S. N. Chew, Fabio P. Valente, Hillary J. Wallace, Joo H. Tan, Suzanah E. Temple, and Patricia Price*	**55**
Chapter 6	MHC, Viral Infection and Immunoinformatics *Maurício Menegatti Rigo, Dinler Amaral Antunes, Marialva Sinigaglia, José Artur Bogo Chies and Gustavo Fioravanti Vieira*	**69**
Chapter 7	HLA-G: Biology, Functions and Roles in Disease *Wei-Hua Yan and Aifen Lin*	**87**
Chapter 8	Non Classical Major Histocompatibility Class I in Health and Disease *Ayman Antoun*	**119**
Chapter 9	HLA Class II Presentation of HLA Class I Binding Antigenic 9mer Peptides *Mingjun Wang, Susanne Rasmussen and Mogens H. Claesson*	**139**

Chapter 10 Immunoregulatory Effect of the Syngeneic Serum Conditioned by Donor-Like sMHC Class I Proteins **153**
Natalya V. Semiletova

Index **175**

PREFACE

This book represents original findings and observations that were made recently on the role and function of MHC proteins in different laboratories around the globe. The articles in this book cover topics from the importance of MHC diversity to the health of the wildlife to intimate molecular mechanisms of MHC exchange between cells. This book will be useful to a wide range of scientists and clinicians who are working in the field of immunology, transplantation and cancer research.

Chapter 1 - Adult T-cell leukemia-lymphoma (ATL) is an aggressive peripheral T-cell neoplasm with a poor prognosis that develops after long-term infection with human T-cell leukemia virus-1 (HTLV-1). Multiple factors (*e.g.* virus, host cells, epigenetic aberrations and immune factors) have been implicated in the development of ATL, although the mechanisms underlying leukemogenesis are not fully understood. Despite recent progress in both chemotherapy and supportive care, the prognosis for ATL is still poor; the overall survival at 3 years is only 24%. Thus, new strategies for the treatment and prophylaxis of ATL (*e.g.* vaccines and novel molecular target agents) are needed. This article reviews new strategies for ATL treatment that target HTLV-1-specific cytotoxic T-lymphocytes (CTLs). HTLV-1-specific CTLs play a critical role in host immune responses against HTLV-1. We describe the decreased frequency and function of HTLV-1-specific CD8+ T cells in ATL patients, and the efficient induction of HTLV-1-specific CTL responses in human leukocyte antigen-A*0201-transgenic mice by the HTLV-1/hepatitis B core chimeric particle and oligomannose-coated liposomes encapsulating HTLV-1 epitopes without adjuvant. The data suggest that efficient antigen delivery systems and CTL induction can be exploited to develop a prophylactic vaccine model against tumors and infectious diseases. These studies suggest that inducing anti-tumor immunity using vaccines may provide a new prophylactic and therapeutic approach for ATL.

Chapter 2 - Tumors are able to evolve survival strategies to “blind” the immune system, so that they could escape from immune elimination and malignancies are progressively developed. A variety of tactics have been utilized by the tumors to exert selective pressure on the local or systemic microenvironment. Up to now, among the reported mechanisms of the tumor immune escape, alterations in the expression of major histocompatibility complex (MHC) class I molecules play a crucial role in the tumor development. MHC class I antigen is involved in the antigen recognition and presentation to T lymphocytes; meanwhile it also indispensably participates in the immune surveillance and regulation of the function of natural killer cells. The loss or down-regulated expression of MHC class I molecules is a customary mechanism for experimental and spontaneous tumors to escape recognition and destruction by T lymphocytes. In this chapter, the most recent studies on the effects of MHC class I antigen in the tumor escape, as well as the important implications for the corresponding design of immunotherapeutic strategies to the cancer, are summarized.

Chapter 3 - The main function of MHC molecules is to present antigenic peptides to T cells in order to evoke an immune response. This is the main mechanism which enables the body's defence system to distinguish between self and non self, in order to fend off invading pathogens. In organ transplantation, this recognition of non-self results in rejection. Recent advances have shown that this view may be over simplistic, as cells can exchange their surface molecules with each other, blurring the boundary between self and non-self. In infection, this may result in non-infected cells presenting foreign peptides to the immune system, which potentially can serve to amplify the process of antigen presentation. In organ transplantation, exchange of MHC molecules between donor and recipient cells results in an added layer of complexity to the immunological response against the donor graft as some cells can express both recipient and donor MHC molecules on their cell surface. The functional consequences of this phenomenon remain to be fully eludicated, but it is likely to have a significant role in the control of the immune system. It may serve as a yet un-recognised tool with which the immune system co-ordinates its response. Here, we describe work to date that demonstrates the extent to which intercellular MHC exchange occurs *in vitro* and *in vivo*, discuss the mechanisms of MHC transfer and the possible consequences. Its implications in different fields within immunology, such as organ transplantation and viral infection, are also highlighted.

Chapter 4 - Genetic variation at the Major Histocompatibility Complex (MHC) plays a key role in defense against infectious diseases. Levels of MHC diversity in wild populations provide an indirect measure of the immunological fitness of that population. Bottlenecked populations with low MHC diversity have limited capability to respond to changes in the environment, especially emergence of new diseases. The recent emergence of a contagious cancer in Tasmanian devils provides a stark example of the effects loss of genetic diversity can have on wildlife species. Devil facial tumor disease (DFTD) is a transmissible cancer that has caused severe population decline in the Tasmanian devil in recent years and is threatening to wipe out the entire species from the wild. DFTD tumor cells are transferred between individuals as allografts without inducing immune rejection. Tumors and devils share the same MHC antigens and hence devils are not able to recognize DFTD cells as non-self. Here we will review our current understanding of the role of the MHC in transmissible cancer and discuss its implications for managing MHC diversity for wildlife conservation.

Chapter 5 - The region spanning the tumor necrosis factor (TNF) cluster in the human major histocompatibility complex (MHC) has been implicated in susceptibility to numerous immunopathological and inflammatory diseases. However, strong linkage disequilibrium in the region creates conserved TNF block haplotypes; hampering identification of specific polymorphisms responsible for disease phenotypes. Here the authors review studies investigating TNF block haplotypes and their links with cytokine production and inflammatory disease risk. Recent work has done much to characterize TNF block haplotypes in different ethnicities and their associations with the larger overall structure of MHC ancestral haplotypes. There have also been studies examining the effects of TNF block haplotypes on levels of inflammatory cytokine production, with others investigating haplotype association with diseases risk. Carriage of specific TNF block haplotypes have been associated with increased risk of Type II Diabetes, Chronic Venous Leg Ulceration and Nucleoside Reverse Transcriptase-associated Sensory Neuropathy, all conditions where the underlying pathogenesis lies in a dysregulated inflammatory response. Despite this, no one haplotype was associated with susceptibility to all these diseases, inferring the TNF block region is involved in the multiple pathways of inflammatory dysregulation leading to disease phenotype. The central MHC on human chromosome 6 spans more than 700 kilobases of DNA and contains in excess of 60 genes, making it one of the most gene-dense regions in the human chromosome. A number of diseases, many of them immunopathological in character, have been associated with variations in MHC genes marked by alleles of the HLA loci. It is thought that whilst there are associations with the HLA class II region of the MHC there are also genes within the central MHC which act in conjunction with the class II genes to mediate susceptibility to these diseases. Some of the genes within the central MHC are well known and characterised. These include the complement genes, the heat shock protein 70 (HSP70) cluster and the tumour necrosis factor (TNF) cluster. Disease pathogenesis may most obviously be influenced by the gene encoding TNF-α. TNF-α confers both protection against infections, but is also implicated in pathological conditions, such as transplant rejection, septic shock, viral replication, rheumatoid arthritis, bacterial infections and Type 1 Diabetes Mellitus (T1DM) depending on the timing, localization and extent of release. Hence anti-TNFα antibodies (Infliximab) are effective in treating rheumatoid arthritis and Crohn's disease, but promote more severe tuberculosis. Inflammatory diseases such as inflammatory bowel disease, multiple sclerosis, rheumatoid arthritis, systemic lupus erythematosus and T1DM show a potential association with TNFα levels. This pro-inflammatory cytokine is an essential component of inflammatory and immune responses, but may be harmful in excess. An interesting example is the 8.1 ancestral haplotype (AH) [HLA -A1, B8, TNFA-308*2, DR3, DQ2]. The broad spectrum of diseases affected by this haplotype [eg: IgA deficiency, T1DM, rapid HIV disease, inclusion body myositis, coeliac disease, myasthenia gravis, Graves disease] suggests it has non-specific immunomodulatory effects. Although the disorders are triggered by different genetic and environmental stimuli and have diverse manifestations, they all involve elevated levels of inflammatory mediators (eg: TNFα). However other diseases with an immunopathological basis associate with other *TNF* haplotypes. Unfortunately the precise gene(s) or polymorphism(s) responsible for these complex disease phenotypes remain unknown, because linkage disequilibrium (LD) creates conserved haplotypes within and across the MHC. Comparisons between haplotypes associated with a disease in multiple ethnic populations may narrow the list of candidate polymorphisms that warrant more detailed study.

Chapter 6 - The immunologic surveillance is performed by several molecules (e.g. antibodies and complement system) and cells (e.g. T lymphocytes, Natural Killer cells) which are triggered depending on the type of infection. In the specific context of the viral infection, a special set of molecules, named Major Histocompatibility Complex of class I (MHC-I), which is represented by the Human Leukocyte Antigen (HLA) genes in humans, perform an essential role. These molecules are responsible for the presentation of small peptides from viruses, parasites, bacteria or even from human proteins to the T Cell Lymphocytes, which will or will not trigger an immune response, through the T Cell Receptor (TCR) interaction. There are two classes of MHC: MHC-I and MHC-II. The MHC-I is responsible for the presentation of small peptides (8-12 amino acids long) generated by endogenous processing, while the MHC-II presents longer peptides (up to 30 amino acids) from exogenous environment. Regarding MHC-I presentation it is known that topologies and electrostatics patterns of the peptide:MHC (pMHC) interacting region are important for TCR recognition. Also, the affinity and stability between the peptide (epitope) and the MHC (receptor) play a crucial role, especially on what concerns electrostatics and non-hydrophobic interactions between the MHC and anchor residues of the peptide. All these features stand for the peptide immunogenicity. The knowledgment of issues regarding peptide affinity by MHC cleft and the stability of resulting complex is pivotal for vaccine development field. Nowadays, there are several immunoinformatics tools available to assist the resolution of this task. For instance, peptide binding affinity could be predicted through several computational methods (i.e. using tools that consider amino acid sequence composition and preferential anchor residues occurrence). There are also bioinformatics tools that are not specific for immunological issues, but can be used for this purpose, such as molecular docking and molecular dynamics. The latter can be used to assess pMHC complex stability, one of the main factors involved in peptide presentation. In the present chapter we intend to review basic molecular aspects regarding the MHC-I molecule and its interaction with different epitopes. Also, the use of immunoinformatics aiming to understand the different levels of MHC-I interaction will be discussed.

Chapter 7 - Human leukocyte antigen G (HLA-G) is a non-classic major histocompatibility complex (MHC) class I molecule that functions as an immune suppressive molecule. HLA-G has direct inhibitory effects on natural killer cells (NK), dendritic cells (DC), T cells by binding to its receptors expressed on these immune cells, and has long-term indirect tolerogenic effects by inducing regulator T cells (Treg) and DCs. HLA-G has been reported to be involved in various physio-pathological conditions such as reproduction, transplantation, autoimmunity, infectious and malignant diseases. Given its tolerant properties, HLA-G expression in the fetal maternal interface during pregnancy and in transplant grafts are of beneficial significance for allogenic fetus and grafts acceptance. On the other hand, induced HLA-G expression in virus infected cells and malignant cells are of harmful outcome for the infection and tumor patients. In the context of clinical aspects, expression of HLA-G in malignant diseases including hematological and solid tumors, infectious diseases and transplantation has been extensively investigated and its relevance to clinico-parameters and potential significance in diagnosis, prognosis and immune target therapy has been postulated. In this chapter, the authors summarized the biology, functions and relevance of HLA-G in disease.

Chapter 8 - Major Histocompatibility Complex (MHC) class I molecules are divided into two major groups, the classical class I (MHC class Ia), which present peptides to T-cells and have a major role in discriminating self from non-self and the non-classical (MHC class Ib) molecules. MHC class Ia and class Ib molecules are similar in their mechanisms of peptide binding and presentation to T-cells. MHC class Ia are considered the most polymorphic molecules in the immune system and direct T cells to kill cells infected with viruses or intracellular bacteria. On the other hand, MHC class Ib are mostly conservative and include several members such as Human leukocyte antigen-E (HLA-E), Human leukocyte antigen-F (HLA-F) and Human leukocyte antigen-G (HLA-G). These molecules act as a bridge between innate and acquired immunity and are characterised by a limited diversity of presented antigens which leads to constraints on the interactions of these molecules with pathogens. They are not only recognized by pathogen-specific T cells but also serve as immune-regulatory molecules by stimulating distinct non-conventional T cell subsets. In this review, the authors examine their expression level and their immunological functions. HLA-E is highly conserved in evolution and we have previously investigated HLA-E gene polymorphisms in three ethnic groups using a polymerase chain reaction-sequence-specific primer method in genomic DNA. They found only two positions in HLA-E to be confirmed as polymorphic (1114 and 1446). These polymorphic positions result in two isoforms proteins expressed by human individuals. The two non-synonymous alleles differ at position 107 and are known as HLA-E^R and HLA-E^G; they differ in their relative peptide affinity and interestingly HLA-E^G expression is higher than that of HLA-E^R. How HLA-E modulates the immune response through interaction with CD94/NKG2 receptors on NK and T-cells will be discussed. HLA-G was initially shown to play a major role in feto–maternal tolerance and it has now been established that HLA-G, as a tolerogenic molecule, participates in the control of the immune response. Finally, the possible role during pregnancy of HLA-F, the least studied member of this family, will be discussed. An overview of the interplay of these non-classical MHC in both health and disease will be elucidated as emerging evidence that they could influence the prognosis of several malignancies.

Chapter 9 - Identification of new antigenic peptides, derived from infectious agents, which bind to human leukocyte antigen (HLA) class I molecules, is of importance for the development of new effective vaccines capable of activating the cellular arm of the immune response. In a search for HLA class I restricted antigenic $CD8^+$ T cell (CTL) epitopes, a computer-based program was used to screen and predict the peptide binding affinity for the recently identified twelve HLA class I supertypes. Peptides derived from *mycobacterium tuberculosis*, vaccinia virus and influenza A protein sequences with a predicted high binding affinity were synthesized, and the binding was biochemically verified and quantified using a recombinant HLA class I molecule-based system.

Chapter 10 - The major histocompatibility complex antigens (MHC) can exist in several forms as membrane complex on all nucleated cells and as soluble form in physiological fluids like blood, tears, saliva, and urine. The three forms of soluble MHC (sMHC) were found in the blood serum: whole heavy chains of class I MHC; MHC molecules lacking the transmembrane and intracellular parts; and molecules merely missing a cytoplasmic tail. Solid organ transplantation stimulates MHC shedding from recipient and donor cellular membranes and it was shown that concentrations of certain forms of sMHC depend on the immunological state of the graft and clinical condition of recipient. Understanding the role of sMHC antigens in the immunoregulation and development of graft chronic rejection is one of the principal goals of organ transplantation. Therapy with donor-like sMHC class I proteins, in conjunction with the short course of CsA, prolonged cardiac graft survival and averted development of chronic rejection in the rat cardiac model of heart transplantation. The tolerant state was characterized by the deviation of alloantibody (allo-Abs) response. This study examines the immunoregulatory effect of the singeneic serum conditioned with sMHC class I proteins on the development of vascular transplant injuries in the MHC disparate cardiac allografts and emergence of protective donor allo-Abs.

In: Major Histocompatibility Complex
Editor: Natalya V. Semiletova

ISBN: 978-1-61942-999-4

Chapter 1

PROPHYLACTIC AND THERAPEUTIC APPROACH FOR ADULT T-CELL LEUKEMIA BASED ON TARGETING ANTI-TUMOR IMMUNITY

Tomohiro Kozako,[1,2*] Shinya Hirata,[3] Makoto Yoshimitsu[4] and Naomichi Arima[2]

[1] Department of Biochemistry, Faculty of Pharmaceutical Sciences, Fukuoka University, Fukuoka, Japan
[2] Division of Hematology and Immunology, Center for Chronic Viral Diseases, Graduate School of Medical and Dental Sciences, Kagoshima University, Kagoshima, Japan
[3] Department of Immunogenetics, Graduate School of Medical Sciences, Kumamoto University, Kumamoto, Japan
[4] Department of Hematology and Immunology, Kagoshima University Hospital, Kagoshima, Japan

ABSTRACT

Adult T-cell leukemia-lymphoma (ATL) is an aggressive peripheral T-cell neoplasm with a poor prognosis that develops after long-term infection with human T-cell leukemia virus-1 (HTLV-1). Multiple factors (*e.g.* virus, host cells, epigenetic aberrations and immune factors) have been implicated in the development of ATL, although the mechanisms underlying leukemogenesis are not fully understood. Despite recent progress in both chemotherapy and supportive care, the prognosis for ATL is still poor; the overall survival at 3 years is only 24%. Thus, new strategies for the treatment and prophylaxis of ATL (*e.g.* vaccines and novel molecular target agents) are needed. This article reviews new strategies for ATL treatment that target HTLV-1-specific cytotoxic T-lymphocytes (CTLs). HTLV-1-specific CTLs play a critical role in host immune responses against HTLV-1. We describe the decreased frequency and function of HTLV-1-specific CD8+ T cells in ATL patients, and the efficient induction of HTLV-1-specific CTL responses in

* Corresponding author: Tomohiro Kozako, PhD; Department of Biochemistry, Faculty of Pharmaceutical Sciences, Fukuoka University; 8-19-1 Nanakuma, Jonan-ku, Fukuoka 814-0180, Japan; Tel: +81-92-871-6631; Fax: +81-92-862-4431; E-mail: kozako@fukuoka-u.ac.jp

human leukocyte antigen-A*0201-transgenic mice by the HTLV-1/hepatitis B core chimeric particle and oligomannose-coated liposomes encapsulating HTLV-1 epitopes without adjuvant. The data suggest that efficient antigen delivery systems and CTL induction can be exploited to develop a prophylactic vaccine model against tumors and infectious diseases. These studies suggest that inducing anti-tumor immunity using vaccines may provide a new prophylactic and therapeutic approach for ATL.

INTRODUCTION

Adult T-cell leukemia/lymphoma (ATL)(Hinuma et al., 1981; Poiesz et al., 1980; Tsukasaki et al., 2009), an aggressive malignancy of mature peripheral T-lymphocytes, and human T-cell lymphotropic virus type I (HTLV-1)-associated myelopathy/tropical spastic paraparesis (HAM/TSP)(Casseb, 2009; Gessain et al., 1985; Osame et al., 1986), a chronic inflammatory disease, are two of the most important diseases associated with long term infection by HTLV-1. HTLV-1 has infected 10–20 million people worldwide, particularly in Equatorial Africa, the Caribbean basin, South America, Melanesia, and southern Japan (Proietti et al., 2005). The lifetime risk of developing ATL or HAM/TSP is estimated to be approximately 2.5%–5% and 0.3%–2%, respectively. The different patterns of clinical disease are thought to be linked to host immunogenetic factors. HTLV-1 is also associated with a variety of autoimmune disorders, including T cell alveolitis, myopathy, uveitis, arthritis, and Sjögren's syndrome (Nishioka et al., 1989; Sugimoto et al., 1987; Terada et al., 1994; Vernant et al., 1988), although the precise relationship between these disorders and HTLV-1 infection remains unclear. Despite recent progress in both chemotherapy and supportive care for hematological malignancies, the median survival time is still only about 13 months (Taylor and Matsuoka, 2005; Tsukasaki et al., 2007; Yamada et al., 2001). Therefore, new strategies for the therapy and prophylaxis of ATL (*e.g.* vaccines and novel molecular target agents) are urgently needed.

Induction of antigen-specific cytotoxic T-lymphocytes (CTLs) is an attractive immunotherapeutic strategy for the treatment of hematologic malignancies and other cancers (Albert et al., 1998; Kawakami et al., 2008). The difficulty in inducing antigen-specific CTLs in individual patients vitiates a more widespread use of adoptive T cell therapy. HTLV-1-specific CTLs also play an important role in suppressing the proliferation of HTLV-1-infected or transformed T-cells *in vitro* (Bangham, 2008; Jacobson et al., 1990). Impaired host CTL function abrogates protection against the accumulation of HTLV-1-transformed cells; thus, circumventing this hurdle may provide an effective immune strategy against leukemogenesis (Harashima et al., 2004; Yasunaga et al., 2001).

The onset of ATL after HTLV-1 infection appears to require a long latency period as the median age at diagnosis ranges from 40 to 60 years in most endemic regions in which mother-child viral transmission is common (Matsuoka and Jeang, 2007). ATL is important with regard to the host immune system in chronic infection and virus-induced malignancy in humans. In this study, we investigated new strategies for ATL treatment based on targeting HTLV-1-specific CTLs.

Decreased Frequency and Function of HTLV-1-Specific CTLs in ATL

Frequency and Function of HTLV-1-Specific CD8+ T-Cell in HTLV-1-Related Diseases

HTLV-1-specific CTLs play an important role in suppressing the proliferation of HTLV-1-infected or transformed T cells *in vitro* (Jacobson et al., 1991; Kannagi et al., 1991). As such, they may prevent the development of ATL (Arnulf et al., 2004; Kannagi et al., 2005). It is possible that CTLs fail to function in a fraction of HTLV-1 carriers with a specific immunogenetic background (Sonoda et al., 1996). Yashiki *et al.* identified the HTLV-1 Tax epitopes recognized by human leukocyte antigen (HLA) class I molecules using peripheral blood mononuclear cells (PMBCs) isolated from asymptomatic HTLV-1 carriers (ACs) and reported that the frequency of HLA alleles lacking epitope anchor motifs (HLA-A*26, HLA-B*4002, HL-B*4006, and HLA-B*4801) was higher in ATL patients than in ACs. These findings suggested that insufficient generation of CTLs allowed the outgrowth of HTLV-1-transformed cells in the host (Yashiki et al., 2001) and that anti-HTLV-1 Tax CTLs may play a key role of in preventing ATL leukemogenesis. However, the *in vivo* condition of anti-HTLV-1 CTLs, both before and after the development of ATL, has yet to be determined.

To characterize anti-HTLV-1 CTLs in ACs and ATL patients, we analyzed the frequency and diversity of HTLV-1-specific CD8+ T-cells within the PBMCs of ACs and ATL patients using 16 distinct epitopes derived from HTLV-1 Tax or Env/HLA tetramers. These epitopes were based on previously identified epitopes (Table 1), along with intracellular cytolytic effector molecules (interferon–gamma (IFN-γ), perforin, and granzyme B). In ACs, 73% of CTLs were Tax11-19/HLA-A*0201-specific tetramer+ and 94% were Tax301-309/HLA-A*2402-specific tetramer+ (Table 1). Some ACs recognized more than one epitope. In contrast, CTLs from ATL patients recognized only Tax 11–19 with HLA-A*0201, and Tax301–309 with HLA-A*2402, at frequencies of 33% and 52%, respectively. Overall, the frequency of Tax-specific CD8+ T-cells was significantly lower in ATL patients than in ACs (57% *vs.* 96%, $p < 0.001$), whereas the difference in the frequency of Env-specific CD8+ T-cells was not significant (Table 2). There was also a significant difference between ACs and ATL patients in terms of the percentage of cells binding Tax11-19/HLA-A*0201 and Tax301-309/HLA-A*2402 tetramers (Figure 1). In contrast, expression of perforin and granzyme B by the anti-HTLV-1 CD8+ T-cells from ATL patients was significantly lower than that of ACs (Kozako et al., 2006). The frequency of Tax-specific CD8+ T-cells was related to the proviral load in ACs carrying HLA-A*0201. These results suggest that decreased frequency, diversity, and function of anti-HTLV-1 Tax CD8+ T-cell clones may be one of the risk factors for ATL development.

To date, there is no report regarding the repertoire of HTLV-1-specific $CD8^+$ T-cells in HAM/TSP patients or carriers with autoimmune diseases (CCs), both of which are characterized by an abnormal immune state. Therefore, to characterize HTLV-1-specific $CD8^+$ T-cells in ACs, HAM/TSP patients and CCs, we examined the frequency and diversity of HTLV-1-specific $CD8^+$ T-cells using HTLV-1 tetramers. HTLV-1 Env-specific $CD8^+$ T-cells were significantly more frequent in HAM/TSP and CCs than in ACs, while the frequency of HTLV-1 Tax-specific $CD8^+$ T-cells was not significantly different (Table 1).

The number of $CD8^+$ cells binding to HTLV-1 Tax tetramers in CCs was significantly less than that in HAM/TSP patients (Fig. 1). These results demonstrate the importance of $CD8^+$ T-cell recognition of HTLV-1 Env-tetramers in HAM/TSP patients and CCs, and suggest that the diversity, frequency and repertoire of HTLV-1 Env-specific $CD8^+$ T-cell clones may be related to the hyper-immune responses in these individuals, although different immunological mechanisms may mediate hyper-immunity in these conditions (Akimoto et al., 2007; Kozako et al., 2011a).

Dysfunction of HTLV-1-Specific CD8+ T-Cells in ATL Patients Mediated *via* the PD-1/PD-L1 Pathway

T cell receptor costimulatory pathways assist in regulating T cell activation and tolerance (Blank and Mackensen, 2007; Greenwald et al., 2005; Sharpe et al., 2007). Membership of the B7-CD28 superfamily has been expanded to include costimulatory and inhibitory T cell receptors such as CD28 and programmed death-1 (PD-1)(Greenwald et al., 2005). Indeed, studies in PD-1-deficient mice indicate that PD-1 serves as a negative regulator of immune responses (Nishimura et al., 1998). The negative regulatory PD-1/programmed death-ligand 1 (PD-L1) pathway has been implicated in the induction of CTL exhaustion during chronic viral infection and tumor escape from host immunity. Studies also suggest that the PD-1/PD-L1 pathway may be operating in virus-specific CD8+ T cells during chronic HIV infection (Day et al., 2006). However, there are no reports regarding PD-1 expression by tumor-associated antigen-specific CTLs in humans. To determine whether the PD-1/PD-L1 pathway is involved in establishing persistent HTLV-1 infection and immune evasion in ATL patients, we examined PD-1/PD-L1 expression in cells from ACs and ATL patients and compared it with that in cells from healthy donors (HDs). The results showed that PD-1 expression by HTLV-1-specific CTLs from ACs and ATL patients was dramatically increased (Figure 2A).

Table 1. Diversity of HTLV-1 epitopes recognized by CTL in ACs, ATL patients, HAM/TSP patients and CCs

Tetramers	HLA allele	HTLV-1 peptide	ACs	ATL	HAM/TSP	CCs
T11	A*0201	Tax11-19	73% (8 / 11)[a]	33% (3 / 9) **	90% (9 / 10)	58% (7 / 12)
T123	A*0201	Tax123-131	9% (1 / 11)	0% (0 / 9)	20% (2 / 10)	42% (5 / 12)
T155	A*0201	Tax155-163	0% (0 / 11)	0% (0 / 9)	10% (1 / 10)	0% (0 / 12)
T178	A*0201	Tax178-186	9% (1 / 11)	0% (0 / 9)	20% (2 / 10)	17% (2 / 12)
T307	A*0201	Tax307-315	9% (1 / 11)	0% (0 / 9)	0% (0 / 10)	0% (0 / 12)
E175	A*0201	Env175-183	0% (0 / 11)	0% (0 / 9)	0% (0 / 10)	8% (1 / 12)
E239	A*0201	Env239-247	0% (0 / 11)	0% (0 / 9)	10% (1 / 10)	17% (2 / 12)
E442	A*0201	Env442-450	0% (0 / 11)	0% (0 / 9)	0% (0 / 10)	17% (2 / 12)
T12	A*2402	Tax12-20	11% (2 / 18)	0% (0 / 23)	13% (2 / 15)	26% (5 / 19)
T187	A*2402	Tax187-195	11% (2 / 18)	0% (0 / 23)	7% (1 / 15)	16% (3 / 19)
T289	A*2402	Tax289-297	0% (0 / 18)	0% (0 / 23)	13% (2 / 15)	16% (3 / 19)
T301	A*2402	Tax301-309	94% (17 / 18)	52% (12 / 23) **	87% (13 / 15)	79% (15 / 19)
T311	A*2402	Tax311-319	0% (0 / 18)	0% (0 / 23)	7% (1 / 15)	5% (1 / 19)
E11	A*2402	Env11-19	6% (1 / 18)	0% (0 / 23)	40% (6 / 15) #	42% (8 / 19) #
E21	A*2402	Env21-29	0% (0 / 18)	0% (0 / 23)	13% (2 / 15)	32% (6 / 19) #
E153	A*2402	Env153-161	0% (0 / 18)	0% (0 / 23)	13% (2 / 15)	21% (4 / 19)
Tax CTL positives			22% (32 / 145)	9% (15 / 160) *	26% (33 / 125)	26% (41 / 155)
Env CTL positives			1% (1 / 87)	0% (0 / 96)	15% (11 / 75) *	25% (23 / 93) *
Total CTL positives			14% (33 / 232)	6% (15 / 256) *	22% (44 / 200) #	26% (64 / 248) **

[a]Epitopes detected by HTLV-1/HLA tetramers/number of tetramers tested.
*, $p<0.001$; **, $p<0.01$; #, $p<0.05$ vs. ACs.

Table 2. The number of subjects positive for HTLV-1-specific CD8+ T cells among ACs, ATL patients, HAM/TSP patients and CCs

HLA allele	Tetramers	ACs	ATL	HAM/TSP	CCs
A*02	Tax	82% (9 / 11)	22% (2 / 9) #	90% (9 / 10)	67% (8 / 12)
A*02	Env	0% (0 / 11)	0% (0 / 9)	10% (1 / 10)	25% (3 / 12)
A*24	Tax	94% (17 / 18)	27% (6 / 22) #	100% (15 / 15)	89% (17 / 19)
A*24	Env	6% (1 / 18)	0% (0 / 22)	40% (6 / 15) #	74% (14 / 19) #
Tax CTL positivities		96% (25 / 26)	57% (16 / 28) #	100% (18 / 18)	81% (22 / 27)
Env CTL positivities		4% (1 / 26)	0% (0 / 28)	50% (9 / 18) #	59% (16 / 27) #

The number of subjects positive for tetramers; tetramer positivity indicates subjects with percentages of HTLV-1/HLA tetramer+ CD8 T cells in the CD8+CD45+ T lymphocytes >0.1%.
#, *p*<0.001 vs. ACs

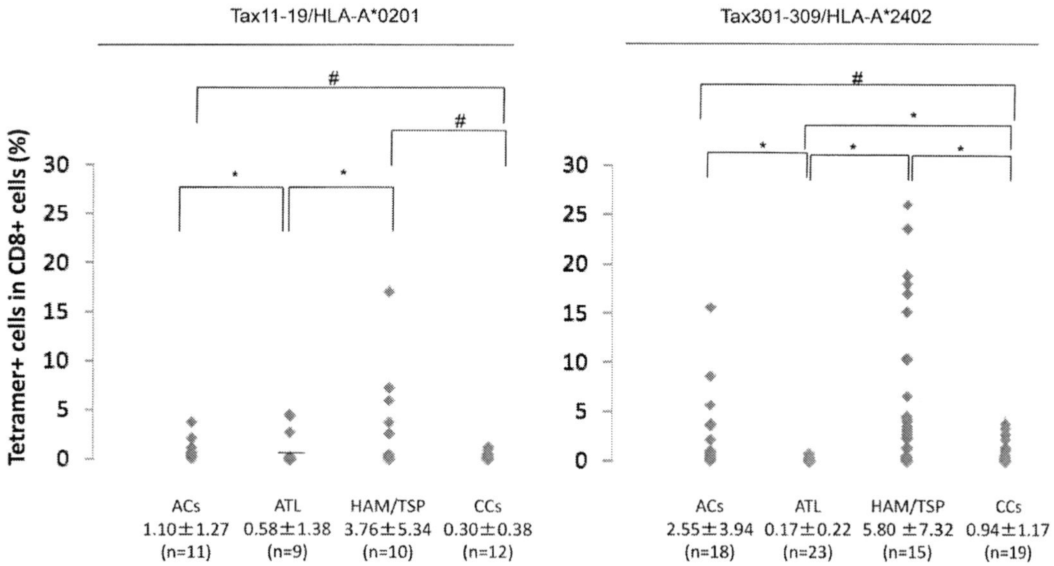

Figure 1. Frequency of Tax11-19/HLA-A*0201 or Tax301-309/HLA-A*0201 tetramer binding CD8+ T cells in ACs, ATL patients, HAM/TSP patients and CCs. The percentage of tetramer+ cells within the CD8+ lymphocyte population from ACs, HAM/TSP patients and CCs. Horizontal bars indicate the mean percentage of tetramer positive cells. The numbers below each subject represent the mean ± SD. *$P < 0.001$; #$P < 0.05$ (Mann-Whitney U test).

In addition, PD-1 expression was significantly higher on CD8+ T-cells (along with cytomegalovirus (CMV)- and Epstein-Barr virus (EBV)-specific CTLs) in ATL patients compared with ACs and HDs. Primary ATL cells in 21.7% of ATL patients expressed PD-L1, but increased expression was not observed in cells from ACs (Kozako et al., 2009b). Finally, in functional studies we observed that an anti-PD-L1 antagonistic antibody up-regulated HTLV-1-specific CD8+ T-cell responses (Figure 2B). These observations suggest that the PD-1/PD-L1 pathway plays a role in fostering persistent HTLV-1 infections, and may support ATL development and facilitate immune evasion by ATL cells.

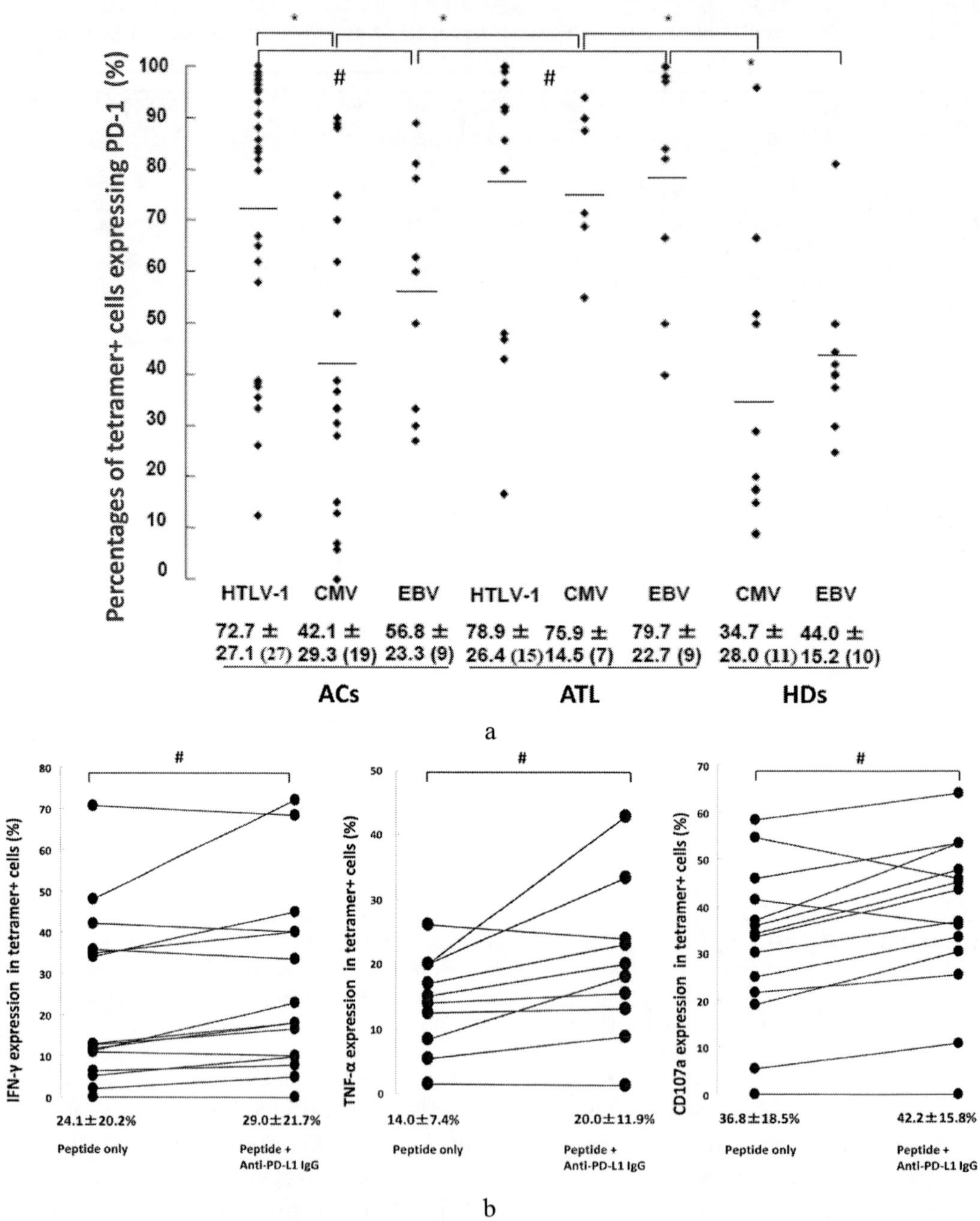

Figure 2. PD-1 expression by virus-specific CD8+ T lymphocytes and blockade of the PD-1/PD-L1 pathway in HTLV-1-specific CD8+ cells. (A) Percentage PD-1 expression by CD8+ lymphocytes from AC, ATL, and HD. Horizontal bars indicate the mean percentage of PD-1-positive cells. The number below each subject represents the mean ± SD. *$P < 0.01$; #$P < 0.05$ (Mann-Whitney U test). (B) Percentage of intracellular cytolytic effector function (IFN-γ and TNF-α) and CD107a —an integral membrane protein in cytolytic granules—expression by HTLV-1-specific CD8+ T lymphocytes treated with peptide or anti-PD-L1 IgG. The numbers represent the mean ± SD. Statistical comparisons were made using the Wilcoxon matched pairs test.

Efficient Induction of HTLV-1-Specific CTLs

Induction of HTLV-1-Specific CTLs by Chimeric Particles without Adjuvant

Antigen-specific CTL induction is an attractive immunotherapeutic strategy for treating hematologic malignancies and other cancers (Albert et al., 1998; Kawakami et al., 2008). The difficulty in inducing antigen-specific CTLs in individual patients supports the more widespread use of adoptive T cell therapy. Whereas free synthetic peptides have proven to be relatively poor immunogens, viral-like particles, such as hepatitis B core (HBc), have been consistently shown to induce strong antibody and CTL responses, even without an adjuvant (Grgacic and Anderson, 2006; Zhang et al., 2009). The HBcAg, a potent immunogen that elicits strong humoral, T-helper and CTL responses that is amenable to a variety of heterologous epitopes without an adjuvant (Milich et al., 1987), is a potentially effective carrier protein for use in T-cell mediated vaccine development (Storni et al., 2002). In the present study, we fused the HTLV-1 Tax11–19 peptide, which is recognized by HLA-A*0201-restricted HTLV-1-specific CD8+ T-cells with high frequency (Kozako et al., 2006), to HBcAg to yield an HTLV-1/HBc chimeric particle (Figures 3A and B).

Immunization of HLA-A*0201 transgenic mice with the chimeric particle induced antigen-specific IFN-γ production as assessed by enzyme-linked immunospot assays, whereas immunization with the epitope peptide alone induced no reaction (Figure 3C). Immunization with the chimeric particle also induced HTLV-1-specific CD8+ T-cells in the spleen and inguinal lymph nodes (Kozako et al., 2009a). Furthermore, dendritic cells (DCs) isolated from HLA-A*0201-transgenic mice exposed to the chimeric particle showed increased expression of CD86, HLA-A02, Toll-like receptor 4 (TLR4) and Major Histocompatibility Complex (MHC) class II (Fig. 4). Also, our results show that HTLV-1-specific CD8+ T cells can be induced by a peptide with HTLV-1/HBc particles from ATL patients, but not by the peptide or HTLV-1/HBc particles alone, and that these HTLV-1-specific CD8+ T cells were able to lyze immune cells presenting the peptide (Kozako et al., 2009a). This suggests that HTLV-1/HBc chimeric particles are capable of inducing strong cellular immune responses without the need for an adjuvant via effective maturation of DCs and is, therefore, potentially useful as an effective carrier for therapeutic vaccines against tumors or infectious diseases.

Oligomannose-Coated Liposomes (OMLs) Efficiently Induce HTLV-1-Specific CTLs

Effective antigen-delivery using OMLs induced the production of T cell helper (Th) subsets and CTLs against ovalbumin antigens encapsulated in the liposomes (Ikehara et al., 2008). OMLs, using human monocytes/macrophages as cellular vehicles, have the potential to target peritoneal micrometastasis in the omentum of gastric cancer patients (Matsui et al., 2010). Thus, OMLs can also be used as an effective antigen delivery system for cancer immunotherapy via activation of CTLs and Th subsets (Fukasawa et al., 1998; Sugimoto et al., 1995). Here, we examined the efficient induction of HTLV-1-specific CD8+ T cell response by OMLs encapsulating the HLA-A*0201-restricted HTLV-1 Tax-epitope (OML/Tax).

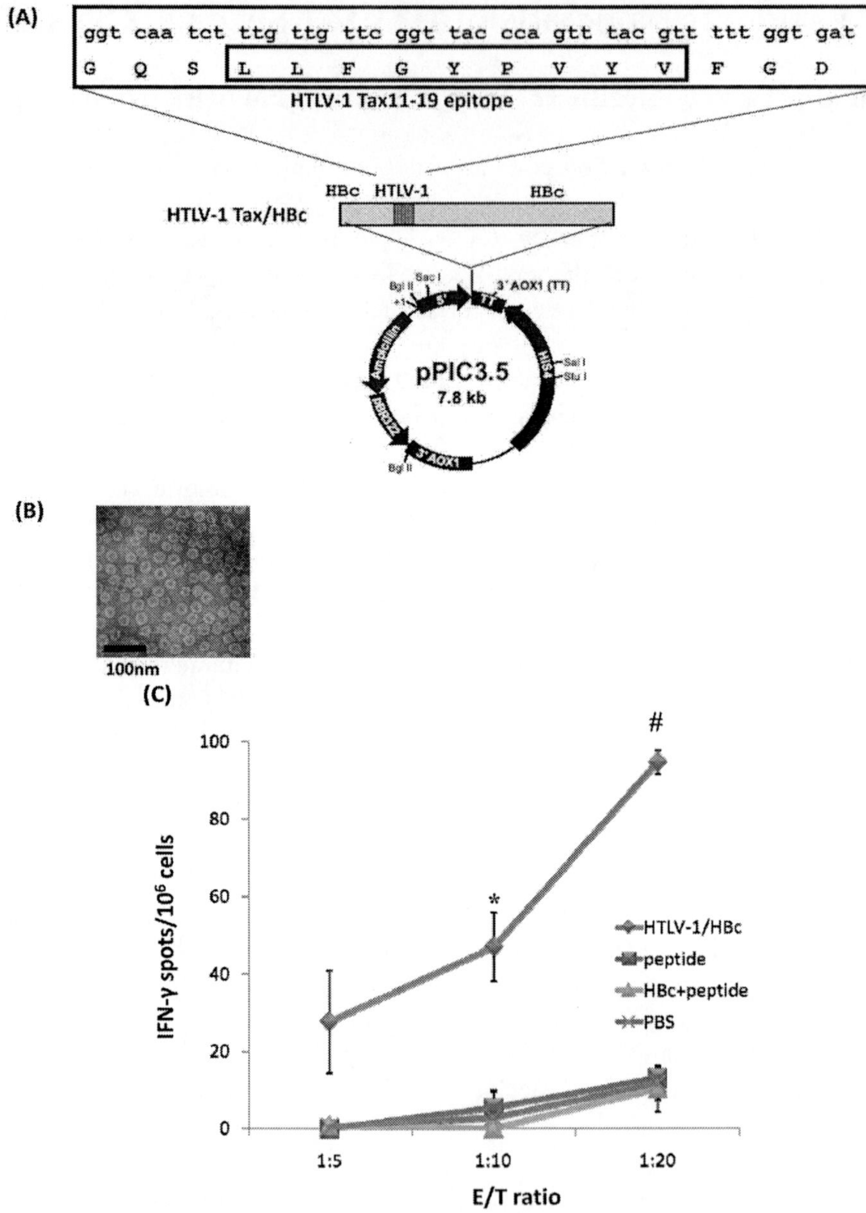

Figure 3. Expression of recombinant HTLV-1/HBc chimeric particles. (A) Construction of the HTLV-1/HBc chimeric protein. (B) Electron micrograph of the HTLV-1/HBc chimeric particle. Original magnification ×100,000. (C) HLA-A*0201 transgenic mice were intradermally immunized twice with HTLV-1/HBc chimeric particles (20 μg), an HTLV-1 peptide (1 μg: LLFGYPVYV), an HTLV-1 peptide (1 μg) plus HBc particles (20 μg), or phosphate buffered saline (PBS) on Day 0 and Day 14. Seven days after the last immunization, the spleens and inguinal lymph nodes were collected. Inguinal lymph node cells (2×10^6/well) were stimulated *in vitro* with the Tax11–19 peptide and, 6 days later, the number of IFN-γ-producing cells per 5, 10, and 20×10^4 inguinal lymph node cells upon stimulation with syngeneic bone marrow derived DCs (1×10^4/well, pulsed with or without each peptide) was determined using an ELISPOT assay. IFN-γ spots were expressed as the number of peptide-loaded to peptide-unloaded target cells. *$P < 0.05$ and #$P < 0.01$ *vs.* PBS group. All experiments were performed in triplicate. Results represent the mean ± S.D. HTLV-1-specific CD8+ T-cell induction from spleen cells.

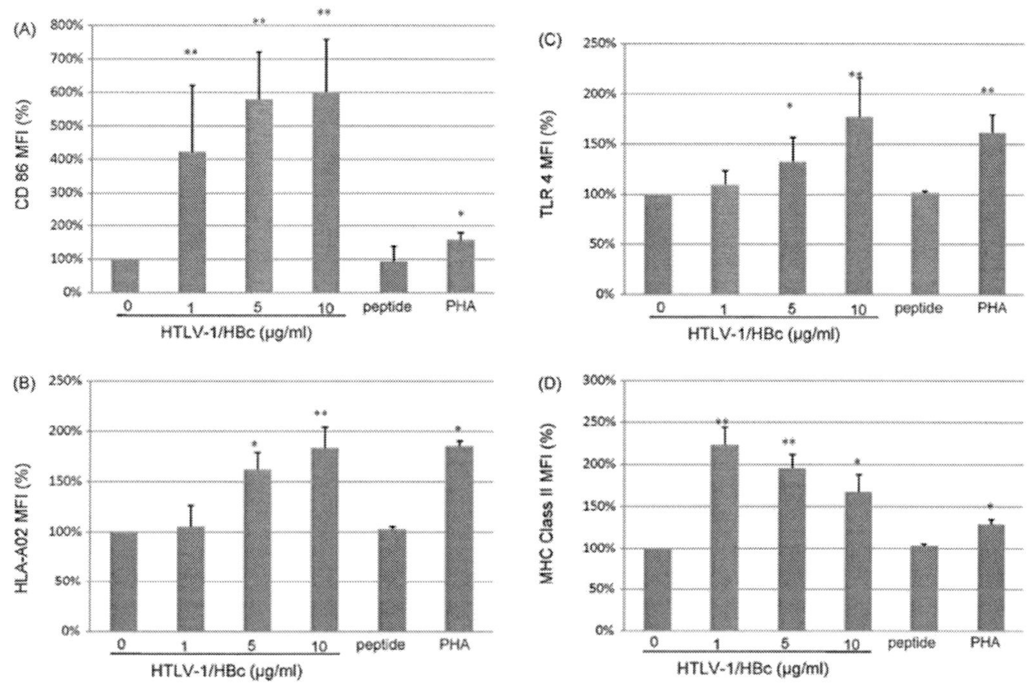

Figure 4. Maturation of DCs induced by HTLV-1/HBc chimeric particles. The maturation of DCs induced by HTLV-1/HBc chimeric particles is illustrated by the expression of CD86 (A), HLA-A02 (B), TLR4 (C) and MHC class II (D) on the surface of DCs after incubation with antigen. Immature DCs (iDC) were incubated with the indicated concentrations of HTLV-1/HBc chimeric particles, 10 μg/ml of HTLV-1 peptide, or 10 μg/ml of phytohemagglutinin (PHA) at 37°C. Data are expressed as the mean fluorescence intensity for each molecule compared with that of non-pulsed (0 μg/ml) iDC controls. Results represent the mean ± SD from four independent experiments. #*P* < 0.05 and ***P* < 0.01 *vs* non-pulsed iDC controls.

Immunization of HLA-A*0201 transgenic mice with OML/Tax induced HTLV-1-specific IFN-γ production, whereas immunization with the epitope peptide alone did not (Fig. 5A). DCs exposed to OML/Tax showed increased expression of CD86, MHC class I, HLA-A02 and MHC class II expression (Kozako et al., 2011b). In addition, HTLV-1-specific CD8+ T cells were efficiently induced by OML/Tax derived from HTLV-1 carriers compared with the epitope peptide alone (Fig. 5B), and these HTLV-1-specific CD8+ T cells were able to lyse immune cells presenting the peptide. These results suggest that OML/Tax induces antigen-specific cellular immune responses without the need for adjuvants and may be an effective vaccine carrier for prophylaxis in tumors and infectious diseases (Kozako et al., 2011b).

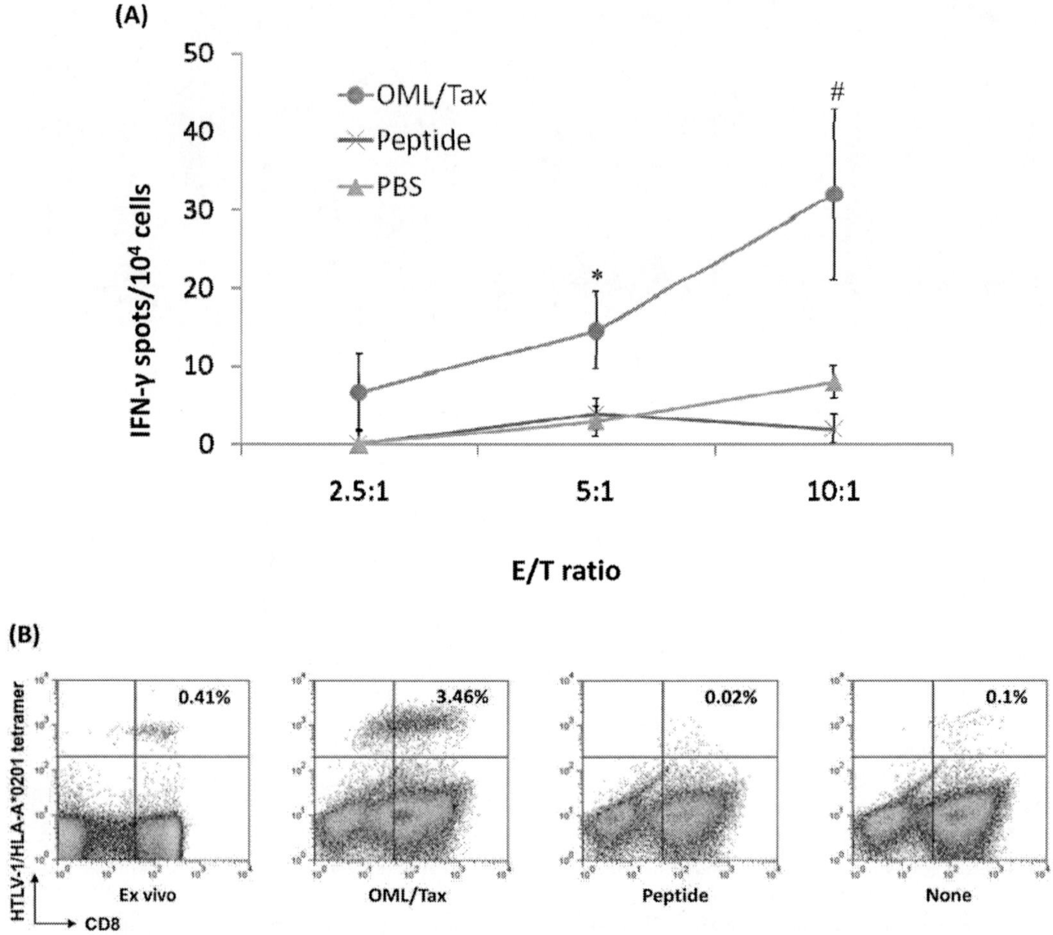

Figure 5. Induction of cellular immunity by intradermal immunization with OML/Tax. (A) HLA-A*0201 transgenic mice ($n = 5$ per group) were intradermally immunized twice with OML/Tax, HTLV-1 peptide (LLFGYPVYV), or PBS on Days 0 and 14. Seven days after the last immunization, the spleens and inguinal lymph nodes were collected. Inguinal lymph node cells (2×10^6/well) were stimulated *in vitro* with HTLV-1 peptide. Six days later, the number of IFN-γ-producing cells per 2.5, 5 or 10×10^4 inguinal lymph node cells upon stimulation with syngeneic bone marrow derived-DCs (1×10^4/well, pulsed with or without each peptide) were determined using an ELISPOT assay. IFN-γ spots were expressed as the number of peptide-loaded to peptide-unloaded target cells. *$P < 0.05$ and #$P < 0.01$ *vs.* PBS group. All experiments were performed in triplicate. Values represent the average from five mice. Results represent the mean ± S.D. (B) Freshly isolated or cryopreserved PBMCs from HTLV-1 carriers were cultured with OML/Tax, peptide alone, or without antigen. The tetramer assay was performed using fresh (*ex vivo*) or cultured PBMCs. The numbers in the upper right quadrants represent the percentage of tetramer+CD8+ T cells within the T lymphocyte population.

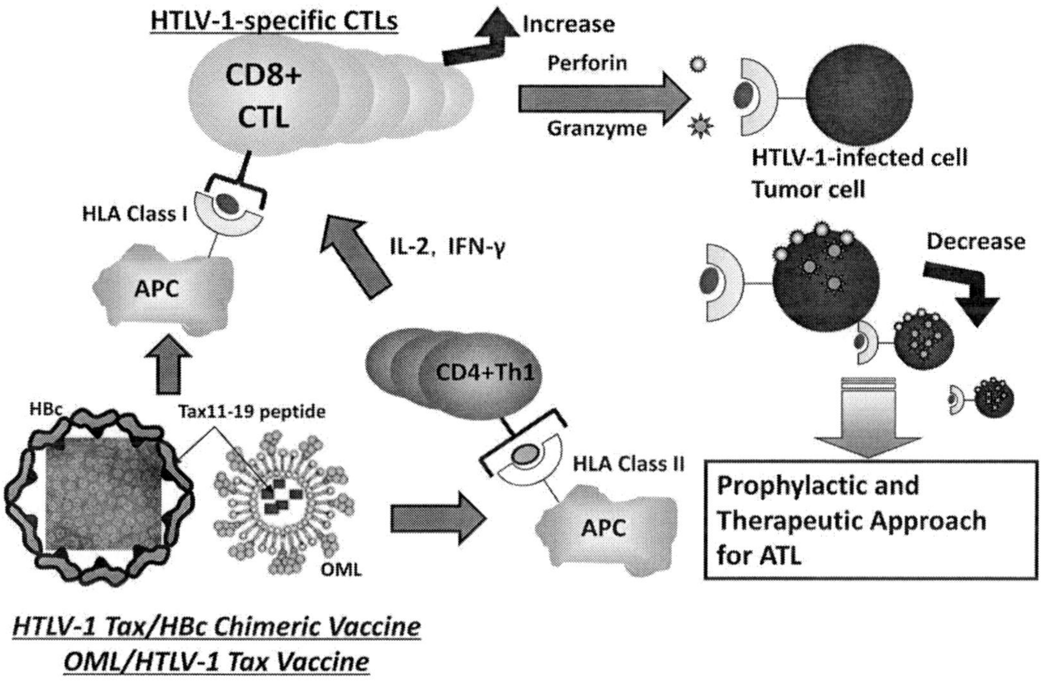

Figure 6. Strategies targeted at inducing anti-tumor immunity for the therapy and prophylaxis of ATL. HTLV-1/HBc chimeric particles and OML/Tax capable of inducing strong cellular immune responses without the need for adjuvants are potentially useful as effective carriers for the prophylaxis and treatment of infectious diseases and tumors, including HTLV-1-infected cells and ATL cells. APC, antigen presenting cell. Th, T cell helper.

Conclusion

The study of ATL is important with regard to human host immune responses during chronic infection and virus-induced malignancy. Although the clinical discovery of ATL was made three decades ago, the results of conventional cytotoxic chemotherapy remain dismal. This is mainly because of low response rates and lack of long-term efficacy. New experimental treatments for ATL now under investigation include hematopoietic stem cell transplantation and molecular targeting by anti-CCR4 antibodies. In addition to these new approaches, inducing anti-tumor immunity using vaccines may provide a new prophylactic and therapeutic approach for ATL.

Acknowledgments

I would like to express my thanks to Dr. Kino Y. and Dr. Fukada K. from The Chemo-Sero-Therapeutic Research Institute (Kumamoto, Japan), Dr. Suzuki S. and Mr. Toji S. from Medical and Biological Laboratories Co. Ltd (Nagoya, Japan), Dr. Sato Y. and Dr. Shimizu Y. from BioMedCore Inc. (Yokohama, Japan) and Dr. Sonoda S. from the Department of International Island and Community Medicine, Kagoshima University (Kagoshima, Japan).

This work was supported in part by a Grant-in-Aid for Scientific Research from the Japan Society for the Promotion of Science and the Japan Leukemia Research Fund.

References

Akimoto M., Kozako T., Sawada T., Matsushita K., Ozaki A., Hamada H., Kawada H., Yoshimitsu M., Tokunaga M., Haraguchi K., Uozumi K., Arima N. and Tei C. (2007) Anti-HTLV-1 tax antibody and tax-specific cytotoxic T lymphocyte are associated with a reduction in HTLV-1 proviral load in asymptomatic carriers. *J. Med. Virol.* 79, 977-86.

Albert M. L., Sauter B. and Bhardwaj N. (1998) Dendritic cells acquire antigen from apoptotic cells and induce class I-restricted CTLs. *Nature.* 392, 86-9.

Arnulf B., Thorel M., Poirot Y., Tamouza R., Boulanger E., Jaccard A., Oksenhendler E., Hermine O. and Pique C. (2004) Loss of the ex vivo but not the reinducible CD8+ T-cell response to Tax in human T-cell leukemia virus type 1-infected patients with adult T-cell leukemia/lymphoma. *Leukemia.* 18, 126-32.

Bangham C. R. (2008) HTLV-1 infection: role of CTL efficiency. *Blood.* 112, 2176-7.

Blank C. and Mackensen A. (2007) Contribution of the PD-L1/PD-1 pathway to T-cell exhaustion: an update on implications for chronic infections and tumor evasion. *Cancer Immunol. Immunother.* 56, 739-45.

Casseb J. (2009) Is human T cell lymphotropic type 1 (HTLV-1)-associated myelopathy/tropical spastic paraparesis (HAM/TSP) syndrome a neglected disease? *PLoS. Negl. Trop Dis.* 3, e487.

Day C. L., Kaufmann D. E., Kiepiela P., Brown J. A., Moodley E. S., Reddy S., Mackey E. W., Miller J. D., Leslie A. J., DePierres C., Mncube Z., Duraiswamy J., Zhu B., Eichbaum Q., Altfeld M., Wherry E. J., Coovadia H. M., Goulder P. J., Klenerman P., Ahmed R., Freeman G. J. and Walker B. D. (2006) PD-1 expression on HIV-specific T cells is associated with T-cell exhaustion and disease progression. *Nature.* 443, 350-4.

Fukasawa M., Shimizu Y., Shikata K., Nakata M., Sakakibara R., Yamamoto N., Hatanaka M. and Mizuochi T. (1998) Liposome oligomannose-coated with neoglycolipid, a new candidate for a safe adjuvant for induction of CD8+ cytotoxic T lymphocytes. *FEBS Lett.* 441, 353-6.

Gessain A., Barin F., Vernant J. C., Gout O., Maurs L., Calender A. and de The G. (1985) Antibodies to human T-lymphotropic virus type-I in patients with tropical spastic paraparesis. *Lancet.* 2, 407-10.

Greenwald R. J., Freeman G. J. and Sharpe A. H. (2005) The B7 family revisited. *Annu. Rev. Immunol.* 23, 515-48.

Grgacic E. V. and Anderson D. A. (2006) Virus-like particles: passport to immune recognition. *Methods.* 40, 60-5.

Harashima N., Kurihara K., Utsunomiya A., Tanosaki R., Hanabuchi S., Masuda M., Ohashi T., Fukui F., Hasegawa A., Masuda T., Takaue Y., Okamura J. and Kannagi M. (2004) Graft-versus-Tax response in adult T-cell leukemia patients after hematopoietic stem cell transplantation. *Cancer Res.* 64, 391-9.

Hinuma Y., Nagata K., Hanaoka M., Nakai M., Matsumoto T., Kinoshita K. I., Shirakawa S. and Miyoshi I. (1981) Adult T-cell leukemia: antigen in an ATL cell line and detection of antibodies to the antigen in human sera. *Proc. Natl. Acad. Sci. U.S.A.* 78, 6476-80.

Ikehara Y., Shiuchi N., Kabata-Ikehara S., Nakanishi H., Yokoyama N., Takagi H., Nagata T., Koide Y., Kuzushima K., Takahashi T., Tsujimura K. and Kojima N. (2008) Effective induction of anti-tumor immune responses with oligomannose-coated liposome targeting to intraperitoneal phagocytic cells. *Cancer Lett.* 260, 137-45.

Jacobson S., Reuben J. S., Streilein R. D. and Palker T. J. (1991) Induction of CD4+, human T lymphotropic virus type-1-specific cytotoxic T lymphocytes from patients with HAM/TSP. Recognition of an immunogenic region of the gp46 envelope glycoprotein of human T lymphotropic virus type-1. *J. Immunol.* 146, 1155-62.

Jacobson S., Shida H., McFarlin D. E., Fauci A. S. and Koenig S. (1990) Circulating CD8+ cytotoxic T lymphocytes specific for HTLV-I pX in patients with HTLV-I associated neurological disease. *Nature.* 348, 245-8.

Kannagi M., Harada S., Maruyama I., Inoko H., Igarashi H., Kuwashima G., Sato S., Morita M., Kidokoro M., Sugimoto M. and et al. (1991) Predominant recognition of human T cell leukemia virus type I (HTLV-I) pX gene products by human CD8+ cytotoxic T cells directed against HTLV-I-infected cells. *Int. Immunol.* 3, 761-7.

Kannagi M., Harashima N., Kurihara K., Ohashi T., Utsunomiya A., Tanosaki R., Masuda M., Tomonaga M. and Okamura J. (2005) Tumor immunity against adult T-cell leukemia. *Cancer. Sci* 96, 249-55.

Kawakami Y., Fujita T., Kudo C., Sakurai T., Udagawa M., Yaguchi T., Hasegawa G., Hayashi E., Ueda Y., Iwata T., Wang Q., Okada S., Tsukamoto N., Matsuzaki Y. and Sumimoto H. (2008) Dendritic cell based personalized immunotherapy based on cancer antigen research. *Front. Biosci.* 13, 1952-8.

Kozako T., Akimoto M., Toji S., White Y., Suzuki S., Arima T., Suruga Y., Matsushita K., Shimeno H., Soeda S., Kubota R., Izumo S., Uozumi K. and Arima N. (2011a) Target epitopes of HTLV-1 recognized by class I MHC-restricted cytotoxic T lymphocytes in patients with myelopathy and spastic paraparesis and infected patients with autoimmune disorders. *J. Med. Virol.* 83, 501-9.

Kozako T., Arima N., Toji S., Masamoto I., Akimoto M., Hamada H., Che X. F., Fujiwara H., Matsushita K., Tokunaga M., Haraguchi K., Uozumi K., Suzuki S., Takezaki T. and Sonoda S. (2006) Reduced frequency, diversity, and function of human T cell leukemia virus type 1-specific CD8+ T cell in adult T cell leukemia patients. *J. Immunol.* 177, 5718-26.

Kozako T., Fukada K., Hirata S., White Y., Harao M., Nishimura Y., Kino Y., Soeda S., Shimeno H., Lemonnier F., Sonoda S. and Arima N. (2009a) Efficient induction of human T-cell leukemia virus-1-specific CTL by chimeric particle without adjuvant as a prophylactic for adult T-cell leukemia. *Mol. Immunol.*

Kozako T., Hirata S., Shimizu Y., Satoh Y., Yoshimitsu M., White Y., Lemonnier F., Shimeno H., Soeda S. and Arima N. (2011b) Oligomannose-coated liposomes efficiently induce human T-cell leukemia virus-1-specific cytotoxic T lymphocytes without adjuvant. *FEBS J.*

Kozako T., Yoshimitsu M., Fujiwara H., Masamoto I., Horai S., White Y., Akimoto M., Suzuki S., Matsushita K., Uozumi K., Tei C. and Arima N. (2009b) PD-1/PD-L1 expression in human T-cell leukemia virus type 1 carriers and adult T-cell leukemia/lymphoma patients. *Leukemia.* 23, 375-82.

Matsui M., Shimizu Y., Kodera Y., Kondo E., Ikehara Y. and Nakanishi H. (2010) Targeted delivery of oligomannose-coated liposome to the omental micrometastasis by peritoneal macrophages from patients with gastric cancer. *Cancer Sci.*

Matsuoka M. and Jeang K. T. (2007) Human T-cell leukaemia virus type 1 (HTLV-1) infectivity and cellular transformation. *Nat. Rev. Cancer.* 7, 270-80.

Milich D. R., McLachlan A., Thornton G. B. and Hughes J. L. (1987) Antibody production to the nucleocapsid and envelope of the hepatitis B virus primed by a single synthetic T cell site. *Nature.* 329, 547-9.

Nishimura H., Minato N., Nakano T. and Honjo T. (1998) Immunological studies on PD-1 deficient mice: implication of PD-1 as a negative regulator for B cell responses. *Int. Immunol.* 10, 1563-72.

Nishioka K., Maruyama I., Sato K., Kitajima I., Nakajima Y. and Osame M. (1989) Chronic inflammatory arthropathy associated with HTLV-I. *Lancet.* 1, 441.

Osame M., Usuku K., Izumo S., Ijichi N., Amitani H., Igata A., Matsumoto M. and Tara M. (1986) HTLV-I associated myelopathy, a new clinical entity. *Lancet.* 1, 1031-2.

Poiesz B. J., Ruscetti F. W., Gazdar A. F., Bunn P. A., Minna J. D. and Gallo R. C. (1980) Detection and isolation of type C retrovirus particles from fresh and cultured lymphocytes of a patient with cutaneous T-cell lymphoma. *Proc. Natl. Acad. Sci. U. S. A.* 77, 7415-9.

Proietti F. A., Carneiro-Proietti A. B., Catalan-Soares B. C. and Murphy E. L. (2005) Global epidemiology of HTLV-I infection and associated diseases. *Oncogene.* 24, 6058-68.

Sharpe A. H., Wherry E. J., Ahmed R. and Freeman G. J. (2007) The function of programmed cell death 1 and its ligands in regulating autoimmunity and infection. *Nat. Immunol.* 8, 239-45.

Sonoda S., Fujiyoshi T. and Yashiki S. (1996) Immunogenetics of HTLV-I/II and associated diseases. *J. Acquir. Immune Defic. Syndr. Hum. Retrovirol.* 13 Suppl 1, S119-23.

Storni T., Lechner F., Erdmann I., Bachi T., Jegerlehner A., Dumrese T., Kundig T. M., Ruedl C. and Bachmann M. F. (2002) Critical role for activation of antigen-presenting cells in priming of cytotoxic T cell responses after vaccination with virus-like particles. *J. Immunol.* 168, 2880-6.

Sugimoto M., Nakashima H., Watanabe S., Uyama E., Tanaka F., Ando M., Araki S. and Kawasaki S. (1987) T-lymphocyte alveolitis in HTLV-I-associated myelopathy. *Lancet.* 2, 1220.

Sugimoto M., Ohishi K., Fukasawa M., Shikata K., Kawai H., Itakura H., Hatanaka M., Sakakibara R., Ishiguro M., Nakata M. and et al. (1995) Oligomannose-coated liposomes as an adjuvant for the induction of cell-mediated immunity. *FEBS Lett.* 363, 53-6.

Taylor G. P. and Matsuoka M. (2005) Natural history of adult T-cell leukemia/lymphoma and approaches to therapy. *Oncogene.* 24, 6047-57.

Terada K., Katamine S., Eguchi K., Moriuchi R., Kita M., Shimada H., Yamashita I., Iwata K., Tsuji Y., Nagataki S. and et al. (1994) Prevalence of serum and salivary antibodies to HTLV-1 in Sjogren's syndrome. *Lancet.* 344, 1116-9.

Tsukasaki K., Hermine O., Bazarbachi A., Ratner L., Ramos J. C., Harrington W., Jr., O'Mahony D., Janik J. E., Bittencourt A. L., Taylor G. P., Yamaguchi K., Utsunomiya A., Tobinai K. and Watanabe T. (2009) Definition, prognostic factors, treatment, and response criteria of adult T-cell leukemia-lymphoma: a proposal from an international consensus meeting. *J. Clin. Oncol.* 27, 453-9.

Tsukasaki K., Utsunomiya A., Fukuda H., Shibata T., Fukushima T., Takatsuka Y., Ikeda S., Masuda M., Nagoshi H., Ueda R., Tamura K., Sano M., Momita S., Yamaguchi K., Kawano F., Hanada S., Tobinai K., Shimoyama M., Hotta T. and Tomonaga M. (2007) VCAP-AMP-VECP compared with biweekly CHOP for adult T-cell leukemia-lymphoma: Japan Clinical Oncology Group Study JCOG9801. *J. Clin. Oncol.* 25, 5458-64.

Vernant J. C., Buisson G., Magdeleine J., De Thore J., Jouannelle A., Neisson-Vernant C. and Monplaisir N. (1988) T-lymphocyte alveolitis, tropical spastic paresis, and Sjogren syndrome. *Lancet.* 1, 177.

Yamada Y., Tomonaga M., Fukuda H., Hanada S., Utsunomiya A., Tara M., Sano M., Ikeda S., Takatsuki K., Kozuru M., Araki K., Kawano F., Niimi M., Tobinai K., Hotta T. and Shimoyama M. (2001) A new G-CSF-supported combination chemotherapy, LSG15, for adult T-cell leukaemia-lymphoma: Japan Clinical Oncology Group Study 9303. *Br. J. Haematol.* 113, 375-82.

Yashiki S., Fujiyoshi T., Arima N., Osame M., Yoshinaga M., Nagata Y., Tara M., Nomura K., Utsunomiya A., Hanada S., Tajima K. and Sonoda S. (2001) HLA-A*26, HLA-B*4002, HLA-B*4006, and HLA-B*4801 alleles predispose to adult T cell leukemia: the limited recognition of HTLV type 1 tax peptide anchor motifs and epitopes to generate anti-HTLV type 1 tax CD8(+) cytotoxic T lymphocytes. *AIDS Res. Hum. Retroviruses.* 17, 1047-61.

Yasunaga J., Sakai T., Nosaka K., Etoh K., Tamiya S., Koga S., Mita S., Uchino M., Mitsuya H. and Matsuoka M. (2001) Impaired production of naive T lymphocytes in human T-cell leukemia virus type I-infected individuals: its implications in the immunodeficient state. *Blood.* 97, 3177-83.

Zhang S., Cubas R., Li M., Chen C. and Yao Q. (2009) Virus-like particle vaccine activates conventional B2 cells and promotes B cell differentiation to IgG2a producing plasma cells. *Mol. Immunol.* 46, 1988-2001.

In: Major Histocompatibility Complex
Editor: Natalya V. Semiletova
ISBN: 978-1-61942-999-4

Chapter 2

MHC CLASS I ANTIGENS AND TUMOR IMMUNE ESCAPE

***Ping Yu*[1*] *and Chi Lu*[2]**
[1] Metabolism Branch, National Cancer Institute,
National Institutes of Health, Bethesda, MD, US
[2] Department of Electrical and Computer Engineering and Center for Nanoscale Science and Engineering, University of Kentucky,
Lexington, KY, US

ABSTRACT

Tumors are able to evolve survival strategies to "blind" the immune system, so that they could escape from immune elimination and malignancies are progressively developed. A variety of tactics have been utilized by the tumors to exert selective pressure on the local or systemic microenvironment. Up to now, among the reported mechanisms of the tumor immune escape, alterations in the expression of major histocompatibility complex (MHC) class I molecules play a crucial role in the tumor development. MHC class I antigen is involved in the antigen recognition and presentation to T lymphocytes; meanwhile it also indispensably participates in the immune surveillance and regulation of the function of natural killer cells. The loss or down-regulated expression of MHC class I molecules is a customary mechanism for experimental and spontaneous tumors to escape recognition and destruction by T lymphocytes. In this chapter, the most recent studies on the effects of MHC class I antigen in the tumor escape, as well as the important implications for the corresponding design of immunotherapeutic strategies to the cancer, are summarized.

Keywords: Major histocompatibility complex (MHC); tumor immunology; immune escape; epigenetic regulations

* Corresponding author: Ping Yu, M.D., Ph. D.; Building 10, Room 4N112; 10 Center Drive, Bethesda, MD 20892-1374; TEL: (301) 435-8322; FAX: (301) 496-9956; E-mail: yuping2@mail.nih.gov

Introduction

Accumulated evidence has indicated that the occurrence of tumor, at least in early stages of tumor development, is not due to the existence of a deteriorated immune system but rather to the newly developed genetic and phenotypic characteristics, using which the cancer cells could escape anti-tumor immune responses [1-3]. One of the general mechanisms that tumors adopt to escape from T-cell-mediated immune attack is the down-regulation of surface expression of major histocompatibility complex (MHC) class I molecules. This has been regarded as a common obstacle to the development of effective antitumor immunotherapy or vaccination. Therefore, approaches considering distinct cell surface expression of the MHC class I molecules on the tumors are essential and critical in order to achieve optimal therapeutic effects.

Major Histocompatibility Complex Class I Molecules

MHC class I molecules bind antigens in the form of peptides that are presented to cytotoxic T-lymphocytes (CTL) on the surface of tumor or virus-infected cells. MHC class I molecules include the classical (class Ia) human leukocyte antigens (HLA)-A, -B, and -C antigens in humans and H-2K, D, and L in mice, as well as the nonclassical (class Ib) E, F, and G in humans and Qa and Tla antigens in mice [4]. They form a tri-molecular complex consisting of a 45-kDa heavy chain, a peptide antigen, and a non-polymorphic 12-kDa β2-microglobulin (β2-m) light chain. The HLA-A, -B, and -C and the H-2K, D, and L are highly polymorphic [5]. In humans, MHC class I molecules are encoded by genes located within the MHC region on chromosome 6, whereas β2-m is encoded by a gene mapped on chromosome 15. In mice, these antigens are encoded in chromosome 17 and chromosome 2, respectively. The classical HLA/H-2 class I molecules are expressed on the surface of most mammalian cells with only a few exceptions [6]. It is estimated that there are up to 250,000 of each HLA class I molecule on the surface of a somatic cell [7].

Major Histocompatibility Complex Class I Molecule Down-Regulation as a Mechanism of Tumor Cell Escape from Immune Defenses

Tumor cells with high level of MHC class I expression are targets being attacked by adaptive immune response mediated by CD8 T cells. Studies concerning HLA class I expression in surgically removed tumors have strongly supported that the majority of the tumor cells, including both primary and metastatic tumors, may escape from immune-surveillance by down-regulating MHC class I expression and this could represent a general mechanism by which cells escape from specific $CD8^+$ T-cell mediated immune responses [8-12]. In a study on endometrial cancers, MHC class I down-modulation was correlated with worse disease-specific survival and, importantly, with poorly differentiated or undifferentiated tumors [13].

On the other hand, while down-regulation of MHC class I molecule could escape from CD8-T cells lysis, the complete MHC class I-deficient tumors have to deal with innate immune responses owing to the 'missing self' recognition. Natural killer (NK) cells have both activation and inhibition receptors on the surface and thus the fate of MHC class I-deficient tumor cells depends on the ratio of positive to negative signals received by NK cells. In other words, the involvement of MHC class I-restricted and unrestricted effectors depends not only on the cell surface expression levels of activators and inhibitors but also on their ratios [14]. Furthermore, the growing tumors may not be infiltrated by NK cells in sufficient numbers to initiate effective immune response [15]. In general, growing tumors may therefore represent variants that escape from innate immunity and specific adaptive immunity mediated by CD8 T-cells [16].

INDUCTION OF MAJOR HISTOCOMPATIBILITY COMPLEX CLASS I EXPRESSION AND EPIGENETIC REGULATIONS

Since a significant proportion of MHC class I defects on tumor cells are caused by silencing the relevant genes rather than by the deletion or aberration, approaches that could induce the MHC class I molecule re-expression on the tumor cells might be optimal to cope with the down-regulation of MHC class I molecules by tumors [15]. This can be achieved by immunotherapy or some chemotherapeutic approaches, or gene therapy. Next we will summarize certain immunotherapies against the down-regulation MHC class I molecule on the tumors.

In both preclinical and clinical studies, it has been suggested that the MHC class I expression on the tumor cells can be induced by administrating cytokines. Unfortunately, systemic provision of cytokines will lead to severe adverse effects and the clinical application is therefore restricted. Further studies have reported that only low doses of cytokine administration could be considered for patient treatments. Since IFN-gamma is the most powerful cytokine mediating MHC class I up-regulation, potential benefits from MHC class I up-regulation by low doses of IFN-gamma have been demonstrated in preclinical studies on mice [17] as well as in patients with metastatic malignant melanoma [18]. The mechanism that IFN-gamma up-regulates MHC class I expression is due to that IFN-gamma can induce multiple gene expressions that are related to MHC class I antigen processing and presentation. In brief, controlled IFN-gamma binds to IFN receptors, and then activates JAK1/JAK2/STAT1 signal transduction via phosphorylation of JAK and STAT1 in cells. Sequentially, phosphorylated STAT1 initiates the expression of interferon regulatory factor 1 (IRF-1) and IRF-1 triggers the MHC class I antigen presentation-associated gene to up-regulate MHC class I molecule on the surface. Through activating JAK/STAT1 signal transduction pathway, IFN-gamma effectively up-regulates MHC class I antigen expression on the tumor cells [19-22].

Meanwhile, along with IFN-gamma, some other cytokines, such as IL-2 or IL-12, could function indirectly through the activation of immune cells, which subsequently produce IFN-gamma. B16 melanoma cells produced by IL-2 is able to activate NK cells or tumor-associated macrophages, and then up-regulate MHC class I expression on tumor cells by mechanisms involving IFN-gamma production [23, 24]. Several studies have demonstrated the efficacy of cellular vaccines based on tumor cells engineered to produce GM-CSF, IL-12 or TNF-alpha cytokines, in a prophylactic setting in murine models [25-28].

Besides MHC class I up-regulation, cytokine is also capable of inducing NKG2D ligand expression, up-regulating expression of MHC class II molecules, as well as increasing co-stimulatory molecules or adhesive molecules, to enhance antigen presentation and immune response [29, 30]. Improvements in the tumor microenvironment could increase NK and CTL cell infiltration, finally leading to the improvement of antitumor effects.

For MHC class I-deficient tumor cells, the immune responses against tumors depend on the levels of residual expression of the MHC class I molecules on tumor cells and the inducibility of MHC class I expression, as well as on the expression of ligands for NK-cell receptors. Expression of co-stimulatory molecules on tumor cells is also crucial for the development of an efficient antitumor response against poorly immunogenic MHC class I-deficient tumors. In the murine tumor model, CD70/CD80-transfected tumor cells were effectively rejected compared to parental tumor cells; the co-administration of CD70/CD80 gene-modified tumor cells with the IL-12-producing cells appeared to be effective against parental MHC class I-deficient B16F10 tumors [31].

In the clinic, radiotherapy has been widely used to against variable tumors. The irradiation not only eliminates tumor cells directly, but also substantially increases the sensitivity of tumor cells to T cell cytotoxic effects. It has been reported that irradiation induces long-lasting MHC class I expression on human melanoma cell line in a dose-dependent manner [32]. Moreover, irradiation leads to cell damages, which would generate altered intracellular peptide pools and increase the antigen processing and presentation.

In brief, multiple therapeutic pathways have beneficial impacts on anti-tumor activities through up-regulating MHC class I on the tumor cells. Both the experimental and clinical studies have strongly suggested the importance of this MHC class I up-regulation, especially in combined chemo-immunotherapy.

Conclusion

It is of particular interest to develop immunotherapeutic strategies against various tumors regardless of their MHC class I expression status. Data from preclinical and clinical studies have emphasized the critical role that MHC class I molecules play on the tumor cells in tumors escaping from immune responses. Meanwhile, therapeutic strategies including immunotherapies and chemotherapies, which lead to robust immune responses, are required to cope with weakly immunogenic tumors in spite of their MHC class I status. Up-regulation of MHC class I expression through the administration of cytokine as well as epigenetic regulations may become an attractive modality to achieve enhanced efficacy against tumors.

Reviewed by

Yizhen Chen, Ph.D.
Baylor College of Medicine, Dept. of Molecular and Cellular Biology,
Mail Stop: BCM130, Room: BCMD-325D,One Baylor Plaza, Houston, Texas 77030

REFERENCES

[1] Mareel M, van Roy FM, de Baetseiller P. The invasive phenotypes. *Cancer Metastasis Rev. 1990,* **9**, 45–62.

[2] Seymour K, Pettit S, O'Flaherty E, Charnley RM, Kirby JA. Selection of metastatic tumor phenotypes by host immune system. *Lancet* 1999, **353**, 1989–1991.

[3] Villunger A, Strasser A. The great escape: Is evasion required for tumour progression? *Nat. Med. 1999,* **5**, 874–875.

[4] Bjorkman PJ, Saper MA, Samraoui B, Bennett WS, Strominger JL, Wiley DC. Structure of the human class I histocompatibility antigen, HLA-A2. *Nature 1987,* **329**, 506–512.

[5] Bjorkman PJ, Parham P. Structure, function, and diversity of class I major histocompatibility complex molecules. *Annu. Rev. Biochem.* 1990, **59**, 253–288.

[6] Le Bouteiller P. HLA class I chromosomal region, genes, and products: Facts and questions. *Crit. Rev. Immunol. 1994,* **14**, 89–129.

[7] Parham P, Ohta T. Population biology of antigen presentation by MHC class I molecules. *Science* 1996, **272**, 67–74.

[8] Hicklin DJ, Marincola FM, Ferrone S. HLA class I antigen downregulation inhuman cancers: T-cell immunotherapy revives an old story. *Mol. Med. Today* 1999, *5*, 178–186.

[9] Garrido F, Ruiz-Cabello F, Cabrera T, Pérez-Villar JJ, López-Botet M, Duggan-Keen M, Stern PL. Implications for immunosurveillance ofaltered HLA class I phenotypes in humantumours. *Immunol. Today* 1997, *18*, 89–95.

[10] Khong HT, Restifo NP. Natural selection of tumor variants in the generation of "tumor escape" phenotypes. *Immunology* 2002, *3*, 999–1005.

[11] Seliger B, Ritz U, Ferrone S. Molecular mechanisms of HLA class I antigen abnormalities following viral infection and transformation. *Int. J. Cancer* 2006, *118*, 129–138.

[12] Bubeník J. Prospects for immunotherapy of MHC class I-deficient tumours. *Folia. Biol. (Praha)* 2002, *49*, 95–99.

[13] Bijen CB, Bantema-Joppe EJ, de Jong RA, Leffers N, Mourits MJ, Eggink HF, van der Zee AG, Hollema H, de Bock GH, Nijman HW. The prognostic role of classical and nonclassical MHC class I expression in endometrial cancer. *Int. J. Cancer* 2010, *126*, 1417–1427.

[14] Reinis M. Immunotherapy of MHC class I-deficient tumors. *Future Oncol.* 2010, *6*, 1577–1589.

[15] Menon AG, Janssen-van Rhijn CM, Morreau H, Putter H, Tollenaar RA, van de Velde CJ, Fleuren GJ, Kuppen PJ. Immune system and prognosis in colorectal cancer: a detailed immunohistochemical analysis. *Lab. Invest.* 2004, *84*, 493–501.

[16] Bubenik J. Tumor MHC class I downregulation and immunotherapy. *Oncol. Rep.* 2003, *10*, 2005–2008.

[17] Martini M, Testi MG, Pasetto M, Picchio MC, Innamorati G, Mazzocco M, Ugel S, Cingarlini S, Bronte V, Zanovello P, Krampera M, Mosna F, Cestari T, Riviera AP, Brutti N, Barbieri O, Matera L, Tridente G, Colombatti M, Sartoris S. IFN-gamma-mediated up-modulation of MHC class I expression activates tumor-specific immune response in a mouse model of prostate cancer. *Vaccine* 2010, *28*, 3548–3557.

[18] Propper DJ, Chao D, Braybrooke JP, Bahl P, Thavasu P, Balkwill F, Turley H, Dobbs N, Gatter K, Talbot DC, Harris AL, Ganesan TS. Low-dose IFN-g induces tumor MHC expression in metastatic malignant melanoma. *Clin. Cancer Res.* 2003, *9*, 84–92.

[19] Fruh K, Yang Y. Antigen presentation by MHC class I and its regulation by interferon gamma. *Curr. Opin. Immunol.* 1999, *11*, 76–81.

[20] Baldeon ME, Neece DJ, Nandi D, Monaco JJ, Gaskins HR. Interferon-gamma independently activates the MHC class I antigen processing pathway and diminishes glucose responsiveness in pancreatic beta-cell lines. *Diabetes* 1997, *46*, 770–778.

[21] Fujimaki H, Hikawa N, Nagoya M, Nagata T, Minami M. IFN-gamma induces expression of MHC class I molecules in adult mouse dorsal root ganglion neurones. *NeuroReport* 1996, *7*, 2951–2955.

[22] Fang Z. Molecular mechanisms of IFN-γ to up-regulate MHC class I antigen processing and presentation. *Int. Rev. Immunol.* 2009, *28*, 239–260.

[23] Kijima M, Saio M, Oyang GF, Suwa T, Miyauchi R, Kojima Y, Imai H, Nakagawa J, Nonaka K, Umemura N, Nishimura T, Takami T. Natural killer cells play a role in MHC class I in vivo induction in tumor cells that are MHC negative in vitro. *Int. J. Oncol.* 2005, *26*, 679–684.

[24] Ouyang GF, Saio M, Suwa T, Imai H, Nakagawa J, Nonaka K, Umemura N, Kijima M, Takami T. Interleukin-2 augmented activation of tumor associated macrophage plays the main role in MHC class I in vivo induction in tumor cells that are MHC negative in vitro. *Int. J. Oncol.* 2006, *28*, 1201–1208.

[25] Grant JF, Iwasawa T, Sinn HW, Siemens DR, Griffith TS, Takacs EB, Ratliff TL. Induction of protective immunity to RM-1 prostate cancer cells with ALVAC-IL-2/ IL-12/TNF-a combination therapy. *Int. J. Cancer* 2006, *119*, 2632–2641.

[26] Nanni P, Rossi I, De Giovanni C, Landuzzi L, Nicoletti G, Stoppacciaro A, Parenza M, Colombo MP, Lollini PL. Interleukin 12 gene therapy of MHC negative murine melanoma metastases. *Cancer Res.* 1998, *58*, 1225–1230.

[27] Levitsky HI, Lazenby A, Hayashi RJ, Pardoll DM. *In vivo* priming of two distinct antitumor effector populations: the role of MHC class I expression. *J. Exp. Med.* 1994, *179*, 1215–1224.

[28] Lasek W, Mackiewicz A, Czajka A, Switaj T, Goł b J, Wiznerowicz M, Korczak-Kowalska G, Bakowiec-Iskra EZ, Gryska K, Izycki D, Jakóbisiak M. Antitumor effects of the combination therapy with TNF-a gene-modified tumor cells and interleukin 12 in a melanoma model in mice. *Cancer Gene Ther.* 2000, *7*, 1581–1590.

[29] Tomasi TB, Magner WJ, Khan AN. Epigenetic regulation of immune escape genes in cancer. *Cancer Immunol. Immunother.* 2006, *55*, 1159–1184.

[30] Cheng WF, Hung CF, Lin KY, Ling M, Juang J, He L, Lin CT, Wu TC. CD8+ T cells, NK cells and IFN-g are important for control of tumor with downregulated MHC class I expression by DNA vaccination. *Gene Ther.* 2003, *10*, 1311–1320.

[31] Douin-Echinard V, Bornes S, Rochaix P, Tilkin AF, Peron JM, Bonnet J, Favre G, Couderc B. The expression of CD70 and CD80 by gene-modified tumor cells induces an antitumor response depending on the MHC status. *Cancer Gene Ther.* 2000, *7*, 1543–1556.

[32] Reits EA, Hodge JW, Herberts CA, Groothuis TA, Chakraborty M, Wansley EK, Camphausen K, Luiten RM, de Ru AH, Neijssen J, Griekspoor A, Mesman E, Verreck FA, Spits H, Schlom J, van Veelen P, Neefjes JJ. Radiation modulates the peptide repertoire, enhances MHC class I expression, and induces successful antitumor immunotherapy. *J. Exp. Med.* 2006, *203*, 1259–1271.

In: Major Histocompatibility Complex
Editor: Natalya V. Semiletova
ISBN: 978-1-61942-999-4

Chapter 3

MHC Exchange between Cells and its Functional Consequences

Kathryn Brown and Wilson Wong*
MRC Centre for Transplantation, King's College London, School of Medicine at Guy's, King's and St. Thomas' Hospitals, London, UK

Abstract

The main function of MHC molecules is to present antigenic peptides to T cells in order to evoke an immune response. This is the main mechanism which enables the body's defence system to distinguish between self and non self, in order to fend off invading pathogens. In organ transplantation, this recognition of non-self results in rejection.

Recent advances have shown that this view may be over simplistic, as cells can exchange their surface molecules with each other, blurring the boundary between self and non-self. In infection, this may result in non-infected cells presenting foreign peptides to the immune system, which potentially can serve to amplify the process of antigen presentation. In organ transplantation, exchange of MHC molecules between donor and recipient cells results in an added layer of complexity to the immunological response against the donor graft as some cells can express both recipient and donor MHC molecules on their cell surface.

The functional consequences of this phenomenon remain to be fully eludicated, but it is likely to have a significant role in the control of the immune system. It may serve as a yet un-recognised tool with which the immune system co-ordinates its response. Here, we describe work to date that demonstrates the extent to which intercellular MHC exchange occurs *in vitro* and *in vivo*, discuss the mechanisms of MHC transfer and the possible consequences. Its implications in different fields within immunology, such as organ transplantation and viral infection, are also highlighted.

* Corresponding Author: Dr Wilson Wong. MRC Centre for Transplantation, King's College London, School of Medicine at Guy's, King's and St. Thomas' Hospitals, London, UK. Tel: +44(0)2071881522, Fax: +44(0)2071885662. e-mail: wilson.wong@kcl.ac.uk

ABBREVIATIONS

MHC	major histocompatibility complex
DC	dendritic cell
APC	antigen presenting cell
MICA	MHC (HLA) class I chain-related gene A
ICAM-1	intercellular adhesion molecule 1
LFA-1	lymphocyte function-associated antigen 1
NK	natural killer
SMAC	supramolecular activation cluster
SMIC	supramolecular inhibition cluster

INTRODUCTION

The main reason for the development of MHC molecules on the cell surface during evolution is for the presentation of antigenic peptides to T cells in order to evoke an immune response. This is the main mechanism which enables the body's defence system to distinguish between self and non self, in order to fend off invading pathogens. An additional mechanism through which MHC molecules contribute to the differentiation between self and non-self is through MHC class I molecules binding to self NK cells to inhibit killing, described elegantly in the missing self hypothesis (Ljunggren and Karre 1990).

Surface molecules such as ligands andreceptors on cells in the immune system work together to control the immune response. They form a vital component of the communication system, enabling complex communications between individual cells to orchestrate an effective immune response. In addition, they can signal to other cells to inform them of their own status as well as enable the body to distinguish between self and non-self. Immunologists have exploited surface molecules to distinguish one cellular subset from another.

Recently, it has become clear that surface molecules may not be as reliable as traditionally thought when used as markers to distinguish between different cellular subsets. At least some of these molecules, including MHC, can be transferred between cells, suggesting that the system is much more fluid than once thought. Although the mechanisms of this transfer are becoming clearer, whether it has any physiological function under normal circumstances and if so, it's consequences, remains largely unknown. Given the importance of MHC molecules in the immune response, it is likely that exchange of MHC molecules between cells will have important implications. A greater understanding of this process would further our knowledge of cell to cell interactions in the immune system and may provide new therapeutic avenues for intervention.

Transfer of cell surface molecules was first described over 30 years ago, when T cells were shown to acquire surface immunoglobulin molecules from B cells (Hudson and Sprent 1976; Hudson et al. 1974), and antigens from macrophages (Bona et al. 1973). The exchange of both MHC class I and II molecules between cells was first demonstrated in the early 1980's (Lorber et al. 1982; Sharrow et al. 1981; Sharrow et al. 1980). A recent surge in interest, and advances in detection techniques, have confirmed the widespread occurrence of this phenomenon.

EARLY *IN VITRO* STUDIES

Progress in the field of intercellular molecular transfer had been hampered by the lack of a physiologically relevant *in vivo* model. Most data has therefore come from *in vitro* studies. Molecules shown to be transferred *in vitro* include MHC class I and II (Harshyne et al. 2001; Patel et al. 1999; Russo et al. 2000), CD3 (Whale et al. 2006), CD21 (Tabiasco et al. 2003), CD80 (Sabzevari et al. 2001), CD86 (Game et al. 2005), OX40L (Baba et al. 2001), endothelial cell molecules (Brezinschek et al. 1999), inhibitory natural killer (NK) receptors (Sjostrom et al. 2001; Vanherberghen et al. 2004), chemokine receptors (Mack et al. 2000), and GPI-anchored proteins (Anderson et al. 1996; Liu et al. 2002) (table 1). Many cell types have been implicated in this process to different extents – in the case of T cells, uptake of MHC class II is carried out much more efficiently by activated cells (Tsang et al. 2003), but for antigen presenting cells (APC), this transfer occurs in the steady state (Patel and Mannie 2001).

Table 1. Summary of transferred molecules, and cells involved, described to date

Transferred molecule	"donating cell"	"receiving cell"	Reference
MHC class I	DC	DC	(Herrera et al. 2004); (Smyth et al. 2008)
MHC class I	Endothelial cell	DC	(Herrera et al. 2004)
MHC class I	Tumour cell	DC	(Russo et al. 2000)
MHC class I	APC	T cell ($CD4^+$)	(Hao et al. 2007; He et al. 2007; Xiang et al. 2005)
MHC class I	DC	T cell ($CD8^+$)	(Huang et al. 1999; Xia et al. 2006)
MHC class I	Not defined	NK cell	(Sjostrom et al. 2001)
MHC class II	DC	DC	(Herrera et al. 2004)
MHC class II	Tumour cell	DC	(Russo et al. 2000)
MHC class II	Endothelial cell	DC	(Herrera et al. 2004)
MHC class II	Epithelial cell	DC	(Millet et al. 2008)
MHC class II	Epithelial cell	Epithelial cell	(Millet et al. 2008)
MHC class II	APC	T cell ($CD4^+$)	(Arnold and Mannie 1999; Game et al. 2005; Tsang et al. 2003; Undale et al. 2004; Wetzel et al. 2005; Xiang et al. 2005)
MHC class II	APC	T cell ($CD8^+$)	(Undale et al. 2004)
T cell receptor/CD3	T cell ($CD4^+$)	DC	(Busch et al. 2008)

Table 1. (Continued)

Transferred molecule	"donating cell"	"receiving cell"	Reference
B cell receptor	B cell	B cell	(Quah et al. 2008)
IgM	B cell	T cell	(Hudson and Sprent 1976; Hudson et al. 1974)
CD80	APC	T cell ($CD4^+$)	(Game et al. 2005; Hwang et al. 2000; Sabzevari et al. 2001; Tatari-Calderone et al. 2002; Xiang et al. 2005)
CD80	APC	T cell ($CD8^+$)	(Hwang et al. 2000; Xia et al. 2006)
CD86	APC	T cell ($CD4^+$)	(Game et al. 2005; Hwang et al. 2000)
CD86	APC	T cell ($CD8^+$)	(Hwang et al. 2000)
OX40L	Not defined	T cell ($CD4^+$)	(Baba et al. 2001)
CD2	T cell ($CD4^+$)	DC	(Busch et al. 2008)
MICA	Target cell	NK cell	(McCann et al. 2007)
NKG2D	NK cell	Target cell	(Roda-Navarro et al. 2006)
CCR5	PBMC	Monocytes	(Mack et al. 2000)
CD31	Endothelial cell	T cell ($CD4^+$)	(Brezinschek et al. 1999)
CD49d	Endothelial cell	T cell ($CD4^+$)	(Brezinschek et al. 1999)

Abbreviations: dendritic cell (DC); antigen presenting cell (APC)

HOW ARE MOLECULES TRANSFERRED BETWEEN CELLS?

Immunological Synapse

The initial immunological synapses described (Monks et al. 1998) are monocentric (stable) synapses which are made up of two main domains – central and peripheral. Monocentric synapses result between interacting T cells and APC, where adhesion molecules e.g. intercellular adhesion molecule-1 (ICAM-1) are excluded from the central supramolecular activation cluster (cSMAC); being found only in the peripheral supramolecular activation cluster (pSMAC), while MHC-peptide are only found in the cSMAC. This arrangement is mirrored by the cognate ligands on the interacting T cell.

Conversely, inhibitory immunological synapses that form during immune surveillance of target cells expressing MHC class I by NK cells have been found to contain MHC I in the peripheral supramolecular inhibition cluster (pSMIC) and adhesion molecules LFA1 in the cSMIC .

As the interface between two cells, the immunological synapse is clearly an important feature of intercellular communication, and therefore the response to invading pathogens, tumour immunology and transplantation. The immunological synapse can also intuitively be expected to be a means by which cells could communicate or effect their function through the intercellular transfer of surface molecules.

The importance of the formation of the immunological synapse in transfer has been shown by the finding that T cells acquire molecules much more efficiently from syngeneic APC i.e. where synapses can be formed (Arnold et al. 1997). Both the TcR and CD28 can acquire their respective ligands during a synapse (Huang et al. 1999; Hwang et al. 2000; Wetzel et al. 2005). Bystander molecules can also be acquired during the synapse, with MHC class I complexes transferred onto $CD4^+$ T cells from APC due to their presence in the immunological synapse (He et al. 2007).

Synapses between other cell types are also associated with uptake of receptor ligands. Tumour cells can transfer molecules through the synapse (Poupot and Fournie 2003). B cells take up antigen from T cells during the synapse between the two cells (Batista et al. 2001). Cytotoxic T cells acquire fragments of plasma membrane from target cells (Hudrisier et al. 2001; Stinchcombe et al. 2001), as do γδ T cells (Espinosa et al. 2002), and NK cells also transfer molecules through the synapse (Carlin et al. 2001; Roda-Navarro et al. 2006; Tabiasco et al. 2002).

Transfer of cell surface molecules can begin within minutes after the formation of the synapse (Huang et al. 1999; Tabiasco et al. 2002; Wetzel et al. 2005). Adsorption of receptor ligands onto the cell surface is in most cases followed by internalisation of the ligand-receptor pair, but it is clear that in some cases the adsorbed molecule either remains on, or is returned to, the cell surface in a functional form.

Wetzel and colleagues visualised transfer of MHC molecules to T cells during the dissolution of the immunological synapse, but also observed the transfer of these molecules after cell contact without the formation of a mature synapse (Wetzel et al. 2005). Therefore, transfer of molecules through the synapse is not the only method of molecular transfer. Cell surface molecules, with their strong anchors in the plasma membrane, are not in all likelihood removed alone. A portion of membrane, including proteins, is transferred as a whole, a process known as trogocytosis (Joly and Hudrisier 2003). DC have also been shown to acquire membrane from surrounding cells in this way, a process that may involve the class A scavenger receptor present on DC (Harshyne et al. 2001; Harshyne et al. 2003). In addition, T cells acquire membrane fragments including cell surface proteins from endothelial cells during transendothelial migration (Brezinschek et al. 1999).

Exosomes

In addition to being transferred during cell contact, molecules can also be transferred between cells by the release of vesicles called exosomes from one cell and the uptake of these by another cell. Exosomes (reviewed in (Fevrier and Raposo 2004)) are 50-90nm vesicles contained within multivesicular bodies within the cell and are secreted when the multivesicular body fuses with the cell membrane. Exosomes are formed from the plasma membrane of the cell and thus express many of the cell surface molecules present on the cell they derive from.

Exosomes are secreted from APC (Arnold and Mannie 1999), including DC (Zitvogel et al. 1998) and B cells (Raposo et al. 1996), activated T cells (Blanchard et al. 2002), and intestinal epithelial cells (van Niel et al. 2001), amongst others. Directions of exosome transfer demonstrated so far include DC to DC (van Niel et al. 2001), APC to T cells (Arnold and Mannie 1999), and tumour cells to DC (Wolfers et al. 2001). Exosomes are released from both immature and mature DC, with the phenotype of the exosome reflecting the maturation status of the parent cell (Segura et al. 2005a).

Exosomes have been shown to include in their repertoire MHC (both class I and II) and co-stimulatory molecules (Zitvogel et al. 1998), and have been shown to stimulate $CD8^+$ T cell responses (Hwang et al. 2003; Zitvogel et al. 1998), although there is evidence to suggest that these exosomes in $CD4^+$ T cell responses do not directly activate T cells but instead act to deliver MHC class II to DC through integration into the DC membrane (Thery et al. 2002).

This integration of exosomes into the plasma membrane occurs following capture through the integrin LFA-1 on the recipient cell binding to ICAM-1 on the exosome (Nolte-'t Hoen et al. 2009; Segura et al. 2007; Segura et al. 2005b). Cells with high levels of the active form of LFA-1 (e.g. $CD8^+$ DC and activated T cells) therefore acquire exosomes more effectively than other cell types. Macrophages appear to capture exosomes through phosphatidylserine receptors such as Tim1 and Tim4, which bind phosphatidylserine present on exosomes (Miyanishi et al. 2007; Zakharova et al. 2007). As well as being incorporated into the membrane of recipient DC, exosomes can be endocytosed, processed and presented in the normal manner (Morelli et al. 2004).

Transfer along/through Nanotubes

In addition to being secreted by cells, exosomes may travel between cells within nanotubes. Nanotubular networks (reviewed in (Davis and Sowinski 2008)) are newly discovered connections between various cell types, including DC (Watkins and Salter 2005), macrophages (Onfelt et al. 2006), T cells (Sowinski et al. 2008) and NK cells (Onfelt et al. 2004).

Nanotubes may be formed in two ways. They can form between cells after the demise of the immunological synapse as the cells dissociate (Onfelt et al. 2004), possibly resulting from membrane bridges observed during the cytotoxic T cell/target cell synapse (Stinchcombe et al. 2001). Alternatively, they can be formed through an extension of membrane from one cell fusing with a neighbouring cell membrane (Rustom et al. 2004). As well as carrying vesicles such as exosomes and other cytoplasmic components between cells, cell surface molecules can travel along the membranes of the nanotubes and onto the connected cell (Onfelt et al. 2004; Rustom et al. 2004).

Although most of the work on nanotubes has been performed *in vitro*, these structures have recently been observed *in vivo* between MHC class II^+ cells in the murine cornea, and the incidence of nanotube formation was shown to increase during inflammation, suggesting a possible physiological role (Chinnery et al. 2008).

The different mechanisms of transfer of cell surface molecules are not mutually exclusive. During interactions between DC and T cells, DC have been shown to acquire CD2 from T cells in a cell contact dependent manner, and acquire several other T cell surface molecules, including CD3/TcR and OX40 through exosomes (Busch et al. 2008). CD2 is transferred early after contact, possibly by trogocytosis, while the exosome-delivered molecules are acquired much later. The two groups also differed in terms of the activation state of the T cell, suggesting that the transfer of proteins differs in accordance with the mechanism used for delivery.

DURATION OF SURFACE EXPRESSION

For a transferred molecule to be functional, it would need to remain on the cell surface for a substantial period of time. The stability of transferred molecules has been investigated *in vitro*. MHC molecules have been found to remain on recipient cells for as long as 2 days following transfer (Dolan et al. 2006b), providing ample opportunity for interaction of this molecule with it's ligand. MHC (HLA) class I chain-related gene A (MICA), after transfer onto NK cells, survives long enough on the cell surface to be subsequently transferred onto a different NK cell (McCann et al. 2007). Not all molecules have stable expression after transfer however. The co-stimulatory molecules CD80 and OX40L are present for only 4 and 12 hours respectively (Baba et al. 2001; Hwang et al. 2000).

The difference in the duration of surface expression of a transferred molecule may depend on the mechanism of transfer. Busch *et al.* lowered the pH of recipient cells and showed that CD2, transferred through cell contact, enjoyed stable expression on the recipient cell, whilst molecules such as CD3, OX40 and PD-1, transferred via exosomes, were removed at low pH (Busch et al. 2008). This stability in the membrane, related to the mechanism of transfer, may be reflected in the length of time the molecule is expressed.

FUNCTIONALITY OF TRANSFERRED MOLECULES

The transfer of molecules between cells is only important if the molecule remains functional on its host cell, and influences its function or the way that it interacts with other cells. This has shown to be the case in many circumstances. DC can stimulate allogeneic T cells after acquisition of foreign MHC (Russo et al. 2000), and can effectively stimulate both $CD8^+$ and $CD4^+$ T cells through acquired MHC class I and II respectively (Dolan et al. 2006a, b; Xiang et al. 2005). MHC class II/peptide complexes transferred from T cells to DC and B cells are also functional (Nolte-'t Hoen et al. 2004). The functionality of MHC and co-stimulatory molecules such as CD80, CD86 and OX40L transferred to T cells was demonstrated by these cells' subsequent ability to stimulate naïve T cells, and thus dispense with services of APC (Baba et al. 2001; Game et al. 2005; Sabzevari et al. 2001; Tatari-Calderone et al. 2002; Zhou et al. 2005). Presentation of acquired MHC class II/peptide complexes by T cells can also induce hyporesponsiveness (Tsang et al. 2003) and confer regulatory ability upon these cells (LeMaoult et al. 2007). Inhibitory NK receptors, GPI-anchored proteins, and MHC class II taken up by polymorphonuclear cells have all been found to be functional following transfer (Anderson et al. 1996; Sjostrom et al. 2001; Whale et al. 2006). This functional viability of cell surface molecules following transfer suggests that they may have a physiological role.

Consequences

The consequences of transfer appear to be many and varied, at least under the *in vitro* conditions where this process has been investigated.

The most basic consequence of this process may be that it allows cells in an immune synapse to dissociate, with the transfer of a receptor from one cell to the other removing the bond between the two cells. This is especially true of high avidity interactions.

APC to APC Transfer

B cells appear to use transfer to amplify the immune response, as activated B cells can transfer their B cell receptors to surrounding B cells, enabling uptake of that specific antigen by non-antigen specific neighbouring B cells (Quah et al. 2008). This allows a significant immune response to be generated despite the very low numbers of B cells of each specificity.

Antigen spreading is also the result of MHC transfer in the thymus, between thymic epithelial cells, and from thymic epithelial cells to DC. This may allow rare antigens to be more widely expressed and increase the chances of contact with a developing T cell, which can then be positively or negatively selected as appropriate (Millet et al. 2008). It has also been suggested that different populations of DC may be responsible for the tasks of antigen processing, and stimulation of T cells. So DC in the periphery may transfer MHC to allow antigen to be presented by the correct cell type in the correct place (Smith and Fazekas de St Groth 1999).

Regulatory T Cells

MHC transfer has been shown to increase the suppressive activity of regulatory T cells. $CD4^+$ Tr1 cells acquired peptide/MHC class I complexes from the DC used in their generation. This uptake resulted in greater suppression of antigen-specific $CD8^+$ T cells responses in comparison to those Tr1 cells which did not acquire peptide/MHC class I. In this situation MHC transfer may be a means to downregulate an ongoing immune response (Hao et al. 2008).

APC to T Cell Transfer

For T cells, it appears that transfer of MHC class II/peptide complexes and co-stimulatory molecules can either allow continuation of an immune response, or its downregulation, presumably depending on the environmental conditions. It is thought that MHC class I uptake can render the T cells sensitive to killing by surrounding T cells with the same specificity, i.e. fratricide (Chai et al. 1998; Cox et al. 2007; Huang et al. 1999). The transfer of MHC from APC to T cells may also act to downregulate the immune response by removing the stimulus available to other T cells (Kedl et al. 2002), although this may have a further consequence of affinity maturation. However, activated $CD4^+$ T cells that have acquired peptide MHC class I complexes via exosomes can then go on to stimulate a naïve (Hao et al. 2007; Xiang et al. 2005), or memory (Shi et al. 2006), $CD8^+$ T cell response. This is not unique to the mechanism of transfer, as T cells that have acquired MHC class II from APC through cell contact can also go on to stimulate a $CD4^+$ T cell response (Undale et al. 2004). Acquisition of CD80 also allows the continuation of the co-stimulatory signal for 24 hours after the dissolution of the synapse (Zhou et al. 2005).

The outcome of transfer probably depends on the balance between all these different effects, with either up- or down- regulation of the immune response occurring as appropriate to the conditions. For example, a T cell may acquire peptide MHC complexes from APC, allowing it to stimulate a neighbouring T cell. If this occurs in the early stages of an immune response, T cells of the same specificity will be rare, and the dispersal of the peptide MHC complex may amplify the immune response. If however, the immune response is well developed, proliferation of antigen-specific T cells may result in the T cell expressing peptide/MHC being surrounded by other T cells, leading to death through fratricide.

The complex nature of MHC transfer is further demonstrated by the transfer of peptide/MHC class I complexes from APC to $CD8^+$ T cells. The consequences of this process appear to be two-fold. Firstly, the $CD8^+$ T cell bearing peptide/MHC class I can stimulate antigen-specific $CD8^+$ memory T cells to enhance the immune response. However, these peptide/MHC class I carrying cells cause the death of antigen-specific APC and other $CD8^+$ T cells that have acquired peptide MHC class I complexes, which acts to downregulate the immune response. In a similar way, DC that acquire CD3/TcR complexes from $CD4^+$ T cells become less able to stimulate a $CD4^+$ T cell response, apparently due to the masking of MHC class II complexes on the DC surface, but retain the ability to stimulate a $CD8^+$ T cell response (Busch et al. 2008). Although this seems contradictory, these differing outcomes may be carefully controlled to allow the stimulation of the correct immune response (in these cases cytotoxic T lymphocyte responses), whilst removing the stimulus from APC and so preventing the response from becoming out of control, a situation which could easily arise given the ability of MHC to move between cells. These data reveal that MHC transfer is a complicated and structured process, rather than a random redistribution of cell surface molecules between cells.

Regulation of Molecular Transfer

There are many examples of the regulation of MHC transfer. B cell receptors can only be transferred to other B cells, and in a similar way exosomes can only be captured by cells expressing certain receptors. Exosome transfer is further regulated by the make-up of these vesicles. Busch *et al.* found that several co-stimulatory molecules, such as CD28 and CD4, were not transferred through exosomes from T cells to DC, suggesting that an active sorting process takes place (Busch et al. 2008), and the increased levels of tetraspan proteins on B cell exosomes, compared to for example the transferrin receptor, a marker for plasma membranes, provides further evidence for this (Escola et al. 1998).

Nanotubes often form between cells that have been in cell contact (the duration of which must be over 4 minutes (Sowinski et al. 2008)), and therefore the sharing of information is restricted by this initial contact, as in the case of molecular transfer during a synapse. The direction of transport along nanotubes can also be controlled, with unidirectional (Rustom et al. 2004) or bidirectional (Onfelt et al. 2006) transfer being observed depending on the cell types involved.

The stability of expression of the transferred molecules can also provide a means for regulation. As described above, MHC molecules have been found to remain on recipient cells much longer than co-stimulatory molecules following transfer (Baba et al. 2001; Dolan et al. 2006b; Hwang et al. 2000). After loss of co-stimulatory molecules, cells that have acquired MHC molecules will no longer be able to stimulate T cells and may instead downregulate the immune response through the induction of anergy.

In contrast to the tight regulation of co-stimulatory molecules, NK cells acquire MICA from target cells, and this molecule can then be transferred between NK cells, during which time it remains functional (McCann et al. 2007). Again, the differences seen regarding the transfer of different surface molecules suggests a complicated and organised process.

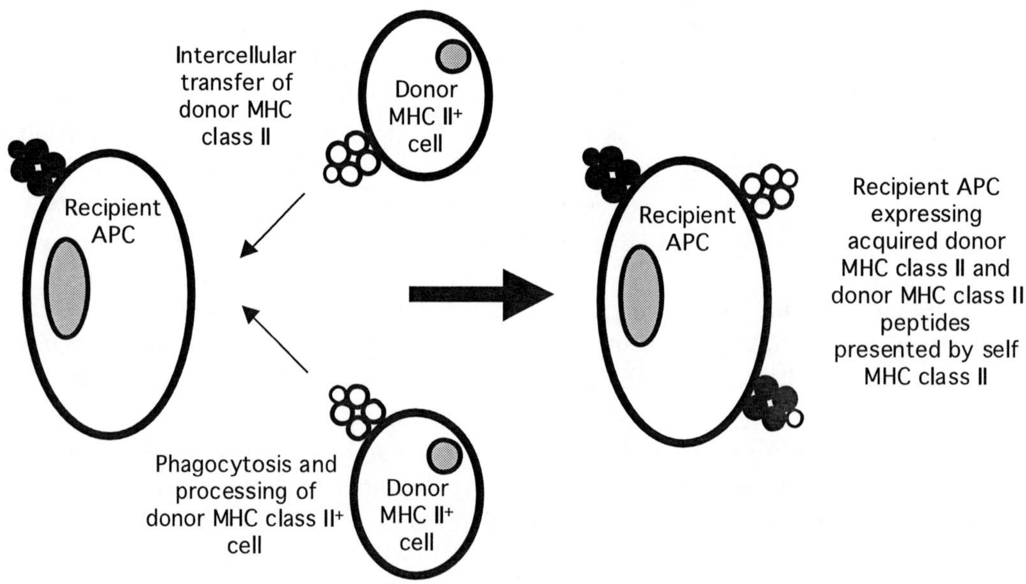

Figure 1. In the context of transplantation, transfer of MHC class II molecules from donor APC would allow recipient APC to present antigen through the direct antigen presentation pathway, as well as the conventional indirect pathway, whereby donor cells are processed, and donor MHC peptides are presented by recipient MHC class II molecules. This has been termed the "semi-direct" pathway of alloantigen presentation.

In Vivo Relevance of Intercellular Transfer of Molecules

Most of the experimental evidence discussed above has been obtained *in vitro* or under artificial conditions *in vivo* such as injection of allogeneic cells. This has led to scepticism as to whether intercellular molecular exchange takes place under normal physiological conditions. Millet and colleagues transplanted bone marrow from MHC null mice into allogeneic wild type recipients, and showed that in the thymus, donor DC had acquired MHC class II from recipient epithelial cells, which was expressed at 5% of normal levels. When the strain combination was reversed, recipient MHC-deficient epithelial cells did not acquire MHC class II from wild type donor cells, demonstrating the unilateral nature of this transfer (Millet et al. 2008).

Transplantation is the only example where foreign MHC molecules are deliberately introduced. Our laboratory has demonstrated that following allogeneic heart or kidney transplantation in mice, cells can be found within the recipient spleen which express both donor and recipient MHC class II molecules. This transfer was extensive and bidirectional - recipient cells can acquire MHC molecules from donor cells and *vice versa* (Brown et al. 2008). The bidirectional nature of DC to DC transfer of MHC class II molecules had previously been shown upon injection of allogeneic DC (de Heusch et al. 2007). One interesting observation is that it takes place only within the spleen of the recipient but not with the graft itself. The reason for this is still unclear.

Physiological Significance of Intercellular Transfer of Molecules

The physiological significance of MHC transfer is yet to be elucidated, but this process may have consequences for transplantation, autoimmunity and the anti-tumour response. The extent of molecular transfer, with the large number of molecules transferred and the wide variety of cells able to participate in this process, suggests a physiological consequence.

Transfer is difficult to study, as it is difficult to distinguish between transfer of molecules from one cell to another and *de novo* expression. However, transplantation is an ideal model in which to study this. Our laboratory has shown that transfer of MHC class II molecules does occur after transplantation in vivo (Brown et al. 2008). A possible mechanism for this was suggested by Montecalvo *et al.*, who showed that graft infiltrating leukocytes contain exosomes which are released *ex vivo* (Montecalvo et al. 2008). The expression by recipient APC of not only recipient MHC class II presenting donor peptides, but also donor-derived MHC class II peptide complexes would allow the stimulation of both the direct and indirect alloresponse, and this has been termed the 'semi-direct' antigen presentation pathway (Herrera et al. 2004) (figure 1).

The unravelling of the physiological effects of MHC transfer will increase our understanding of the immune system and may open a new avenue for therapeutic intervention in the above-mentioned conditions.

Conclusions

A recent surge in interest in intercellular MHC transfer has resulted in significant advances over the past few years. Although circumstantial evidence suggests that it is a controlled process, the aspects of this control and the feedback mechanisms, if any, are poorly understood. Evidence for MHC transfer in physiologically relevant, real life situations have added credence to the phenomenon. The next step would be to determine to what extent intercellular molecular transfer take place *in vivo* and its functional relevance under normal and pathological conditions. It is likely that this process forms a novel mechanism of interaction in the immune system. Understanding the fundamental principles that governs it will have implications on diverse fields in immunology such as infection, autoimmunity, transplantation and tumour immunity.

REFERENCES

Anderson, SM, Yu, G, Giattina, M and Miller, JL (1996) Intercellular transfer of a glycosylphosphatidylinositol (GPI)-linked protein: release and uptake of CD4-GPI from recombinant adeno-associated virus-transduced HeLa cells. *Proc Natl Acad Sci U S A* 93: 5894-5898.

Arnold, PY, Davidian, DK and Mannie, MD (1997) Antigen presentation by T cells: T cell receptor ligation promotes antigen acquisition from professional antigen-presenting cells. *Eur J Immunol* 27: 3198-3205.

Arnold, PY and Mannie, MD (1999) Vesicles bearing MHC class II molecules mediate transfer of antigen from antigen-presenting cells to CD4+ T cells. *Eur J Immunol* 29: 1363-1373.

Baba, E, Takahashi, Y, Lichtenfeld, J, et al. (2001) Functional CD4 T cells after intercellular molecular transfer of 0X40 ligand. *J Immunol* 167: 875-883.

Batista, FD, Iber, D and Neuberger, MS (2001) B cells acquire antigen from target cells after synapse formation. *Nature* 411: 489-494.

Blanchard, N, Lankar, D, Faure, F, et al. (2002) TCR activation of human T cells induces the production of exosomes bearing the TCR/CD3/zeta complex. *J Immunol* 168: 3235-3241.

Bona, C, Robineaux, R, Anteunis, A, Heuclin, C and Astesano, A (1973) Transfer of antigen from macrophages to lymphocytes. II. Immunological significance of the transfer of lipopolysaccharide. *Immunology* 24: 831-840.

Brezinschek, RI, Oppenheimer-Marks, N and Lipsky, PE (1999) Activated T cells acquire endothelial cell surface determinants during transendothelial migration. *J Immunol* 162: 1677-1684.

Brown, K, Sacks, SH and Wong, W (2008) Extensive and bidirectional transfer of major histocompatibility complex class II molecules between donor and recipient cells in vivo following solid organ transplantation. *Faseb J* 22: 3776-3784.

Busch, A, Quast, T, Keller, S, et al. (2008) Transfer of T cell surface molecules to dendritic cells upon CD4+ T cell priming involves two distinct mechanisms. *J Immunol* 181: 3965-3973.

Carlin, LM, Eleme, K, McCann, FE and Davis, DM (2001) Intercellular transfer and supramolecular organization of human leukocyte antigen C at inhibitory natural killer cell immune synapses. *J Exp Med* 194: 1507-1517.

Chai, JG, Bartok, I, Scott, D, Dyson, J and Lechler, R (1998) T:T antigen presentation by activated murine CD8+ T cells induces anergy and apoptosis. *J Immunol* 160: 3655-3665.

Chinnery, HR, Pearlman, E and McMenamin, PG (2008) Cutting edge: Membrane nanotubes in vivo: a feature of MHC class II+ cells in the mouse cornea. *J Immunol* 180: 5779-5783.

Cox, JH, McMichael, AJ, Screaton, GR and Xu, X-N (2007) CTLs Target Th Cells That Acquire Bystander MHC Class I-Peptide Complex from APCs. *J Immunol* 179: 830-836.

Davis, DM and Sowinski, S (2008) Membrane nanotubes: dynamic long-distance connections between animal cells. *Nat Rev Mol Cell Biol* 9: 431-436.

de Heusch, M, Blocklet, D, Egrise, D, et al. (2007) Bidirectional MHC molecule exchange between migratory and resident dendritic cells. *J Leukoc Biol* 82: 861-868.

Dolan, BP, Gibbs, KD, Jr. and Ostrand-Rosenberg, S (2006a) Dendritic cells cross-dressed with peptide MHC class I complexes prime CD8+ T cells. *J Immunol* 177: 6018-6024.

Dolan, BP, Gibbs, KD, Jr. and Ostrand-Rosenberg, S (2006b) Tumor-specific CD4+ T cells are activated by "cross-dressed" dendritic cells presenting peptide-MHC class II complexes acquired from cell-based cancer vaccines. *J Immunol* 176: 1447-1455.

Escola, JM, Kleijmeer, MJ, Stoorvogel, W, et al. (1998) Selective enrichment of tetraspan proteins on the internal vesicles of multivesicular endosomes and on exosomes secreted by human B-lymphocytes. *J Biol Chem* 273: 20121-20127.

Espinosa, E, Tabiasco, J, Hudrisier, D and Fournie, JJ (2002) Synaptic transfer by human gamma delta T cells stimulated with soluble or cellular antigens. *J Immunol* 168: 6336-6343.

Fevrier, B and Raposo, G (2004) Exosomes: endosomal-derived vesicles shipping extracellular messages. *Curr Opin Cell Biol* 16: 415-421.

Game, DS, Rogers, NJ and Lechler, RI (2005) Acquisition of HLA-DR and costimulatory molecules by T cells from allogeneic antigen presenting cells. *Am J Transplant* 5: 1614-1625.

Hao, S, Yuan, J and Xiang, J (2007) Nonspecific CD4(+) T cells with uptake of antigen-specific dendritic cell-released exosomes stimulate antigen-specific CD8(+) CTL responses and long-term T cell memory. *J Leukoc Biol* 82: 829-838.

Hao, S, Yuan, J, Xu, S, et al. (2008) Antigen specificity acquisition of adoptive CD4+ regulatory T cells via acquired peptide-MHC class I complexes. *J Immunol* 181: 2428-2437.

Harshyne, LA, Watkins, SC, Gambotto, A and Barratt-Boyes, SM (2001) Dendritic cells acquire antigens from live cells for cross-presentation to CTL. *J Immunol* 166: 3717-3723.

Harshyne, LA, Zimmer, MI, Watkins, SC and Barratt-Boyes, SM (2003) A role for class A scavenger receptor in dendritic cell nibbling from live cells. *J Immunol* 170: 2302-2309.

He, T, Zong, S, Wu, X, Wei, Y and Xiang, J (2007) CD4+ T cell acquisition of the bystander pMHC I colocalizing in the same immunological synapse comprising pMHC II and costimulatory CD40, CD54, CD80, OX40L, and 41BBL. *Biochem Biophys Res Commun* 362: 822-828.

Herrera, OB, Golshayan, D, Tibbott, R, et al. (2004) A novel pathway of alloantigen presentation by dendritic cells. *J Immunol* 173: 4828-4837.

Huang, JF, Yang, Y, Sepulveda, H, et al. (1999) TCR-Mediated internalization of peptide-MHC complexes acquired by T cells. *Science* 286: 952-954.

Hudrisier, D, Riond, J, Mazarguil, H, Gairin, JE and Joly, E (2001) Cutting edge: CTLs rapidly capture membrane fragments from target cells in a TCR signaling-dependent manner. *J Immunol* 166: 3645-3649.

Hudson, L and Sprent, J (1976) Specific adsorption of IgM antibody onto H-2-activated mouse T lymphocytes. *J Exp Med* 143: 444-449.

Hudson, L, Sprent, J, Miller, JF and Playfair, JH (1974) B cell-derived immunoglobulin on activated mouse T lymphocytes. *Nature* 251: 60-62.

Hwang, I, Huang, JF, Kishimoto, H, et al. (2000) T cells can use either T cell receptor or CD28 receptors to absorb and internalize cell surface molecules derived from antigen-presenting cells. *J Exp Med* 191: 1137-1148.

Hwang, I, Shen, X and Sprent, J (2003) Direct stimulation of naive T cells by membrane vesicles from antigen-presenting cells: distinct roles for CD54 and B7 molecules. *Proc Natl Acad Sci U S A* 100: 6670-6675.

Joly, E and Hudrisier, D (2003) What is trogocytosis and what is its purpose? *Nat Immunol* 4: 815.

Kedl, RM, Schaefer, BC, Kappler, JW and Marrack, P (2002) T cells down-modulate peptide-MHC complexes on APCs in vivo. *Nat Immunol* 3: 27-32.

LeMaoult, J, Caumartin, J, Daouya, M, et al. (2007) Immune regulation by pretenders: cell-to-cell transfers of HLA-G make effector T cells act as regulatory cells. *Blood* 109: 2040-2048.

Liu, T, Li, R, Pan, T, et al. (2002) Intercellular transfer of the cellular prion protein. *J Biol Chem* 277: 47671-47678.

Ljunggren, HG and Karre, K (1990) In search of the 'missing self': MHC molecules and NK cell recognition. *Immunol Today* 11: 237-244.

Lorber, MI, Loken, MR, Stall, AM and Fitch, FW (1982) I-A antigens on cloned alloreactive murine T lymphocytes are acquired passively. *J Immunol* 128: 2798-2803.

Mack, M, Kleinschmidt, A, Bruhl, H, et al. (2000) Transfer of the chemokine receptor CCR5 between cells by membrane-derived microparticles: a mechanism for cellular human immunodeficiency virus 1 infection. *Nat Med* 6: 769-775.

McCann, FE, Eissmann, P, Onfelt, B, Leung, R and Davis, DM (2007) The activating NKG2D ligand MHC class I-related chain A transfers from target cells to NK cells in a manner that allows functional consequences. *J Immunol* 178: 3418-3426.

Millet, V, Naquet, P and Guinamard, RR (2008) Intercellular MHC transfer between thymic epithelial and dendritic cells. *Eur J Immunol* 38: 1257-1263.

Miyanishi, M, Tada, K, Koike, M, et al. (2007) Identification of Tim4 as a phosphatidylserine receptor. *Nature* 450: 435-439.

Monks, CR, Freiberg, BA, Kupfer, H, Sciaky, N and Kupfer, A (1998) Three-dimensional segregation of supramolecular activation clusters in T cells. *Nature* 395: 82-86.

Montecalvo, A, Shufesky, WJ, Stolz, DB, et al. (2008) Exosomes as a short-range mechanism to spread alloantigen between dendritic cells during T cell allorecognition. *J Immunol* 180: 3081-3090.

Morelli, AE, Larregina, AT, Shufesky, WJ, et al. (2004) Endocytosis, intracellular sorting, and processing of exosomes by dendritic cells. *Blood* 104: 3257-3266.

Nolte-'t Hoen, EN, Buschow, SI, Anderton, SM, Stoorvogel, W and Wauben, MH (2009) Activated T cells recruit exosomes secreted by dendritic cells via LFA-1. *Blood* 113: 1977-1981.

Nolte-'t Hoen, EN, Wagenaar-Hilbers, JP, Peters, PJ, et al. (2004) Uptake of membrane molecules from T cells endows antigen-presenting cells with novel functional properties. *Eur J Immunol* 34: 3115-3125.

Onfelt, B, Nedvetzki, S, Benninger, RK, et al. (2006) Structurally distinct membrane nanotubes between human macrophages support long-distance vesicular traffic or surfing of bacteria. *J Immunol* 177: 8476-8483.

Onfelt, B, Nedvetzki, S, Yanagi, K and Davis, DM (2004) Cutting edge: Membrane nanotubes connect immune cells. *J Immunol* 173: 1511-1513.

Patel, DM, Arnold, PY, White, GA, Nardella, JP and Mannie, MD (1999) Class II MHC/peptide complexes are released from APC and are acquired by T cell responders during specific antigen recognition. *J Immunol* 163: 5201-5210.

Patel, DM and Mannie, MD (2001) Intercellular exchange of class II major histocompatibility complex/peptide complexes is a conserved process that requires activation of T cells but is constitutive in other types of antigen presenting cell. *Cell Immunol* 214: 165-172.

Poupot, M and Fournie, JJ (2003) Spontaneous membrane transfer through homotypic synapses between lymphoma cells. *J Immunol* 171: 2517-2523.

Quah, BJ, Barlow, VP, McPhun, V, et al. (2008) Bystander B cells rapidly acquire antigen receptors from activated B cells by membrane transfer. *Proc Natl Acad Sci U S A* 105: 4259-4264.

Raposo, G, Nijman, HW, Stoorvogel, W, et al. (1996) B lymphocytes secrete antigen-presenting vesicles. *J Exp Med* 183: 1161-1172.

Roda-Navarro, P, Vales-Gomez, M, Chisholm, SE and Reyburn, HT (2006) Transfer of NKG2D and MICB at the cytotoxic NK cell immune synapse correlates with a reduction in NK cell cytotoxic function. *Proc Natl Acad Sci U S A* 103: 11258-11263.

Russo, V, Zhou, D, Sartirana, C, et al. (2000) Acquisition of intact allogeneic human leukocyte antigen molecules by human dendritic cells. *Blood* 95: 3473-3477.

Rustom, A, Saffrich, R, Markovic, I, Walther, P and Gerdes, HH (2004) Nanotubular highways for intercellular organelle transport. *Science* 303: 1007-1010.

Sabzevari, H, Kantor, J, Jaigirdar, A, et al. (2001) Acquisition of CD80 (B7-1) by T cells. *J Immunol* 166: 2505-2513.

Segura, E, Amigorena, S and Thery, C (2005a) Mature dendritic cells secrete exosomes with strong ability to induce antigen-specific effector immune responses. *Blood Cells Mol Dis* 35: 89-93.

Segura, E, Guerin, C, Hogg, N, Amigorena, S and Thery, C (2007) CD8+ dendritic cells use LFA-1 to capture MHC-peptide complexes from exosomes in vivo. *J Immunol* 179: 1489-1496.

Segura, E, Nicco, C, Lombard, B, et al. (2005b) ICAM-1 on exosomes from mature dendritic cells is critical for efficient naive T-cell priming. *Blood* 106: 216-223.

Sharrow, SO, Mathieson, BJ and Singer, A (1981) Cell surface appearance of unexpected host MHC determinants on thymocytes from radiation bone marrow chimeras. *J Immunol* 126: 1327-1335.

Sharrow, SO, Ozato, K and Sachs, DH (1980) Phenotypic expression of I-A and I-E/C subregion determinants on murine thymocytes. *J Immunol* 125: 2263-2268.

Shi, M, Hao, S, Chan, T and Xiang, J (2006) CD4(+) T cells stimulate memory CD8(+) T cell expansion via acquired pMHC I complexes and costimulatory molecules, and IL-2 secretion. *J Leukoc Biol* 80: 1354-1363.

Sjostrom, A, Eriksson, M, Cerboni, C, et al. (2001) Acquisition of external major histocompatibility complex class I molecules by natural killer cells expressing inhibitory Ly49 receptors. *J Exp Med* 194: 1519-1530.

Smith, AL and Fazekas de St Groth, B (1999) Antigen-pulsed CD8alpha+ dendritic cells generate an immune response after subcutaneous injection without homing to the draining lymph node. *J Exp Med* 189: 593-598.

Smyth, LA, Harker, N, Turnbull, W, et al. (2008) The relative efficiency of acquisition of MHC:peptide complexes and cross-presentation depends on dendritic cell type. *J Immunol* 181: 3212-3220.

Sowinski, S, Jolly, C, Berninghausen, O, et al. (2008) Membrane nanotubes physically connect T cells over long distances presenting a novel route for HIV-1 transmission. *Nat Cell Biol* 10: 211-219.

Stinchcombe, JC, Bossi, G, Booth, S and Griffiths, GM (2001) The immunological synapse of CTL contains a secretory domain and membrane bridges. *Immunity* 15: 751-761.

Tabiasco, J, Espinosa, E, Hudrisier, D, et al. (2002) Active trans-synaptic capture of membrane fragments by natural killer cells. *Eur J Immunol* 32: 1502-1508.

Tabiasco, J, Vercellone, A, Meggetto, F, et al. (2003) Acquisition of viral receptor by NK cells through immunological synapse. *J Immunol* 170: 5993-5998.

Tatari-Calderone, Z, Semnani, RT, Nutman, TB, Schlom, J and Sabzevari, H (2002) Acquisition of CD80 by human T cells at early stages of activation: functional involvement of CD80 acquisition in T cell to T cell interaction. *J Immunol* 169: 6162-6169.

Thery, C, Duban, L, Segura, E, et al. (2002) Indirect activation of naive CD4+ T cells by dendritic cell-derived exosomes. *Nat Immunol* 3: 1156-1162.

Tsang, JY, Chai, JG and Lechler, R (2003) Antigen presentation by mouse CD4+ T cells involving acquired MHC class II:peptide complexes: another mechanism to limit clonal expansion? *Blood* 101: 2704-2710.

Undale, AH, van den Elsen, PJ and Celis, E (2004) Antigen-independent acquisition of MHC class II molecules by human T lymphocytes. *Int Immunol* 16: 1523-1533.

van Niel, G, Raposo, G, Candalh, C, et al. (2001) Intestinal epithelial cells secrete exosome-like vesicles. *Gastroenterology* 121: 337-349.

Vanherberghen, B, Andersson, K, Carlin, LM, et al. (2004) Human and murine inhibitory natural killer cell receptors transfer from natural killer cells to target cells. *Proc Natl Acad Sci U S A* 101: 16873-16878.

Watkins, SC and Salter, RD (2005) Functional connectivity between immune cells mediated by tunneling nanotubules. *Immunity* 23: 309-318.

Wetzel, SA, McKeithan, TW and Parker, DC (2005) Peptide-specific intercellular transfer of MHC class II to CD4+ T cells directly from the immunological synapse upon cellular dissociation. *J Immunol* 174: 80-89.

Whale, TA, Beskorwayne, TK, Babiuk, LA and Griebel, PJ (2006) Bovine polymorphonuclear cells passively acquire membrane lipids and integral membrane proteins from apoptotic and necrotic cells. *J Leukoc Biol* 79: 1226-1233.

Wolfers, J, Lozier, A, Raposo, G, et al. (2001) Tumor-derived exosomes are a source of shared tumor rejection antigens for CTL cross-priming. *Nat Med* 7: 297-303.

Xia, D, Hao, S and Xiang, J (2006) CD8+ cytotoxic T-APC stimulate central memory CD8+ T cell responses via acquired peptide-MHC class I complexes and CD80 costimulation, and IL-2 secretion. *J Immunol* 177: 2976-2984.

Xiang, J, Huang, H and Liu, Y (2005) A new dynamic model of CD8+ T effector cell responses via CD4+ T helper-antigen-presenting cells. *J Immunol* 174: 7497-7505.

Zakharova, L, Svetlova, M and Fomina, AF (2007) T cell exosomes induce cholesterol accumulation in human monocytes via phosphatidylserine receptor. *J Cell Physiol* 212: 174-181.

Zhou, J, Tagaya, Y, Tolouei-Semnani, R, Schlom, J and Sabzevari, H (2005) Physiological relevance of antigen presentasome (APS), an acquired MHC/costimulatory complex, in the sustained activation of CD4+ T cells in the absence of APCs. *Blood* 105: 3238-3246.

Zitvogel, L, Regnault, A, Lozier, A, et al. (1998) Eradication of established murine tumors using a novel cell-free vaccine: dendritic cell-derived exosomes. *Nat Med* 4: 594-600.

In: Major Histocompatibility Complex
Editor: Natalya V. Semiletova
ISBN: 978-1-61942-999-4

Chapter 4

MHC DIVERSITY AND WILDLIFE HEALTH: LESSONS FROM TASMANIAN DEVIL FACIAL TUMOR DISEASE

Yuanyuan Cheng and Katherine Belov
Faculty of Veterinary Science, University of Sydney, Sydney, Australia

ABSTRACT

Genetic variation at the Major Histocompatibility Complex (MHC) plays a key role in defense against infectious diseases. Levels of MHC diversity in wild populations provide an indirect measure of the immunological fitness of that population. Bottlenecked populations with low MHC diversity have limited capability to respond to changes in the environment, especially emergence of new diseases. The recent emergence of a contagious cancer in Tasmanian devils provides a stark example of the effects loss of genetic diversity can have on wildlife species. Devil facial tumor disease (DFTD) is a transmissible cancer that has caused severe population decline in the Tasmanian devil in recent years and is threatening to wipe out the entire species from the wild. DFTD tumor cells are transferred between individuals as allografts without inducing immune rejection. Tumors and devils share the same MHC antigens and hence devils are not able to recognize DFTD cells as non-self. Here we will review our current understanding of the role of the MHC in transmissible cancer and discuss its implications for managing MHC diversity for wildlife conservation.

INTRODUCTION

Antigen-Presenting MHC Molecules

The Major Histocompatibility Complex (MHC) is one of the most studied gene regions among vertebrates with MHC genes having been cloned from representatives of all vertebrate classes except agnathan fish (Janeway *et al.* 2001). The strong research interest in the MHC primarily arises from the important role played by MHC genes and their protein products in disease resistance and transplantation success. The MHC is also a good target for genetic research as it is one of the few polymorphic systems where it has been possible to firmly establish a functional significance for the observed genetic variation (Andersson 1996). Based on the structure and function of their encoded proteins, the MHC genes are grouped into three classes (class I, class II and class III), and class I and II genes are further classified by function as classical and nonclassical (Parham & Strominger 1982).

Classical class I and II genes are particularly important in the host defense against infectious diseases as they encode cell surface molecules that are centrally involved in antigen presentation to lymphocytes. Classical class I antigens function in the recognition and destruction of foreign, virus-infected or malignant cells by cytotoxic T cells (reviewed in Cresswell *et al.* 2005). They are also believed to be the major antigens involved in self/nonself discrimination and graft rejection. MHC class II molecules are responsible for intravesicular and extracellular pathogens, including many bacteria and some eukaryotic parasites (Frank 2002). Antigens derived from these pathogens are presented on cell surface by class II molecules to CD4 helper T cells, which produce chemical signals triggering the production of antigen-specific antibodies and inflammatory responses that kill the pathogens (reviewed in Pieters 2000).

MHC Antigen Diversity and Infectious Diseases

There are two main features of MHC class I and II genes that together contribute to the diversity of MHC antigens observed within an individual or in a population at large – polygeny and polymorphism (Janeway *et al.* 2001).

On one hand, in most species, more than one MHC class I or II locus is expressed. These paralogs result from gene duplication events during the evolution of MHC (Trowsdale & Parham 2004; Kelley *et al.* 2005). This polygenic feature enables an individual to express more than two alleles encoding one type of MHC molecules and ensures that even a homozygous individual possesses a variety of MHC molecules with different peptide-binding specificities.

On the other hand, MHC class I and II genes can be highly polymorphic, with up to tens or even hundreds of different alleles recorded at a single locus (e.g. human class I HLA-A and class II DRB1). The peptide-binding properties and interactions with T cells of different MHC molecules are determined by the polymorphic residues in peptide-binding regions and each MHC molecule can present a range of peptides with a specific sequence motif. The polymorphism of MHC antigens expressed in an individual enables the immune system to recognize an extensive range of pathogenic antigens.

Infectious diseases play a central role in the maintenance of MHC variability in a population through balancing selection – a form of natural selection favoring polymorphism. MHC genes evolve to cope with large numbers of pathogens that continuously develop new ways to avoid recognition or elimination. Two types of balancing selection are most widely considered to account for the maintenance of MHC diversity – overdominant selection and frequency-dependent selection (Hughes 1999). The overdominant selection hypothesis proposes that being heterozygous at MHC loci leads to selective advantage over homozygotes as a larger variety of MHC molecules are expressed. The scenario of frequency-dependent selection is that, when the frequency of an allele increases, its fitness decreases due to the co-evolution of pathogens; therefore, no allele predominates in the population. The latter theory is suggested to be more sufficient in explaining the high polymorphism of MHC (De Boer *et al.* 2004; Borghans *et al.* 2007).

Associations between MHC polymorphism and resistance to infectious diseases have been identified in many case studies in human and free-ranging animal populations (reviewed in Sommer 2005). For instance, in humans, certain class II DRB alleles have been proved to be crucial in the clearance of hepatitis B or C virus infection (Thursz *et al.* 1995; Scotto *et al.* 2003). A class I antigen (HLA-Bw53) and a class II haplotype (DRB1*1302-DQB1*0501) have been associated with protection from severe malaria in West African populations (Hill *et al.* 1991). In Soay sheep and several mouse species, having specific class II DRB alleles has been correlated with low faecal egg count values in nematode infections (Paterson *et al.* 1998; Froeschke & Sommer 2005; Meyer-Lucht & Sommer 2005). Similarly, certain class II alleles have been proposed to be associated with high resistance to *Vibrio anguillarum* bacterial infection in Japanese flounder species (Xu *et al.* 2008).

From the wildlife conservation point of view, it is suggested that populations with low MHC diversity have limited capability to respond to changes in the environment, such as the emergence of new diseases (O'Brien & Evermann 1988; Edwards & Potts 1996), which is a straightforward extension of the above theories. However, few examples have been found that show a clear correlation between the level of MHC diversity and wild population fitness. Here, we review the recent case of Tasmanian devil and devil facial tumor disease (DFTD), which provides valuable evidence and demonstrates that the level of MHC diversity is an important indicator of the immunological fitness of wild populations.

THE TASMANIAN DEVIL AND DFTD

The Tasmanian Devil

The Tasmanian devil (*Sarcophilus harrisii*), a 4.5-13.0 kg endemic marsupial on the island of Tasmania, Australia, is the largest remaining marsupial carnivore in the world (Jones 2001). Devils have an average lifespan of 5-6 years in the wild, with females producing one litter of pouch young annually during breeding ages (age 2-4) (Jones *et al.* 2008). The devil once occurred on the mainland Australia, but became restricted to Tasmania at least 400 years ago, probably due to the competition with dingos and human impacts on the mainland (Gill 1971; Archer & Baynes 1972; Jones *et al.* 2003). It has been suggested that the island Tasmanian devil population has undergone three major population crashes since European settlement (Bradshaw & Brook 2005). As a result, the population has an overall low level of genetic diversity (Jones *et al.* 2004). Previous to the outbreak of DFTD, the Tasmanian devil was commonly seen throughout the island, especially abundant in the eastern areas and the northwest coast (McCallum *et al.* 2007).

Emergence and Influences of DFTD

DFTD is a host-specific transmissible fatal cancer, which usually first appears as small lumps in and around the mouth and then develops into large tumors around the face and neck and inside the oral cavity (Figure 1a; Loh *et al.* 2006). Most infected devils die within a few months after the appearance of initial symptoms due to the inability to feed, secondary infections or tumor metastases (Pyecroft *et al.* 2007). The first case of DFTD was reported in 1996 at Mount William National Park in the northeast of Tasmania (Hawkins *et al.* 2006). Analysis of a tumor transcriptome has revealed the likely Schwann cell origin of DFTD primary tumor (Murchison *et al.* 2010). Since the first case report, the disease has rapidly spread south and westwards to over 85% of the original devil distributional range and caused severe population declines. The overall population has dropped by 80% and local declines in northeastern populations is higher than 90% (Figure 1b; Hamede *et al.* 2008). Demographic and genetic evidence suggests that DFTD has led to significant changes in the life history, genetic structure and dispersal patterns in post-disease devil populations (Jones *et al.* 2008; Lachish *et al.* 2011). For instance, in five examined eastern populations, the age structure has been greatly altered after disease arrival, resulting in a much lower proportion of older (3+ years) animals. Meanwhile, responding to the increased adult mortality, early reproduction by 1-year-old females has increased by up to 16 fold in these populations (Jones *et al.* 2008). Furthermore, although change in the overall genetic diversity is not detected due to the low diversity level before the disease outbreak, microsatellite genotyping data demonstrates that DFTD has caused increased inbreeding and induced genetic differentiation among disease-affected populations (Lachish *et al.* 2011). To date, no effective vaccine or treatment has been developed against DFTD. Ongoing population decline in diseased areas has raised considerable concerns of possible regional extinction of devils in the wild (McCallum *et al.* 2009). Due to the threat posed by DFTD, the conservation status of the Tasmanian devil was raised from Low Risk to Vulnerable in 2007 and further to Endangered in 2009.

Transmissibility of DFTD and Low MHC Diversity in the Tasmanian Devil

The DFTD tumor cell is a clonal cell line, which is transmitted between devils as allograft by cellular inoculation (e.g. biting). This allograft theory was first put forward by Pearse and Swift (2006) based on cytogenetic studies where they found that tumors from different individuals share the same karyotype which is dramatically different from the normal devil karyotype. Subsequently, independent lines of evidence have further reinforced the allograft hypothesis (Pyecroft *et al.* 2007; Siddle *et al.* 2007; Murchison *et al.* 2010)

Normally, allograft between genetically different individuals will stimulate humoral and cellular immunity in the recipient and trigger acute immunological rejection, which is due to the recognition by the recipient's T lymphocytes of both foreign MHC antigens expressed on the grafted cells and graft-derived peptides bound to self MHC (Bjorkman *et al.* 1987; Hutchinson 1991). However, to date, no Tasmanian devil has been identified to be naturally capable of rejecting the DFTD tumor. The "grafted" tumor cells can overcome immunological barriers of the host and adapt in unrelated individuals across the whole devil population. Such high transmissibility is unusual for cancer, which is commonly considered a non-infectious disease. There have been rare cases suggesting that some cancer can be transmitted between genetically related individuals, such as mother and fetus, or in laboratory inbred animals (reviewed in O'Neill 2010). The only other naturally occurring contagious cancer that has been documented is the canine transmissible venereal tumor (CTVT) in dogs (Karlson & Mann 1952; Das & Das 2000). CTVT is an infectious venereal tumor that is also found to have a clonal nature and spread by physical transfer of tumor cells, but the life history and host adaptation is different from that of DFTD (reviewed in Murchison 2009). Transplantation experiments have shown that most (over 80%) CTVT tumors go through three phases of growth: an initial progressive phase in which tumor size increases rapidly; a subsequent stable phase when tumor growth markedly slows down; finally and most distinct from DFTD, a spontaneous regressive phase, during which the tumor shrinks and eventually disappears (Epstein & Bennett 1974; Chu *et al.* 2001).

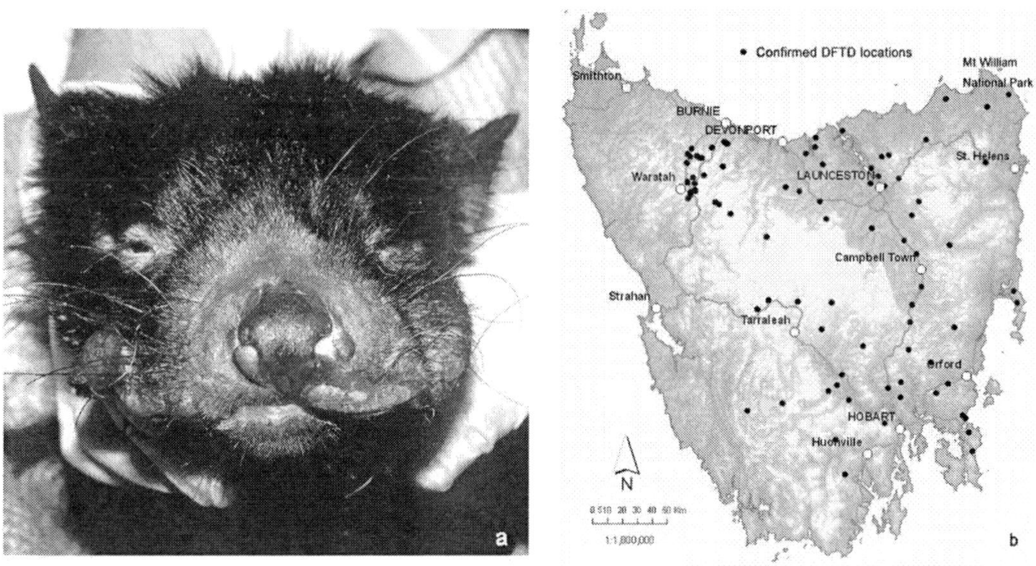

Figure 1. (a) Tasmanian devil with advanced DFTD; (b) Distribution of DFTD in Tasmania by November 2010. (Modified from Save the Tasmanian Devil Program website - http://www.tassiedevil.com.au)

Research on the MHC has led to important insights into the transmissibility of contagious cancers (reviewed in Belov 2011). In CTVT, in spite of the abundant allelic variation of dog MHC, the tumor cells evade immune detection and elimination by T cells and NK cells through downregulating the MHC class I and II gene expression during the progressive growth phase (Murgia *et al.* 2006). It is also found that corresponding to the transition to regressive phase, the normal MHC expression level is resumed under regulation by host cytokines IL-6 and IFN-γ (Murgia *et al.* 2006; Hsiao *et al.* 2008).

In the Tasmanian devil, MHC diversity studies have demonstrated that there is a significant loss of MHC antigen variability in the devil population, which enables DFTD to spread readily (Siddle *et al.* 2007; Siddle *et al.* 2010). In the disease-affected eastern populations, no or extremely low mixed lymphocyte responses were detected (Siddle *et al.* 2007). Single-strand conformation polymorphism (SSCP) analysis conducted on 387 devils across Tasmania revealed 25 types of banding patterns at MHC class I loci (Siddle *et al.* 2010). A high similarity was observed in the eastern devils, with over 30% of individuals sharing the identical SSCP profile as the tumor, whereas the disease-free northwestern population exhibited a slightly higher diversity of MHC types. This has also been further confirmed by sequencing of MHC sequence variants. The genetic variation within the peptide-binding regions of both class I and II molecules is highly limited across the devil population (Siddle *et al.* 2010; Cheng *et al.* 2011). As the host shares essentially the same MHC antigens with the tumor, T cells of the host fail to recognize the DFTD cells as foreign tissue.

Whether there are devils naturally resistant to DFTD remains uncertain. One recent interesting finding is that, based on sequence analysis of MHC class I alleles from eastern and northwestern devils, there could be a variation in the copy number of MHC class I genes between different devil haplotypes (Siddle *et al.* 2010). This raises hopes that some individuals may possess MHC haplotypes that are sufficiently different from those of DFTD to allow immunological recognition of tumor cells. This hypothesis is currently under investigation through construction and sequencing of BAC contigs for different MHC haplotypes (Cheng *et al.* 2011). Another important question to be answered is whether altered expression of MHC antigens occurs in DFTD. Both MHC class I and II complete transcripts have been identified from tumor RNA (Siddle *et al.* 2007), but the expression level and functionality of these molecules require further examination.

DISCUSSION

The disastrous consequences of DFTD on the Tasmanian devil population has provided a striking example of how emerging diseases can cause population declines in short periods of time and be a serious threat to endangered or even common wildlife species. The continuous degradation of global ecosystems, primarily through biological impoverishment, habitat fragmentation and climate change, is leading to increased levels of stress and immunosuppression in wild animals and as a consequence accelerating the emergence of new wildlife diseases (Aguirre & Tabor 2008). These emerging infectious pathogens in wildlife represent an increasing threat to human and domestic animal health. The global spread of avian influenza, the severe acute respiratory syndrome disease outbreak in Asia, the Ebola hemorrhagic fever in Africa, and the Hendra virus outbreaks in Australia are some classical examples of transmission of zoonotic pathogens between wildlife, domestic animals and humans that caused enormous losses (reviewed in Daszak *et al.* 2000; Wang *et al.* 2006; Vandegrift *et al.* 2010). By putting endangered and vulnerable species at risk of extinction, emerging pathogens pose a tremendous threat to biodiversity conservation. Adding to the example of the Tasmanian devil, in 1990s, two emerging diseases, chytridiomycosis and ranaviral disease, caused mass deaths of Amphibian species across the world and led to significant global declines in Amphibian population with local extinctions of multiple species in multiple areas (Daszak *et al.* 1999). Rapid population declines in two common bird species in the UK have been reported recently due to trichomonosis, a protozoal disease newly emerged in 2005 (Robinson *et al.* 2010). In geographic regions of highest disease incidence, the examined bird populations decreased by up to 35% within two years after the disease appeared.

The possibility of new pathogen emergence provides an important incentive to maintain a high MHC antigen variability in wildlife populations. Having a high level of MHC diversity is important for successful defense by the host immune system against pathogens. In order to evade detection by the immune system, pathogens usually evolve in at least one of two possible ways: they can eliminate peptides that can bind MHC molecules by mutations, or they can develop mechanisms to block the pathway of peptide presentation by MHC molecules (Frank 2002). Since different MHC molecules can bind and present different ranges of peptides, increasing the variety of MHC molecules in the population reduces the probability that a pathogen will escape recognition or block antigen presentation by all the them (Trowsdale & Parham 2004). Applying this theory to the scenario when a new pathogen arises, it is reasonable to deduce that having a large collection of diverse MHC antigen variants in a population may increase the chance of recognition of the pathogen by the host immune system and therefore decrease the risk of large-scale outbreak and reduce the deleterious impact of the disease on the population. Moreover, based on the selection theory, an emerging pathogen will post new selective forces on the affected population and alter the genetic structure (e.g. allelic richness, frequency, heterozygosity, etc.) at MHC loci (Hughes 1999). A high MHC diversity may buffer the impact of such purifying selection and reduce the chance of severe selective sweep. Therefore, low MHC diversity represents a major disadvantage to a population threatened by emerging pathogen challenges.

Low MHC diversity can result from a variety of causes. Bottlenecked or small isolated populations suffering from founder effects are vulnerable to the loss of general genetic variation due to evolutionary forces such as genetic drift and inbreeding (George & Brown 1992). The Tasmanian devil, which has an overall low genetic variation, likely belongs to this case (Jones *et al.* 2004; Bradshaw & Brook 2005). Under such circumstances, despite the effect of balancing selection that favors polymorphism, genetic drift can sometimes overwhelm the positive selective force, leading to allelic loss and low genetic variation not only at MHC loci but also across the whole genome. With that being said, one should also note that a low overall genetic diversity does not necessarily imply low MHC diversity. It has been reported that in the San Nicolas Island fox (*Urocyon littoralis dickeyi*), which is monomorphic at a number of hypervariable genetic markers, has remarkably high levels of variation at MHC loci (Aguilar *et al.* 2004). In this case, strong balancing selection is suggested to be the key mechanism to account for such different diversity levels between MHC and neutral loci (Aguilar *et al.* 2004). Using computer simulation models, Ejsmond and Radwan (2011) have recently demonstrated that the extent to which balancing selection can maintain or restore MHC diversity in bottlenecked populations is dependant on the timescales involved, with the balancing selection outweighing drift after ~40 generations of the host after the bottleneck. Another important factor that may cause low MHC variability is purifying selection or selective sweep. Under strong purifying selection, MHC alleles or haplotypes that offer an individual with a significant higher fitness can become predominant in the population and "unfit" alleles can be eliminated. In chimpanzees, evidence has been found that a severe loss of class I gene diversity has been caused by a historical selective sweep, possibly attributed to the chimpanzee-derived simian immunodeficiency virus (De Groot *et al.* 2008).

To date, depleted MHC diversity has been observed in a number of wildlife species. Besides those mentioned above, some other representative examples are cheetah (O'Brien *et al.* 1985), whale (Trowsdale *et al.* 1989), Scandinavian beaver (Ellegren *et al.* 1993), Swedish moose (Mikko & Andersson 1995), Arabian oryx (Hedrick *et al.* 2000), Giant panda (Zhu *et al.* 2007) and Galápagos penguin (Bollmer *et al.* 2007). Here, by revisiting the case of the Tasmanian devil, we stress the importance for conservation biologists to take into account the MHC diversity when assessing the health of wild populations. In some instances, low MHC variability may not have significant impact on population dynamics on a short timescale (Ellegren *et al.* 1993; Halley & Rosell 2002). However, for the long-term survival and health of a population, a low level of MHC diversity should be view as an alarm of compromised capability to respond to environment changes and possible emerging diseases. It is crucial for those who work in conservation and management of such populations to be extra alert to the sign of new disease appearance. We should also keep in mind that only to rely on balancing selection to maintain the diversity of MHC alleles can be insufficient in endangered species (Ejsmond & Radwan 2011). The Save the Tasmanian Devil Program has taken efforts to manage and maintain MHC allelic diversity during the development of the insurance population and breeding strategy. We hope that this will preserve MHC allelic variability in the long term, alleviating loss due to strong selection by DFTD.

ACKNOWLEDGMENTS

Our work is funded by the Australian Research Council, the Save the Tasmanian Devil Appeal and the University of Sydney Veterinary Science Foundation. YC is supported by an Endeavour International Postgraduate Research Scholarship. KB is supported by an ARC Future Fellowship.

REFERENCES

Aguilar A, Roemer G, Debenham S, Binns M, Garcelon D, Wayne RK (2004) High MHC diversity maintained by balancing selection in an otherwise genetically monomorphic mammal. *Proceedings of the National Academy of Sciences*, 101, 3490-3494.

Aguirre AA, Tabor GM (2008) Global Factors Driving Emerging Infectious Diseases. *Annals of the New York Academy of Sciences*, 1149, 1-3.

Andersson L (1996) Major histocompatibility complex evolution. In: *The Major Histocompatibility Complex Region of Domestic Animal Species* (eds Schook LB, Lamont SJ), pp. 1-15, CRC Press, Boca Raton, USA.

Archer M, Baynes A (1972) Prehistoric mammals faunas from two small caves in the extreme southwest of Western Australia. *Journal of The Royal Society of Western Australia*, 55, 80-89.

Belov K (2011) The role of the Major Histocompatibility Complex in the spread of contagious cancers. *Mammalian Genome*, 22, 83-90.

Bjorkman PJ, Saper MA, Samraoui B, Bennett WS, Strominger JL, Wiley DC (1987) The foreign antigen binding site and T cell recognition regions of class I histocompatibility antigens. *Nature*, 329, 512-518.

Bollmer JL, Vargas FH, Parker PG (2007) Low MHC variation in the endangered Galápagos penguin (*Spheniscus mendiculus*). *Immunogenetics*, 59, 593-602.

Borghans J, Keşmir C, De Boer R (2007) MHC diversity in Individuals and Populations. In: *In Silico Immunology* (eds Flower D, Timmis J), pp. 177-196, Springer, New York.

Bradshaw CJA, Brook BW (2005) Disease and the devil: density-dependent epidemiological processes explain historical population fluctuations in the Tasmanian devil. *Ecography*, 28, 181-190.

Cheng Y, Morris K, Taylor R *et al.* (2011) Characterization of the Tasmanian devil MHC. Manuscript in preparation.

Cheng Y, Sanderson C, Siddle HV, Belov K (2011) Loss of genetic diversity at MHC class II loci in the Tasmanian devil. Manuscript in preparation.

Chu RM, Lin CY, Liu CC *et al.* (2001) Proliferation characteristics of canine transmissible venereal tumor. *Anticancer research*, 21, 4017-4024.

Cresswell P, Ackerman AL, Giodini A, Peaper DR, Wearsch PA (2005) Mechanisms of MHC class I-restricted antigen processing and cross-presentation. *Immunological Reviews*, 207, 145-157.

Das U, Das AK (2000) Review of canine transmissible venereal sarcoma. *Vet Res Commun*, 24, 545-556.

Daszak P, Berger L, Cunningham AA, Hyatt AD, Green DE, Speare R (1999) Emerging infectious diseases and amphibian population declines. *Emerging infectious diseases*, 5, 735-748.

Daszak P, Cunningham AA, Hyatt AD (2000) Emerging Infectious Diseases of Wildlife - Threats to Biodiversity and Human Health. *Science*, 287, 443-449.

De Boer RJ, Borghans JA, van Boven M, Keşmir C, Weissing FJ (2004) Heterozygote advantage fails to explain the high degree of polymorphism of the MHC. *Immunogenetics*, 55, 725-731.

De Groot NG, Heijmans CMC, De Groot N *et al.* (2008) Pinpointing a selective sweep to the chimpanzee MHC class I region by comparative genomics. *Molecular Ecology*, 17, 2074-2088.

Edwards SV, Potts WK (1996) Polymorphism of genes in the major histocompatibility complex: implications for conservation genetics of vertebrates. In: *Molecular genetic approaches in conservation* (eds Smith TB, Wayne RK), Oxford University Press, Oxford, UK.

Ejsmond MJ, Radwan J (2011) MHC diversity in bottlenecked populations: a simulation model. *Conservation Genetics*, 12, 129-137.

Ellegren H, Hartman G, Johansson M, Andersson L (1993) Major Histocompatibility Complex Monomorphism and Low Levels of DNA Fingerprinting Variability in a Reintroduced and Rapidly Expanding Population of Beavers. *Proceedings of the National Academy of Sciences*, 90, 8150-8153.

Epstein RB, Bennett BT (1974) Histocompatibility Typing and Course of Canine Venereal Tumors Transplanted into Unmodified Random Dogs. *Cancer Research*, 34, 788-793.

Frank SA (2002) Immunology and Evolution of Infectious Disease. Princeton University Press, Princeton, USA.

Froeschke G, Sommer S (2005) MHC class II DRB variability and parasite load in the striped mouse (*Rhabdomys pumilio*) in the Southern Kalahari. *Molecular Biology and Evolution*, 22, 1254-1259.

George GG, Brown PR (1992) Conservation management of small populations. In: *Australasian Marsupials and Monotremes: An Action Plan for Their Conservation* (eds Kennedy M), International Union for Conservation of Nature, Gland, Switzerland.

Gill ED (1971) The Australian Aborigines and the Tasmanian devil. *Mankind*, 8, 59-60.

Halley DJ, Rosell F (2002) The beaver's reconquest of Eurasia: status, population development and management of a conservation success. *Mammal Review*, 32, 153-178.

Hamede R, McCallum H, Jones ME (2008) Seasonal, demographic and density-related patterns of contact between Tasmanian devils: Implications for transmission of Devil Facial Tumour Disease. *Austral Ecology*, 33, 614-622.

Hawkins CE, Baars C, Hesterman H *et al.* (2006) Emerging disease and population decline of an island endemic, the Tasmanian devil *Sarcophilus harrisii. Biological Conservation*, 131, 307-324.

Hedrick PW, Parker KM, Gutiérrez-Espeleta GA, Rattink A, Lievers K (2000) Major histocompatibility complex variation in the Arabian oryx. *Evolution*, 54, 2145-2151.

Hill AV, Allsopp CE, Kwiatkowski D *et al.* (1991) Common west African HLA antigens are associated with protection from severe malaria. *Nature*, 352, 595-600.

Hsiao YW, Liao KW, Chung TF, Liu CH, Hsu CD, Chu RM (2008) Interactions of host IL-6 and IFN-γ and cancer-derived TGF-β1 on MHC molecule expression during tumor spontaneous regression. *Cancer Immunology, Immunotherapy*, 57, 1091-1104.

Hughes AL (1999) Adaptive Evolution of Genes and Genomes. Oxford University Press, New York, USA.

Hutchinson IV (1991) Cellular mechanisms of allograft rejection. *Current Opinion in Immunology*, 3, 722-728.

Janeway CA, Travers P, Walport M, Shlomchik M (2001) Immunobiology: the immune system in health and disease. Garland Publishing, New York, USA.

Jones ME (2001) Large marsupial carnivores. In: *The Encyclopedia of Mammals* (eds Macdonald DW), pp. 814-817, Oxford University Press, Oxford, UK.

Jones ME, Cockburn A, Hamede R *et al.* (2008) Life-history change in disease-ravaged Tasmanian devil populations. *Proceedings of the National Academy of Sciences*, 105, 10023-10027.

Jones ME, Oakwood M, Belcher CA *et al.* (2003) Carnivore concerns: problems, issues and solutions for conserving Australiasia's marsupial carnivores. In: *Predators with pouches: the biology of carnivorous marsupials* (eds Jones M, Dickman CR, Archer M), pp. 422-434, CSIRO Publishing, Melbourne, Australia.

Jones ME, Paetkau D, Geffen E, Moritz C (2004) Genetic diversity and population structure of Tasmanian devils, the largest marsupial carnivore. *Molecular Ecology*, 13, 2197-2209.

Karlson AG, Mann FC (1952) The transmissible venereal tumor of dogs: observations on forty generations of experimental transfers. *Ann NY Acad Sci*, 54, 1197-1213.

Kelley J, Walter L, Trowsdale J (2005) Comparative genomics of major histocompatibility complexs. *Immunogenetics*, 56, 683-695.

Lachish S, Miller KJ, Storfer A, Goldizen AW, Jones ME (2011) Evidence that disease-induced population decline changes genetic structure and alters dispersal patterns in the Tasmanian devil. *Heredity*, 106, 172-182.

Loh R, Bergfeld J, Hayes D *et al.* (2006) The pathology of Devil Facial Tumor Disease (DFTD) in Tasmanian Devils (*Sarcophilus harrisii*). *Veterinary Pathology*, 43, 896-903.

McCallum H, Jones M, Hawkins C *et al.* (2009) Transmisson dynamics of Tasmanian devil facial tumor disease may lead to disease-induced extinction. *Ecology*, 90, 3379-3392.

McCallum H, Tompkins DM, Jones M *et al.* (2007) Distribution and impacts of Tasmanian devil facial tumor disease. *EcoHealth*, 4, 318-325.

Meyer-Lucht Y, Sommer S (2005) MHC diversity and the association to nematode parasitism in the yellow-necked mouse (*Apodemus flavicollis*). *Molecular Ecology*, 14, 2233-2243.

Mikko S, Andersson L (1995) Low major histocompatiblity complex class II diversity in European and North American moose. *Proceedings of the National Academy of Sciences*, 92, 4259-4263.

Murchison EP (2009) Clonally transmissible cancers in dogs and Tasmanian devils. *Oncogene*, 27, S19-S30.

Murchison EP, Tovar C, Hsu A *et al.* (2010) The Tasmanian Devil Transcriptome Reveals Schwann Cell Origins of a Clonally Transmissible Cancer. *Science*, 327, 84-87.

Murgia C, Pritchard JK, Kim SY, Fassati A, Weiss RA (2006) Clonal Origin and Evolution of a Transmissible Cancer. *Cell*, 126, 477-487.

O'Brien S, Evermann J (1988) Interactive influence of infectious disease and genetic diversity in natural populations. *Trends in Ecology & Evolution*, 3, 254-259.

O'Brien SJ, Roelke ME, Marker L *et al.* (1985) Genetic basis for species vulnerability in the cheetah. *Science*, 227, 1428-1434.

O'Neill ID (2010) Tasmanian devil facial tumor disease: insights into reduced tumor surveillance from an unusual malignancy. *International Journal of Cancer*, 127, 1637-1642.

Parham P, Strominger JL (1982) Histocompatibility Antigens Structure and Function. In: *Receptors and Recognition Series B, Vol.14*, Chapman and Hall, New York.

Paterson S, Wilson K, Pemberton JM (1998) Major histocompatibility complex variation associated with juvenile survival and parasite resistance in a large unmanaged ungulate population (*Ovis aries L.*) *Proceedings of the National Academy of Sciences*, 95, 3714-3719.

Pearse AM, Swift K (2006) Allograft theory: transmission of devil facial-tumour disease. *Nature*, 439, 549.

Pieters J (2000) MHC class II-restricted antigen processing and presentation. *Advances in Immunology*, 75, 159-208.

Pyecroft SB, Pearse AM, Loh R *et al.* (2007) Towards a case definition for Devil Facial Tumour Disease: What is it? *EcoHealth*, 4, 346-351.

Robinson RA, Lawson B, Toms MP *et al.* (2010) Emerging Infectious Disease Leads to Rapid Population Declines of Common British Birds. *PLoS ONE*, 5, e12215.

Scotto G, Fazio V, D'Alessandro G *et al.* (2003) Association between HLA class II antigens and hepatitis C virus infection. *Journal of Biological Regulators & Homeostatic Agents*, 17, 316-321.

Siddle HV, Kreiss A, Eldridge MDB *et al.* (2007) Transmission of a fatal clonal tumor by biting occurs due to depleted MHC diversity in a threatened carnivorous marsupial. *Proceedings of the National Academy of Sciences*, 104, 16221-16226.

Siddle HV, Marzec J, Cheng Y, Jones M, Belov K (2010) MHC gene copy number variation in Tasmanian devils: implications for the spread of a contagious cancer. *Proceedings of the Royal Society B*, 277, 2001-2006.

Sommer S (2005) The importance of immune gene variability (MHC) in evolutionary ecology and conservation. *Frontiers in Zoology*, 2, 16.

Thursz MR, Kwiatkowski D, Allsopp CE, Greenwood BM, Thomas HC, Hill AV (1995) Association between an MHC class II allele and clearance of hepatitis B virus in the Gambia. *The New England journal of medicine*, 332, 1065-1069.

Trowsdale J, Groves V, Arnason A (1989) Limited MHC polymorphism in whales. *Immunogenetics*, 41, 19-24.

Trowsdale J, Parham P (2004) Mini-review: Defense strategies and immunity-related genes. *European Journal of Immunology*, 34, 7-17.

Vandegrift KJ, Sokolow SH, Daszak P, Kilpatrick AM (2010) Ecology of avian influenza viruses in a changing world. *Annals of the New York Academy of Sciences*, 1195, 113-128.

Wang LF, Shi Z, Zhang S, Field H, Daszak P, Eaton BT (2006) Review of bats and SARS. *Emerging infectious diseases*, 12, 1834-1840.

Xu TJ, Chen SL, Ji XS, Tian YS (2008) MHC polymorphism and disease resistance to Vibrio anguillarum in 12 selective Japanese flounder (*Paralichthys olivaceus*) families. *Fish & shellfish immunology*, 25, 213-221.

Zhu L, Ruan XD, Ge YF, Wan QH, Fang SG (2007) Low major histocompatibility complex class II DQA diversity in the Giant Panda (*Ailuropoda melanoleuca*). *BMC Genetics*, 8, 29.

In: Major Histocompatibility Complex
Editor: Natalya V. Semiletova
ISBN: 978-1-61942-999-4

Chapter 5

TNF BLOCK HAPLOTYPES REVEAL DIVERSE PATHWAYS BETWEEN TNF AND DISEASE: IMPLICATIONS FOR UNDERSTANDING NEUROPATHY IN HIV PATIENTS

Constance S. N. Chew[1], Fabio P. Valente[2], Hillary J. Wallace[3], Joo H. Tan[1], Suzanah E. Temple[4], and Patricia Price[1]*

[1]Pathology and Laboratory Medicine, University of Western Australia, Nedlands, Australia
[2]School of Bioinformatics, University of Paris Diderot, Paris, France
[3]Pathology and Laboratory Medicine, University of Western Australia, Fremantle Hospital, Fremantle, Australia
[4]School of Medicine and Pharmacology, University of Western Australia, Perth, Australia

ABSTRACT

The region spanning the tumor necrosis factor (TNF) cluster in the human major histocompatibility complex (MHC) has been implicated in susceptibility to numerous immunopathological and inflammatory diseases. However, strong linkage disequilibrium in the region creates conserved TNF block haplotypes; hampering identification of specific polymorphisms responsible for disease phenotypes. Here we review studies investigating TNF block haplotypes and their links with cytokine production and inflammatory disease risk.

Recent work has done much to characterize TNF block haplotypes in different ethnicities and their associations with the larger overall structure of MHC ancestral

* Corresponding author. Professor Patricia Price, School of Pathology and Laboratory Medicine, University of Western Australia, Nedlands, Australia, 6009. Tel: 618-9224 0378, Fax : 618-9224 0204, email patricia.price@uwa.edu.au.

haplotypes. There have also been studies examining the effects of TNF block haplotypes on levels of inflammatory cytokine production, with others investigating haplotype association with diseases risk. Carriage of specific TNF block haplotypes have been associated with increased risk of Type II Diabetes, Chronic Venous Leg Ulceration and Nucleoside Reverse Transcriptase-associated Sensory Neuropathy, all conditions where the underlying pathogenesis lies in a dysregulated inflammatory response. Despite this, no one haplotype was associated with susceptibility to all these diseases, inferring the TNF block region is involved in the multiple pathways of inflammatory dysregulation leading to disease phenotype.

The central MHC on human chromosome 6 spans more than 700 kilobases of DNA and contains in excess of 60 genes, making it one of the most gene-dense regions in the human chromosome. A number of diseases, many of them immunopathological in character, have been associated with variations in MHC genes marked by alleles of the HLA loci. It is thought that whilst there are associations with the HLA class II region of the MHC there are also genes within the central MHC which act in conjunction with the class II genes to mediate susceptibility to these diseases. Some of the genes within the central MHC are well known and characterised. These include the complement genes, the heat shock protein 70 (HSP70) cluster and the tumour necrosis factor (TNF) cluster. Disease pathogenesis may most obviously be influenced by the gene encoding TNF-α.

TNF-α confers both protection against infections, but is also implicated in pathological conditions, such as transplant rejection, septic shock, viral replication, rheumatoid arthritis, bacterial infections and Type 1 Diabetes Mellitus (T1DM) depending on the timing, localization and extent of release (reviewed in [1]). Hence anti-TNFα antibodies (Infliximab) are effective in treating rheumatoid arthritis and Crohn's disease [2], but promote more severe tuberculosis [3]. Inflammatory diseases such as inflammatory bowel disease, multiple sclerosis, rheumatoid arthritis, systemic lupus erythematosus and T1DM show a potential association with TNFα levels [4]. This pro-inflammatory cytokine is an essential component of inflammatory and immune responses, but may be harmful in excess.

An interesting example is the 8.1 ancestral haplotype (AH) [HLA -A1, B8, TNFA-308*2, DR3, DQ2]. The broad spectrum of diseases affected by this haplotype [eg: IgA deficiency, T1DM, rapid HIV disease, inclusion body myositis, coeliac disease, myasthenia gravis, Graves disease] suggests it has non-specific immunomodulatory effects. Although the disorders are triggered by different genetic and environmental stimuli and have diverse manifestations, they all involve elevated levels of inflammatory mediators (eg: TNFα). However other diseases with an immunopathological basis associate with other *TNF* haplotypes [5].

Unfortunately the precise gene(s) or polymorphism(s) responsible for these complex disease phenotypes remain unknown, because linkage disequilibrium (LD) creates conserved haplotypes within and across the MHC. Comparisons between haplotypes associated with a disease in multiple ethnic populations may narrow the list of candidate polymorphisms that warrant more detailed study.

1. The Distribution of TNF Block Haplotypes Varies with Ethnicity

TNF block haplotypes were first studied in a West African population recruited in Gambia [6]. Twenty five single nucleotide polymorphisms (SNPs) spanning ~80kb near *TNF* yielded 22 haplotypes accounting for 80% of the sample. Subsequently, Allcock *et al* investigated 19 SNPs spanning 45kb around *TNF* and found only 17 distinct haplotypes in a mixed European population from Western Australia [7]. We built on this work to characterize TNF block haplotypes. DNA from 999 healthy donors from European, Asian (Bidayuh, Chinese, Indian, Jehai, Malay, Temuan) and Australian Aboriginal populations was genotyped at 38 loci to provide a framework which subsequent disease association studies could refer to. The polymorphisms were primarily in coding and promoter regions over a 60kb region spanning seven genes near *TNF* (*MCCD1, BAT1, ATP6V1G2, IKBL, LTA, TNF* and *LST1*).

31 TNF block haplotypes were observed (out of 2^{38} possible haplotypes) in all populations combined, with 19 or less in any single population (Table 1, reproduced with permission from Valente *et al*). The number of reconstructed haplotypes in the European populations was similar (18 and 15), whilst the Asian and Indian cohorts had fewer haplotypes (8 to 15). Some haplotypes were observed at a high frequency in the Asian and Indian groups as an artefact arising from the small sample sizes or due to derivation from a small ancestral pool. Despite variations in the frequencies of haplotypes in each ethnicity, four to eight TNF block haplotypes exist across all ethnicities and hence must pre-date the divergence of these populations from a common ancestor >160,000 years ago.

TNF block haplotypes could be separated in a hierarchical structure with five distinct clusters. Some haplotypes were unique to isolated populations but they did not contain unique SNP. In a phylogenic analysis, each population grouping had haplotypes in all five clusters and no cluster was specific to one population. Hence they reflect restricted migration and/or extinction of some families rather than *de novo* mutation. This highlights the need to study relationships between the haplotypes found in each ethnic population.

The study addressed the pitfalls of using non-tag SNPs (see Table1); the FV16 haplotype contains TNFA-308*A (rs1800629), which has been associated with multiple disease phenotypes [8]. BAT1intron10*A (rs9281523) is a tag SNP for FV16 in Northern Indians, Australian Aborigines, South East Asians and Europeans. However carriage of TNFA-308*A without BAT1intron10*A has been observed previously [9] and was characterised here as FV15 and FV17. NFKBIL1-62*A (rs2071592) is associated with susceptibility to rheumatoid arthritis [10] and lies in FV16 and six other haplotypes, so typing this SNP provides little information. Thus it is important to characterize conserved TNF haplotypes to establish a framework for disease association studies.

Associations with MHC genes outside the TNF block also vary with ethnicity. For example HLA-B8 and DR3,DQ2 span FV16 in Europeans (the 8.1 ancestral haplotype (AH)) and FV20 in North Indians (the 8.2AH) [11]. HSP and C4 alleles of the 8.2AH have been described [12].

Table 1. Thirty-one haplotypes explain all populations studied (Table reproduced with the permission of Valente *et al*)

Haplotype	rs3130055	rs9281523	rs1055388	rs1129540	rs2516393	rs3130059	rs2239527	rs2523506	rs2239528	rs2523504	rs2844509	rs2251824	rs2071594	rs2071593	rs3219186	rs2071592	rs2239708	rs2071591	rs7738380	rs6916921	rs2857505	rs2230365	rs3130062	rs4947324	rs2516312	rs2071590	rs2229394	rs1799964	rs4248158	rs1800730	rs1800529	rs361525	rs3093561	rs1799769	rs3093562	rs3093565	rs3093568	rs1052248
FV1	-	-	-	-	-	-	-	-	-	-	2	-	-	-	-	-	-	-	-	-	-	-	-	2	-	-	2	2	-	-	-	2	2	-	2	-	2	2
FV2	-	-	-	-	-	-	-	2	-	-	2	-	-	-	-	-	-	-	-	-	-	-	-	2	-	-	2	2	-	-	-	2	2	-	2	-	2	2
FV3	-	-	-	-	-	-	-	-	-	-	2	-	-	-	-	-	-	-	-	-	-	-	-	2	-	-	2	2	-	-	-	2	2	-	2	-	2	-
FV4	-	-	-	-	-	-	-	-	-	-	2	-	-	-	-	-	-	-	-	-	-	-	-	2	-	-	2	2	-	2	-	2	-	-	2	-	-	-
FV5	-	-	-	-	-	-	-	-	-	-	2	-	-	-	-	-	-	-	-	-	-	-	-	2	-	-	2	-	-	-	-	-	-	-	2	2	-	2
FV6	-	-	-	-	-	-	-	2	-	-	-	2	-	-	-	-	-	-	-	-	-	-	-	-	-	-	2	2	2	-	-	-	-	-	-	-	-	2
FV7	-	-	-	-	-	-	-	2	-	-	-	2	-	-	2	-	-	-	-	-	-	-	-	-	-	-	2	2	2	-	-	-	-	-	-	-	-	2
FV8	-	-	-	-	-	-	-	2	-	-	-	2	-	-	-	-	-	-	-	-	-	-	-	-	-	-	2	2	-	-	-	-	-	-	-	-	-	2
FV9	-	-	-	-	-	-	-	2	-	-	-	2	-	-	-	-	-	-	-	-	-	2	-	-	-	-	2	2	-	-	-	-	-	-	-	-	-	-
FV10	-	-	-	-	-	-	-	2	-	-	-	2	-	-	-	-	-	-	-	-	-	2	-	-	-	-	2	2	-	-	-	-	-	-	-	-	-	2
FV11	-	-	-	-	-	-	-	-	-	-	2	-	-	-	-	-	-	-	-	2	-	-	-	-	-	2	-	-	-	-	-	-	-	-	-	-	-	-
FV12	-	-	-	-	-	-	-	-	-	-	2	-	-	-	-	-	-	-	-	2	-	-	-	-	-	2	-	2	2	-	-	-	-	-	-	-	-	-
FV13	-	-	-	-	-	-	-	-	-	-	2	-	-	-	-	-	-	-	-	2	-	-	-	-	-	2	-	-	-	-	-	-	-	-	-	-	-	2
FV14	-	-	-	-	-	-	-	-	-	-	2	-	-	-	-	-	-	-	-	-	-	-	-	-	-	2	-	-	-	-	-	-	-	-	-	-	-	-
FV15	-	-	-	-	-	2	2	-	-	-	-	-	2	-	-	2	-	2	-	-	-	-	-	-	-	-	-	-	-	-	2	-	-	2	-	-	-	-
FV16	-	2	-	-	-	2	2	-	-	-	-	-	2	-	-	2	-	2	-	-	-	-	-	-	-	-	-	-	-	-	2	-	-	-	-	-	-	-
FV17	-	-	-	-	-	2	2	-	-	-	-	-	2	-	-	2	-	2	-	-	-	-	-	-	-	-	-	-	-	-	2	-	-	-	-	-	-	-
FV18	-	-	-	-	-	2	2	-	-	-	-	-	2	-	-	2	-	2	-	-	-	-	-	-	-	-	-	-	-	-	-	-	-	-	-	-	-	-
FV19	2	-	2	-	-	2	2	-	-	-	-	-	2	-	-	2	-	2	-	-	-	-	-	-	-	-	-	-	-	-	-	-	-	-	-	-	-	-
FV20	-	-	-	-	-	2	-	-	-	-	-	-	2	-	-	2	-	2	-	-	-	-	-	-	-	-	-	-	-	-	-	-	-	-	-	-	-	2
FV21	-	-	-	-	-	2	2	-	-	-	-	-	2	-	-	2	-	2	-	-	-	-	-	-	-	-	-	-	-	-	-	-	-	-	-	-	-	2
FV22	-	-	-	-	-	2	2	-	-	-	-	-	2	-	-	-	-	2	-	-	-	-	-	-	-	-	-	-	-	-	-	-	-	-	-	-	-	-
FV23	-	-	-	-	-	2	2	-	-	-	-	-	2	-	-	-	-	2	-	-	2	-	-	-	-	-	-	-	-	-	-	-	-	-	-	-	-	-
FV24	-	-	-	-	-	-	2	-	-	-	-	-	2	-	-	-	-	-	-	-	-	2	-	-	-	-	2	2	-	-	-	-	-	-	-	-	-	2
FV25	2	-	2	-	-	-	-	-	2	2	-	-	-	2	-	-	2	-	-	-	2	2	-	-	-	-	-	-	-	-	-	-	-	-	-	-	-	2
FV26	2	-	2	-	-	-	-	-	2	2	-	-	-	2	-	-	2	-	-	-	2	2	-	-	-	-	-	-	-	-	-	-	2	-	-	-	-	2
FV27	2	-	2	2	2	-	-	-	2	2	-	-	-	-	2	-	-	-	-	-	2	-	-	-	-	2	-	-	-	-	-	-	-	-	-	-	-	-
FV28	2	-	2	2	2	-	-	-	2	2	-	-	-	-	2	-	-	-	-	-	2	-	2	-	-	2	-	-	-	-	-	-	-	-	-	-	-	-
FV29	2	-	2	2	2	-	-	-	2	2	-	-	-	-	2	-	-	-	-	-	2	-	-	-	-	2	-	-	-	-	-	-	2	-	-	-	-	-
FV30	2	-	2	2	2	-	-	-	2	2	-	-	-	-	-	-	-	-	2	-	-	-	-	-	2	2	-	-	-	-	-	-	-	-	-	-	-	-
FV31	-	-	2	-	-	-	-	-	2	2	-	-	-	2	-	-	-	-	-	-	-	-	-	2	-	-	2	-	-	-	-	-	-	-	-	-	-	-

Haplotype	Population Frequencies									
	Busselton	Perth	Australian Aboriginal	North Indian	South Indian	Bidayuh	Chinese	Jehai	Malay	Temuan
FV1	3.86%	4.50%	1.18%	4.68%	5.85%	NF	NF	NF	NF	NF
FV2	NF	NF	NF	NF	0.03%	NF	NF	NF	1.00%	NF
FV3	NF	NF	0.51%	NF	NF	0.16%	2.04%	NF	3.00%	NF
FV4	1.38%	0.49%	1.03%	NF	NF	NF	NF	NF	NF	NF
FV5	1.81%	2.19%	0.76%	NF	NF	NF	NF	NF	NF	NF
FV6	1.81%	1.50%	**19.3%**	**3.50%**	**20.1%**	0.49%	9.42%	NF	3.22%	NF
FV7	NF	NF	0.13%	NF	NF	15.6%	NF	NF	3.83%	NF
FV8	4.66%	4.74%	1.89%	11.0%	6.68%	1.22%	NF	NF	5.24%	3.41%
FV9	NF	NF	0.06%	NF	NF	NF	4.08%	2.31%	1.00%	NF
FV10	9.36%	12.8%	6.70%	5.11%	3.34%	10.2%	2.74%	16.0%	8.47%	24.7%
FV11	5.74%	7.56%	14.3%	14.1%	18.9%	NF	**14.3%**	3.06%	3.00%	3.99%
FV12	NF	NF	NF	1.95%	NF	NF	NF	NF	0.95%	NF
FV13	0.49%	0.45%	1.66%	0.03%	NF	NF	NF	NF	NF	NF
FV14	8.12%	9.63%	2.39%	1.73%	0.03%	NF	3.06%	NF	1.00%	NF
FV15	4.14%	4.63%	0.88%	1.15%	NF	NF	NF	NF	0.54%	NF
FV16	**14.2%**	12.4%	4.85%	6.42%	NF	8.16%	15.7%	4.79%	8.24%	6.37%
FV17	0.06%	NF	0,52%	3.17%	3.66%	NF	1.04%	0.04%	0.51%	0.21%
FV18	11.6%	13.3%	8.57%	12.3%	13.4%	13.3%	**29.2%**	8.34%	26.9%	22.8%
FV19	NF	NF	NF	0.16%	NF	NF	7.12%	NF	2.00%	NF
FV20	1.04%	NF	NF	7.81%	3.08%	NF	NF	NF	NF	NF
FV21	NF	NF	0,27%	2.09%	0.77%	NF	NF	NF	NF	0.02%
FV22	2.29%	1.71%	2.19%	NF	NF	NF	NF	NF	NF	NF
FV23	NF	NF	0,50%	NF	NF	NF	NF	19.4%	5.00%	5.98%
FV24	NF	NF	NF	NF	NF	NF	NF	NF	NF	**1.07%**
FV25	5.68%	2.35%	10.4%	13.3%	6.87%	7.10%	3.06%	5.10%	11.0%	9.94%
FV26	NF	NF	NF	NF	NF	**13.3%**	NF	NF	NF	NF
FV27	8.92%	7.56%	9.33%	**4.68%**	9.87%	16.8%	8.15%	**40.8%**	12.6%	17.9%
FV28	6.05%	7.56%	4.10%	NF	NF	NF	NF	NF	NF	NF
FV29	NF	NF	NF	NF	NF	**11.3%**	NF	NF	NF	NF
FV30	2.23%	0.73%	NF	NF	0.61%	NF	NF	NF	NF	0.54%
FV31	2.80%	2.68%	1.16%	1.12%	0.73%	NF	NF	NF	NF	NF
Cumulative Frequency	95.8%	95.1%	89.1%	94.2%	91.7%	97.0%	99.8%	99.8%	95.5%	96.2%
2n	386	410	386	256	66	98	98	98	100	100
Number of Haplotypes > 1%	18	15	15	16	10	9	12	8	15	9

Frequencies were defined by PHASE program [Stephens and Donnelly, 2003] such that values reflect the probability of a given haplotypic assignment in each individual of that population. A dash "-" represents the major allele and "2" represents the minor allele. NF = not found in the samples tested. Red indicates SNP which tag haplotypes in all cohorts and grey represents population-specific tag SNP.

Table 2. Population frequencies of haplotypes carrying TNF-1031*2 (rs1799964) in HIV+ SN patients and controls

Panel A	*Bat1*	*Bat1*	*Bat1*	*NFKIBL*	*TNF*	*TNF*	Malay			Chinese			Caucasian		
Haplotype	rs9281523	rs2523506	rs2844509	rs2230365	rs1799964	rs1800629	HIV+ SN+ (n=21)	HIV+ SN- (n=43)	Healthy controls (n=136)	HIV+ SN+ (n=19)	HIV+ SN- (n=55)	Healthy controls (n=99)	HIV+ SN+ (n=17)	HIV+ SN- (n=20)	Healthy controls (n=193)
TNF-1031*2	NI	NI	NI	NI	2	NI	47.7%	36.6%	48.1%	55.6%	34.4%	31.3%	47.3%	45.0%	41.4%
FVa 1, 3, 4, 12	1	1	2	1	2	1	0%	0%	5.2%	0%	5.5%	3.0%	5.9%	5.0%	11.0%
FVa 6, 7, 8	1	2	1	1	2	1	33.3%	14.0%	32.6%[b,c]	21.1%[a]	3.6%	12.1%	11.8%	5.0%	10.5%
FVa 9, 10	1	2	1	2	2	1	14.3%	7.0%	11.1%[b,c]	31.6%	18.2%	23.2%	38.9%	19.0%	18.8%
FVa 24	1	1	1	2	2	1	0%	2.3%	0%	0%	0%	0%	0%	0%	0%
Cumulative Frequency							47.6%	23.3%	48.7%	52.7%	27.3%	38.3%	56.6%	29.0%	40.3%
2n							42	86	272	38	110	198	34	40	362

Panel B	Malay			Chinese			Caucasian		
Variable	p	OR	95% CI	p	OR	95% CI	p	OR	95% CI
Age (years)	0.02	1.18	1.02 - 1.36	0.06	1.04	1.00 - 1.10	0.005	1.21	1.06 -1.38
Height (cm)	0.01	1.11	1.03 - 1.21	NS	NS	NS	NA	NA	NA
FVa6,7,8	0.03	5.02	1.19 - 21.0	0.03	7.68	1.18 - 50.0	0.16	8.69	0.74 -1130
Overall model p-value	0.002			0.01			0.001		

Bivariate analysis suggested FVa6,7,8 may affect SN status (Panel A). Multivariate analysis comparing genotyping and age, height and FVa6,7,8 between stavudine-exposed HIV patients with and without sensory neuropathy yielded a significant model in Chinese and Malays ($p=0.007$, $p=0.02$ respectively) (Panel B). Haplotypes not found in any populations were omitted.

NI denotes SNPs not included in analyses.

The major allele at each SNP is denoted '1' and the rare allele at each SNP is denoted '2'.

NS denotes $p \geq 0.2$ in bivariate analyses and therefore excluded from the multivariate model.

NA denotes incomplete data.

[a] Indicates $p < 0.05$ using Fisher's exact test comparing HIV+ SN+ with HIV+ SN- cohorts.

[b] Indicates $p < 0.05$ using Fisher's exact test comparing Healthy Malay controls with Healthy Chinese controls.

[c] Indicates $p < 0.05$ using Fisher's exact test comparing Healthy Malay controls with Healthy Caucasian controls.

[Note: The cumulative FVa haplotype and rs1799964 minor allele frequencies were measured by carriage. In some cases, a few donors were homozygous for the minor allele of rs1799964 but carried two different FVa haplotypes, accounting for the lower values recorded for rs1799964. A few carriers of rs1799964 had no resolvable haplotype, accounting for some instances where the allele frequencies were higher than haplotype frequencies.]

2. Venous Leg Ulcers are Caused by Excess Production of TNF and Correlate with a Known Disease-Associated Haplotype Spanning the TNF Block

Venous leg ulcers, chronic wounds of the lower leg, are the most severe clinical outcome of individuals with chronic venous insufficiency. Chronic venous insufficiency is caused by primary varicose diseases and secondary effects of deep venous thrombosis (post-thrombotic syndrome) and the incidence of ulceration increases with age. Impaired venous return facilitates the beginning of the inflammatory cascade, but the mechanism of impaired healing remains largely uncharacterized [13]. Persistent inflammation is a key feature of chronic venous leg ulcers (CVLU) and initiation of healing is associated with the decline of TNF-α protein levels in wound fluid [14, 15].

Wallace *et al* [11] used conserved FV-series of TNF block haplotypes to examine their associations with susceptibility to CVLU in elderly Caucasian donors. 171 patients with confirmed CVLU were compared with 173 age/gender-matched controls, excluding individuals with T1DM) or rheumatoid arthritis. 194 healthy subjects formed a separate population-based control group. Samples were typed for TNF Block SNP, HLA-B and HLA-DRB1 alleles. TNF haplotypes were derived using the PHASE algorithm and assigned numbers (FVx) as defined by Valente *et al* [11].

The CVLU cases and age/gender-matched controls shared 16 TNF block haplotypes (frequency >1%). The cases cohort had two additional haplotypes (FV5 and FV6). Carriage of FV16 and/or certain MHC ancestral haplotypes (AH) (8.1AH, 62.1AH and 60.3AH) was more common in patients with CVLU than controls. Recombinant mapping implicated FV16 as the critical portion of the 8.1AH. Associations were slightly different when cases were compared to the population-based controls, probably reflecting subtle changes in haplotype frequencies due to the exclusion of individuals with T1DM or rheumatoid arthritis.

3. TNF Haplotypes May Contribute to Associations between HLA-DR/DQ and Type 1 Diabetes Mellitus

The clearest genetic markers of susceptibility to T1DM are HLA class II haplotypes marked by HLA-DRB1*0301 (DR3) and –DRB1*0401 (DR4) [16, 17]. Amongst Caucasians, HLA-DR3 occurs most commonly on a single MHC class II haplotype HLA-DRB1*0301, DQA1*0501, DQB1*0201. This is usually carried as part of the 8.1 AH (HLA-A1,B8,DR3,DQ2) in Northern Europeans or on the 18.2 AH (HLA-A30, B18, DR3, DQ2) in Southern Europeans. We have mapped additional susceptibility determinants carried by the 8.1 AH to putative immunoregulatory genes in the central MHC [5, 18], and shown that these modify the effects of the associated class II alleles. Other groups have used microsatellite alleles to demonstrate susceptibility loci telomeric of the class II region [19]. Associations with alleles of *MICA* [20] and *TNFA* [21] microsatellites and a single nucleotide polymorphism (SNP) in *RAGE* [22] have been demonstrated, with plausible arguments that alleles of these genes could influence pathogenesis. Studies of NOD mice confirm a role for MHC genes other than the class II genes (IA^{g7}) in susceptibility. Alleles linked to *H-2D* were implicated [23]. This fits with the concept that the induction of inflammation requires a "danger signal", as well as antigen recognition.

An interesting observation is the association between T1DM and the 8.2AH (HLA-A26,B8, DR3, DQ2) in the Northern Indian population [24]. It is unclear whether these individuals carry diabetogenic genes in the central MHC in addition to the class II alleles, since their TNF block haplotype is FV20 (compared with FV16 in the 8.1AH) [11]. Alleles shared by FV16 and FV20 warrant further investigation.

In contrast to HLA-DR3 (DRB1*0301), several sub-types of HLA-DR4 are common and have divergent affects on T1DM. T1DM susceptibility has been associated with HLA-DRB1*0401, -DRB1*0402 and -DRB1*0405 alleles in several Caucasian cohorts. Conversely HLA-DRB1*0403, and in some studies -DRB1*0404, marked resistance. Strong linkage disequilibrium between HLA-DR and -DQ complicates identification of critical class II alleles. We addressed whether the MHC associations reflect linkage disequilibrium with the true susceptibility locus by studying broader MHC haplotypes marked by alleles of *HLA-B*, *IKBL* (adjacent to *TNFA*) and complement *C4.* At that time we had used 19 SNP spanning the TNF cluster including IKBL+446(C/T) (rs2230365) to define 17 haplotypes describing 90% of a Caucasian population [7]. Haplotypes containing HLA-DRB1*0401 and -DRB1*0404 were distinguished by several alleles including IKBL+446.

HLA-DRB1*0401 and HLA-DRB1*0405 marked susceptibility to T1DM [25]. In Caucasians, *DRB1*0401* occurs predominantly in the 44.1 AH (HLA-A2,B44, DRB1*0401,DQB1*0301) and the 62.1AH (HLA-A2,B15[62], DRB1*0401,DQB1*0302). We then screened alleles characteristic of the 62.1AH (C4B3, IKBL+446*T and HLA-A2,B15) in donors pre-selected for *HLA-DRB1*0401. C4B3* was associated with T1DM, consistent with a diabetes gene telomeric of MHC class II. Unfortunately increases in carriage of IKBL+446*T and HLA-A2,B15 were marginal, as too few control subjects were available with the diabetogenic alleles. However with these tools, selection of HLA-DRB1*0401, DQB1*0302 donors who are positive and negative for *C4B3* will allow bi-directional mapping of diabetes genes in the central MHC.

4. Disease-associated Haplotypes do not Affect Production of TNF and LTA in Short Term Cultures

Tan *et al* [26] used the 31 TNF block haplotypes (denoted FV1-31) identified in Caucasians, Asians and Australian Aboriginals [11]. TNF-α and lymphotoxin alpha (LTA) protein production by peripheral blood mononuclear cells were examined in samples from 205 healthy Caucasian subjects, following *in vitro* stimulation with *Streptococcus pneumoniae* (*S.pneumoniae;* Gram positive bacteria), *Escherichia coli* (*E coli;* Gram negative bacteria) or TNF-α over 4, 8 and 24 hours.

Fifteen haplotypes were present at >1%, accounting for 94.5% of the cohort. Following stimulation, cells from carriers of the FV10 haplotype produced less LTA than non-FV10 carriers. Carriers of the FV18 haplotype produced more LTA than other donors. Induction of TNF-α by *S.pneumoniae* following 24h stimulation was also greater in donors with FV18. The FV18 haplotype associated with the 44.1 AH (HLA-A2, C5, B44, DRB1*0401, DQB1*0301) which has few disease associations. FV16 occurred in the 8.1 AH (HLA-A1,

B8, DR3) associated with multiple immunopathological diseases. FV16 did not affect TNF-α or LTA levels. The findings suggest that many genetic variations critical *in vivo* are not effectively modelled by short term cultures.

5. TNF Block Haplotypes Incorporating TNFA-1031 Increase risk of Sensory Neuropathy (SN) in HIV Patients on Antiretroviral Therapy

Given that TNF haplotypes affect several inflammatory diseases, we considered their role in the pathogenesis of SN. Antiretroviral therapy has lengthened the life expectancy of patients with HIV [27] and prompted a shift in focus to the patients' quality of life. The incidence of most neurological complications of HIV has declined following the introduction of antiretroviral therapy. In contrast, the prevalence of SN has increased, exceeding 40% in some cohorts [28, 29]. Studies of risk factors associated with SN are hampered by the lack of a "gold standard" definition. SN is typically characterized by pain in the feet described as 'aching', 'painful numbness' or 'burning'[30]. Patients may also have reduced or absent ankle reflexes, hyperalgesia and allodynia. SN may be promoted by exposure to nucleoside analogue reverse transcriptase inhibitors (NRTI), notably stavudine (d4T) [29]. NRTI-associated sensory neuropathy (NRTI-SN) is clinically and histologically similar to distal sensory polyneuropathy (DSP), a subset of SN directly caused by HIV. NRTI-SN is distinguished from other forms of SN by a temporal relationship between symptom onset and exposure to NRTIs [31].

The neurotoxicity of NRTIs d4T, ddI and ddC is well recognized. From the time they were introduced into phase 1 clinical trials, SN was the dose-limiting toxicity of all these agents [32] and since then SN has been associated with exposure to NRTIs in multiple cohorts. Stavudine (d4T) is still widely used in the developing world as it is cheap and effective in the control of HIV replication.

The pathogenesis of DSP involves disordered local inflammation in the dorsal route and ganglia. Immunopathological studies have shown macrophage infiltration and cytokine production, with TNF-α observed around peripheral nerves in affected patients [33, 34]. Neuronal dysfunction may result from excessive production of neurotoxic cytokines by activated macrophages [34, 35]. As regulators of inflammation, cytokines may play a role in SN. Elevated serum levels of TNFα are documented in Guillain-Barre syndrome, chronic inflammatory demyelinating polyneuropathy and multifocal motor neuropathy [36-38]. There is *in vivo* and *in vitro* evidence that aberrant host inflammatory responses underpin painful neuropathies in non-HIV associated neuropathies [39].

T1DM patients with diabetic neuropathy showed an activation of the TNF-α system [40]. Soluble TNFR1 and TNFR2 receptors were measured in the plasma of patients with >14 years of T1DM who were screened for sensory neuropathy. A 2.8- and 1.6-fold increased risk for diabetic neuropathy was observed for each 1ug/l increase in sTNFR1 and sTNFR2, respectively. The finding remained significant after adjusting for potential confounders in a multivariate analysis. This supports previous studies reporting diabetic nephropathy and retinopathy were associated with activation of the TNF-α pathway [41, 42].

In animal models of T1DM, suppression of the TNF-α system has been associated with an improvement of diabetic polyneuropathy [43]. Daily oral administration of NAC (a precursor of glutathione) dose-dependently inhibited LPS-induced serum levels of TNF-α in diabetic rats. Diabetic rats dosed with TNF-α had decreased motor nerve conduction velocity in the sciatic nerve, although the same effect was not observed in non-diabetic rats. Treatment with NAC improved the decreased motor nerve conduction velocity in diabetic rats previously given TNF-α. NAC administration did not affect metabolic changes associated with T1DM, so the beneficial effects of NAC on diabetic nerve probably reflect inhibition of the TNF-α pathway.

In a 2007 study of non-HIV SN, Uceyler *et al* observed patients with painful neuropathy had 2- fold higher blood IL-2 and TNF mRNA levels than patients with painless neuropathy and healthy controls [39]. This mirrored similar trends in TNF-α protein levels. In contrast patients with painless neuropathy had about two-fold higher levels of anti-inflammatory cytokine IL-10 compared to patients with painful neuropathy or controls [39]. This supports the likely hyperalgesic function of TNF-α in animal models of pain, where TNF-α applied to nerve fibres *in vitro* or *in vivo* increases electrical activity [44, 45]. Applied to patients, this implies increased levels of TNF-α in blood and the endoneurial environment would increase c-fibre activity and thus elicit sensations of pain. At a local level, pro-inflammatory cytokine levels may be higher than circulatory levels. Sural nerve biopsies of patients with inflammatory and non-inflammatory neuropathies show a positive correlation between locally elevated TNF-α levels and pain [46]. The authors suggested two hypotheses; the first implies TNF-α production is a result of neuropathy and not a factor in disease pathogenesis, whilst the second attributes a direct role to TNF-α in pathogenesis via increased microvascular permeability, hypercoagulability or direct nerve damage.

Expression of *TNF* is regulated at the transcriptional level so polymorphisms in the promoter region modulate *TNF* gene expression. Carriage of the minor alleles of *TNF* promoter region single nucleotide polymorphism TNFA-308*A (rs1800629) and TNFA-857*C (rs1799724) have been associated with increased circulating TNF-α levels [47, 48] though the studies did not consider linkage disequilibrium. The effects of TNF block haplotypes on TNF-α levels were covered previously (section 4). TNF haplotypes may affect SN as TNFA-308*A occurred at a higher frequency in Caucasian and African American HIV-infected adults with dementia, than in HIV-infected adults without dementia or a healthy control group [49, 50]. We had associated SNP within the TNF block, including TNFA-1031*C, with NRTI-SN risk in Australian Caucasian patients exposed to potentially neurotoxic NRTI [51]. This SNP also associated with SN in stavudine-exposed Indonesian HIV patients [52].

Valente *et al* defined the FV TNF block haplotype set which could be used to identify SNPs responsible for various disease phenotypes (see Section 1). Eleven haplotypes contained the SN-associated SNP TNFA-1031*C (rs1799964).

We identified a FV haplotype group associated with neuropathy in ethnically Malay (Indonesian and Malaysian), Chinese and Caucasian (Australian) HIV patients. To narrow down the list of SNPs affecting neuropathy, we selected six SNPs which sorted the 11 haplotypes containing TNFA-1031*C into four groups. The SNPs were located in *TNF* promoter regions (rs1799964 and rs1800629), *BAT1* intron and promoter regions (rs9281526, rs2523506 and rs2844509) and *NFKIBL* promoter regions (rs2230365). The four 6-SNP-haplotypes were named FVa1,3,4,12, FVa6,7,8, FVa9,10 and FVa24. Carriage of each FVa haplotype was compared with SN incidence in a univariate analysis (Table 2A). Carriage of FVa9,10 was more common in Caucasian HIV+ SN+ patients compared with healthy controls, but controls and HIV+ SN− patients were otherwise similar. However several ethnic differences were apparent. Carriage of FVa9,10 was less common in Malay HIV patients compared with Caucasian HIV patients; carriage of FVa6,7,8 was more common in Malay than healthy Chinese and Caucasian controls, and more common in Malay HIV patients than in Chinese HIV patients. In bivariate analyses FVa6,7,8 conferred a 7-fold increased risk of NRTI-SN in Chinese patients. Malay and Caucasian patients also displayed similar trends. In general, carriage of FVa6,7,8 was similar in HIV+ SN+ patients and healthy controls, and lower in HIV+ SN− patients. This difference was significant amongst Malays. FVa9,10 appeared to be associated with a reduced risk of SN in Caucasians, but this was not evident in a multivariate analysis. TNFA-1031*C (rs1799964) was the only SNP where carriage of the minor allele differed between patients with and without SN.

Clinical risk factors considered included age, height, gender, nadir and current CD4 T-cell counts. Only age was associated with SN across all ethnicities, and height was associated with SN in Malay patients. Logistic regression modelling showed that FVa6,7,8 was independently associated with NRTI-SN risk in both Malay and Chinese patients after correcting for age and height (Table 2B). It conferred an increased SN risk in Chinese and Malay HIV patients. A similar trend was observed in the Caucasian cohort.

Conclusions

Recent experimental studies imply that genetically-determined increases in the production of TNF-α are involved with the pathogenesis of inflammatory disease. As the SNP responsible have not been identified, these variations are most effectively marked by TNF block haplotypes. Although the haplotypes appear to modulate susceptibility to neuropathy in HIV patients, the underlying mechanisms are unknown. Histochemical studies may provide critical evidence. Genetic analyses of an African population where SN is common [53] will also be revealing.

References

[1] Aggarwal BB. Signalling pathways of the TNF superfamily: a double-edged sword. *Nat Rev Immunol.* 2003;3(9):745-56.

[2] Maini RN, Taylor PC, Paleolog E, Charles P, Ballara S, Brennan FM, *et al.* Anti-tumour necrosis factor specific antibody (infliximab) treatment provides insights into the pathophysiology of rheumatoid arthritis. *Ann Rheum Dis.* 1999 November 1, 1999;58(90001):i56-60.

[3] Keane J, Gershon S, Wise RP, Mirabile-Levens E, Kasznica J, Schwieterman WD, *et al.* Tuberculosis Associated with Infliximab, a Tumor Necrosis Factor {alpha}-Neutralizing Agent. *N Engl J Med.* 2001 October 11, 2001;345(15):1098-104.

[4] Mackay F, Kalled SL. TNF ligands and receptors in autoimmunity: an update. *Current Opinion in Immunology.* 2002;14(6):783-90.

[5] Price P, Witt C, Allcock R, Sayer D, Garlepp M, Chee Choy K, *et al.* The genetic basis for the association of the 8.1 ancestral haplotype (A1, B8, DR3) with multiple immunopathological diseases. *Immunological Reviews.* 1999;167(1):257-74.
[6] Ackerman HC, Ribas G, Jallow M, Mott R, Neville M, Sisay-Joof F, *et al.* Complex haplotypic structure of the central MHC region flanking TNF in a West African population. *Genes Immun.* 2003 Oct;4(7):476-86.
[7] Allcock RJ, Windsor L, Gut IG, Kucharzak R, Sobre L, Lechner D, *et al.* High-Density SNP genotyping defines 17 distinct haplotypes of the TNF block in the Caucasian population: implications for haplotype tagging. *Hum Mutat.* 2004 Dec;24(6):517-25.
[8] Bayley JP, Ottenhoff TH, Verweij CL. Is there a future for TNF promoter polymorphisms? *Genes Immun.* 2004 Aug;5(5):315-29.
[9] Price P, Morahan G, Huang D, Stone E, Cheong KY, Castley A, *et al.* Polymorphisms in cytokine genes define subpopulations of HIV-1 patients who experienced immune restoration diseases. *AIDS.* 2002 Oct 18;16(15):2043-7.
[10] Okamoto K, Makino S, Yoshikawa Y, Takaki A, Nagatsuka Y, Ota M, *et al.* Identification of I kappa BL as the second major histocompatibility complex-linked susceptibility locus for rheumatoid arthritis. *Am J Hum Genet.* 2003 Feb;72(2):303-12.
[11] Valente FP, Tan C, Phipps M, Witt CS, Kaur G, Gut I, *et al.* TNF block haplotypes associated with conserved MHC haplotypes in European, Asian and Australian Aboriginal donors. *Tissue Antigens.* 2009 Jul;74(1):57-61.
[12] Kaur G, Kumar N, Szilagyi A, Blasko B, Fust G, Rajczy K, *et al.* Autoimmune-associated HLA-B8-DR3 haplotypes in Asian Indians are unique in C4 complement gene copy numbers and HSP-2 1267A/G. *Hum Immunol.* 2008 Sep;69(9):580-7.
[13] Abbade LP, Lastoria S. Venous ulcer: epidemiology, physiopathology, diagnosis and treatment. *Int J Dermatol.* 2005 Jun;44(6):449-56.
[14] Wallace HJ, Stacey MC. Levels of tumor necrosis factor-alpha (TNF-alpha) and soluble TNF receptors in chronic venous leg ulcers--correlations to healing status. *J Invest Dermatol.* 1998 Mar;110(3):292-6.
[15] Trengove NJ, Bielefeldt-Ohmann H, Stacey MC. Mitogenic activity and cytokine levels in non-healing and healing chronic leg ulcers. *Wound Repair Regen.* 2000 Jan-Feb;8(1):13-25.
[16] Noble JA, Valdes AM, Cook M, Klitz W, Thomson G, Erlich HA. The role of HLA class II genes in insulin-dependent diabetes mellitus: molecular analysis of 180 Caucasian, multiplex families. *Am J Hum Genet.* 1996 Nov;59(5):1134-48.
[17] She JX. Susceptibility to type I diabetes: HLA-DQ and DR revisited. *Immunol Today.* 1996 Jul;17(7):323-9.
[18] Degli-Esposti MA, Abraham LJ, McCann V, Spies T, Christiansen FT, Dawkins RL. Ancestral haplotypes reveal the role of the central MHC in the immunogenetics of IDDM. *Immunogenetics.* 1992;36(6):345-56.
[19] Hanifi Moghaddam P, de Knijf P, Roep BO, Van der Auwera B, Naipal A, Gorus F, *et al.* Genetic structure of IDDM1: two separate regions in the major histocompatibility complex contribute to susceptibility or protection. Belgian Diabetes Registry. *Diabetes.* 1998 Feb;47(2):263-9.
[20] Gambelunghe G, Ghaderi M, Cosentino A, Falorni A, Brunetti P, Sanjeevi CB. Association of MHC Class I chain-related A (MIC-A) gene polymorphism with Type I diabetes. *Diabetologia.* 2000 Apr;43(4):507-14.
[21] Obayashi H, Nakamura N, Fukui M, Tegoshi H, Fujii M, Ogata M, *et al.* Influence of TNF microsatellite polymorphisms (TNFa) on age-at-onset of insulin-dependent diabetes mellitus. *Hum Immunol.* 1999 Oct;60(10):974-8.

[22] Prevost G, Fajardy I, Fontaine P, Danze PM, Besmond C. Human RAGE GLY82SER dimorphism and HLA class II DRB1-DQA1-DQB1 haplotypes in type 1 diabetes. *Eur J Immunogenet.* 1999 Oct;26(5):343-8.
[23] Mathews CE, Graser RT, Serreze DV, Leiter EH. Reevaluation of the major histocompatibility complex genes of the NOD-progenitor CTS/Shi strain. *Diabetes.* 2000 Jan;49(1):131-4.
[24] Kanga U, Vaidyanathan B, Jaini R, Menon PS, Mehra NK. HLA haplotypes associated with type 1 diabetes mellitus in North Indian children. *Hum Immunol.* 2004 Jan;65(1):47-53.
[25] Windsor L, Puschendorf M, Allcock R, Scott A, Sayer D, Kucharzak R, *et al.* Does a central MHC gene in linkage disequilibrium with HLA-DRB1*0401 affect susceptibility to type 1 diabetes? *Genes Immun.* 2005 Jun;6(4):298-304.
[26] Tan JH, Temple SE, Kee C, Waterer GW, Tan CR, Gut I, *et al.* Characterisation of TNF block haplotypes affecting the production of TNF and LTA. *Tissue Antigens.* Feb;77(2):100-6.
[27] Palella FJ, Jr., Delaney KM, Moorman AC, Loveless MO, Fuhrer J, Satten GA, *et al.* Declining morbidity and mortality among patients with advanced human immunodeficiency virus infection. HIV Outpatient Study Investigators. *N Engl J Med.* 1998 Mar 26;338(13):853-60.
[28] Pettersen JA, Jones G, Worthington C, Krentz HB, Keppler OT, Hoke A, *et al.* Sensory neuropathy in human immunodeficiency virus/acquired immunodeficiency syndrome patients: protease inhibitor-mediated neurotoxicity. *Ann Neurol.* 2006 May;59(5):816-24.
[29] Smyth K, Affandi JS, McArthur JC, Bowtell-Harris C, Mijch AM, Watson K, *et al.* Prevalence of and risk factors for HIV-associated neuropathy in Melbourne, Australia 1993-2006. *HIV Med.* 2007 Sep;8(6):367-73.
[30] So YT, Holtzman DM, Abrams DI, Olney RK. Peripheral neuropathy associated with acquired immunodeficiency syndrome. Prevalence and clinical features from a population-based survey. *Arch Neuro*l. 1988 Sep;45(9):945-8.
[31] Keswani SC, Pardo CA, Cherry CL, Hoke A, McArthur JC. HIV-associated sensory neuropathies. *Aids.* 2002 Nov 8;16(16):2105-17.
[32] Cherry CL, McArthur JC, Hoy JF, Wesselingh SL. Nucleoside analogues and neuropathy in the era of HAART. *J Clin Virol.* 2003 Feb;26(2):195-207.
[33] Nagano I, Shapshak P, Yoshioka M, Xin K, Nakamura S, Bradley WG. Increased NADPH-diaphorase reactivity and cytokine expression in dorsal root ganglia in acquired immunodeficiency syndrome. *J Neurol Sci.* 1996 Mar;136(1-2):117-28.
[34] Wesselingh SL, Glass J, McArthur JC, Griffin JW, Griffin DE. Cytokine dysregulation in HIV-associated neurological disease. *Adv Neuroimmunol.* 1994;4(3):199-206.
[35] Bradley W, Shapshak P, Delgado S, Nagano I, Stewart R, Rocha B. Morphometric analysis of the peripheral neuropathy of AIDS. *Muscle & Nerve.* 1998;21(9):1188-95.
[36] Creange A, Belec L, Clair B, Raphael JC, Gherardi RK. Circulating tumor necrosis factor (TNF)-alpha and soluble TNF-alpha receptors in patients with Guillain-Barre syndrome. *J Neuroimmunol.* 1996 Aug;68(1-2):95-9.
[37] Misawa S, Kuwabara S, Mori M, Kawaguchi N, Yoshiyama Y, Hattori T. Serum levels of tumor necrosis factor-alpha in chronic inflammatory demyelinating polyneuropathy. *Neurology.* 2001 Mar 13;56(5):666-9.
[38] Terenghi F, Allaria S, Nobile-Orazio E. Circulating levels of cytokines and their modulation by intravenous immunoglobulin in multifocal motor neuropathy. *J Peripher Nerv Syst.* 2006 Mar;11(1):67-71.

[39] Uceyler N, Rogausch JP, Toyka KV, Sommer C. Differential expression of cytokines in painful and painless neuropathies. *Neurology.* 2007 Jul 3;69(1):42-9.
[40] Gonzalez-Clemente JM, Mauricio D, Richart C, Broch M, Caixas A, Megia A, *et al.* Diabetic neuropathy is associated with activation of the TNF-alpha system in subjects with type 1 diabetes mellitus. *Clin Endocrinol* (Oxf). 2005 Nov;63(5):525-9.
[41] Zoppini G, Faccini G, Muggeo M, Zenari L, Falezza G, Targher G. Elevated plasma levels of soluble receptors of TNF-alpha and their association with smoking and microvascular complications in young adults with type 1 diabetes. *J Clin Endocrinol Metab.* 2001 Aug;86(8):3805-8.
[42] Tataranni PA, Ortega E. A burning question: does an adipokine-induced activation of the immune system mediate the effect of overnutrition on type 2 diabetes? *Diabetes.* 2005 Apr;54(4):917-27.
[43] Satoh J, Yagihashi S, Toyota T. The possible role of tumor necrosis factor-alpha in diabetic polyneuropathy. *Exp Diabesity Res.* 2003 Apr-Jun;4(2):65-71.
[44] Junger H, Sorkin LS. Nociceptive and inflammatory effects of subcutaneous TNFalpha. *Pain.* 2000 Mar;85(1-2):145-51.
[45] Schafers M, Lee DH, Brors D, Yaksh TL, Sorkin LS. Increased sensitivity of injured and adjacent uninjured rat primary sensory neurons to exogenous tumor necrosis factor-alpha after spinal nerve ligation. *J Neurosci.* 2003 Apr 1;23(7):3028-38.
[46] Empl M, Renaud S, Erne B, Fuhr P, Straube A, Schaeren-Wiemers N, *et al.* TNF-alpha expression in painful and nonpainful neuropathies. *Neurology.* 2001 May 22;56(10):1371-7.
[47] Wilson AG, Symons JA, McDowell TL, McDevitt HO, Duff GW. Effects of a polymorphism in the human tumor necrosis factor alpha promoter on transcriptional activation. *Proc Natl Acad Sci U S A.* 1997 Apr 1;94(7):3195-9.
[48] van Heel DA, Udalova IA, De Silva AP, McGovern DP, Kinouchi Y, Hull J, *et al.* Inflammatory bowel disease is associated with a TNF polymorphism that affects an interaction between the OCT1 and NF(-kappa)B transcription factors. *Hum Mol Genet.* 2002 May 15;11(11):1281-9.
[49] Quasney MW ZQ, Sargent S, Mynatt M, Glass J, McArthur J. Increased frequency of the tumor necrosis factor-alpha-308 A allele in adults with human immunodeficiency virus dementia. *Annual Neurology.* 2001 2001 Aug;50(2):157-62.
[50] Pemberton LA, Stone E, Price P, van Bockxmeer F, Brew BJ. The relationship between ApoE, TNFA, IL1a, IL1b and IL12b genes and HIV-1-associated dementia. *HIV Med.* 2008 Oct;9(8):677-80.
[51] Cherry CL, Rosenow A, Affandi JS, McArthur JC, Wesselingh SL, Price P. Cytokine genotype suggests a role for inflammation in nucleoside analog-associated sensory neuropathy (NRTI-SN) and predicts an individual's NRTI-SN risk. *AIDS Res Hum Retroviruses.* 2008 Feb;24(2):117-23.
[52] Affandi JS, Price P, Imran D, Yunihastuti E, Djauzi S, Cherry CL. Can we predict neuropathy risk before stavudine prescription in a resource-limited setting? *AIDS Res Hum Retroviruses.* 2008 Oct;24(10):1281-4.
[53] Cherry CL, Affandi J, Brew B, Kamerman P, McArthur JC, Price P, *et al.* Ethnicity Is an Independent Predictor of Neuropathy Risk in HIV Patients. *18th Conference on Retroviruses and Opportunistic infections.* 2011.

In: Major Histocompatibility Complex
Editor: Natalya V. Semiletova

ISBN: 978-1-61942-999-4

Chapter 6

MHC, VIRAL INFECTION AND IMMUNOINFORMATICS

Maurício Menegatti Rigo, Dinler Amaral Antunes, Marialva Sinigaglia, José Artur Bogo Chies and Gustavo Fioravanti Vieira
Department of Genetics, Federal University of Rio Grande do Sul, Porto Alegre, Brazil

ABSTRACT

The immunologic surveillance is performed by several molecules (e.g. antibodies and complement system) and cells (e.g. T lymphocytes, Natural Killer cells) which are triggered depending on the type of infection. In the specific context of the viral infection, a special set of molecules, named Major Histocompatibility Complex of class I (MHC-I), which is represented by the Human Leukocyte Antigen (HLA) genes in humans, perform an essential role. These molecules are responsible for the presentation of small peptides from viruses, parasites, bacteria or even from human proteins to the T Cell Lymphocytes, which will or will not trigger an immune response, through the T Cell Receptor (TCR) interaction. There are two classes of MHC: MHC-I and MHC-II. The MHC-I is responsible for the presentation of small peptides (8-12 amino acids long) generated by endogenous processing, while the MHC-II presents longer peptides (up to 30 amino acids) from exogenous environment. Regarding MHC-I presentation it is known that topologies and electrostatics patterns of the peptide:MHC (pMHC) interacting region are important for TCR recognition. Also, the affinity and stability between the peptide (epitope) and the MHC (receptor) play a crucial role, especially on what concerns electrostatics and non-hydrophobic interactions between the MHC and anchor residues of the peptide. All these features stand for the peptide immunogenicity. The knowledgment of issues regarding peptide affinity by MHC cleft and the stability of resulting complex is pivotal for vaccine development field. Nowadays, there are several immunoinformatics tools available to assist the resolution of this task. For instance, peptide binding affinity could be predicted through several computational methods (i.e. using tools that consider amino acid sequence composition and preferential anchor residues occurrence). There are also bioinformatics tools that are not specific for immunological issues, but can be used for this purpose, such as molecular docking and molecular dynamics. The latter can be used to assess pMHC complex stability, one of the main factors involved in peptide presentation. In the present chapter we intend to review basic molecular aspects regarding the MHC-I molecule and its interaction with different epitopes. Also, the use of immunoinformatics aiming to understand the different levels of MHC-I interaction will be discussed.

INTRODUCTION

Considered as the most polymorphic and densest (taking into account the number of genes) of all regions of the human genome, widely explored and studied by different approaches, the Major Histocompatibility Complex (MHC) region contains a wide variety of genes involved in immune responses. Among them, the so-called HLA (for Human Leukocyte Antigen) are certainly the better studied and yet most mysterious molecules coded by genes of this region. Classically divided into class I and class II, HLA molecules have as primary function the presentation of antigens to immune cells. Antigen presentation is the special feature that allows T lymphocytes to recognize processed molecules (peptides) bound at the HLA peptide cleft. In a simplified way, it is possible to state that peptides produced within the cells (endogenous) will be presented in the context of HLA class I molecules, and that peptides from the extracellular environment (exogenous) internalized through any process of phagocytosis or endocytosis will be presented in the context of HLA class II molecules. In this way, HLA molecules are responsible by presentation of peptides independently of the self or non-self origin of such peptides. For instance, an "endogenous" peptide can be derived from a self protein or can be derived from a viral protein in an infected cell; and conversely, an "exogenous" peptide presented in the context of HLA class II can be derived from any self or non-self phagocytosed protein. Therefore, the simple presentation of a peptide in a given MHC molecule do not dictates if an immune response should be induced. In this chapter we will discuss the requirements that allow a given MHC cleft to actually accommodate a peptide, forming a pMHC complex that can be potentially recognized by a T lymphocyte. It will become clear, as the players of this game are presented, that specific characteristics are required on any and all molecules involved on antigen presentation. We will focus the discussion on MHC-class I molecules and in its involvement in the presentation of viral-derived peptides. We will also review some bioinformatic and immunoinformatic tools currently used to model peptide/MHC interactions and to predict the ability of a given pMHC complex to induce an immune response.

THE MHC REGION AND THE HLA GENE FAMILY

As previously stated, the most polymorphic genomic region in humans lies in the short arm of chromosome 6 (6p21.3), which is referred as MHC region [1-2]. More than a proper biological meaning, this name is a reference to the clinical context in which this region was discovered, back in the 40s [3]. Moreover, this region is also the densest portion of our genome, presenting an average rate of 8.5 genes for 100 Kb [2, 4]. All these aspects reflects the importance of the MHC, which is largely involved with immune response and susceptibility to several pathologies, especially infectious and autoimmune diseases [2].

The MHC region can be divided into tree *loci*: MHC class I *locus*, MHC class II *locus* and MHC class III *locus* (Figure 1). The former two encode the Human Leukocyte Antigens

(HLA), which are involved with the peptide presentation to the immune system, while the last one encodes cytokines and Complement System proteins [1]. The MHC class II *locus* encodes the HLA class II molecule, an homodimer also called MHC-II, which presents exogenous peptides derived from phagocytized proteins [5]. This pathway is found only in a few specialized cells, such as macrophages, dendritic cells and B lymphocytes. These cells are called professional Antigen Presenting Cells (APCs). The MHC class II *locus* also encodes proteins involved in the endogenous peptide presenting pathway, such as proteasome and transporter TAP subunits.

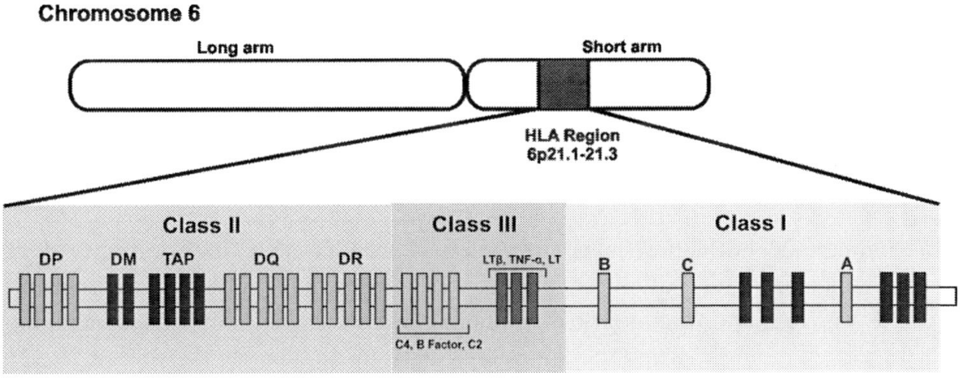

Figure 1. MHC region in humans. The MHC region is located on the chromosome 6 and is subdivided in three main *loci*: Class I, II and III. The class I MHC *locus* encodes molecules that are involved in the endogenous peptides presentation pathway. It should be noted, in yellow, classic alleles (HLA-A, HLA-B and HLA-C). The class II MHC *locus* encodes proteins mainly involved in the presentation of exogenous peptides, while the class III MHC locus encodes molecules that are essential for the immunologic response maintenance. (*Modified from Cellular and Molecular Immunology, 5ª edition [6]*).

The molecule responsible for presenting peptides derived from cytosolic processing is the MHC-I, an heterodimer whose heavy chain is encoded by the MHC class I *locus*. A deeper analysis of the endogenous peptide presenting pathway goes beyond the scope of this chapter. Briefly, this route is found in all nucleated cells and allows the immune system to perform the "surveillance" over the cytoplasmic content of each cell. For this reason, the MHC-I pathway plays a critical role in the defense against intracellular pathogens, mainly viruses, through the triggering of cellular immune response mechanisms.

The MHC class I *locus* can be subdivided in classical and non-classical genes. The classical genes, HLA-A, HLA-B and HLA-C, encode the heavy chain of the MHC-I molecule, which holds the peptide binding cleft [5]. There are more than 1,519 (HLA-A), 2,069 (HLA-B) and 1,016 (HLA-C) described alleles for the human leukocyte antigen genes (IMGT/HLA-http://hla.alleles.org/nomenclature/stats.html), which reflects the great MHC region variability of this *locus*. This huge number of alleles is probably the result of positive selection toward to the maintenance of the variability [7]. Each MHC allele possesses affinity for a specific group of epitopes and, thus, a given peptide will only be presented in the context of some of these MHC alleles [8]. Individuals or populations with greater variability in these genes are able to identify and process a greater number of pathogenic antigens, being potentially better succeeded in a greater range of immunological challenges.

The HLAs nomenclature was also influenced by this increasing number of described alleles, passing through many modifications in the past few years. The current nomenclature stands as the following:

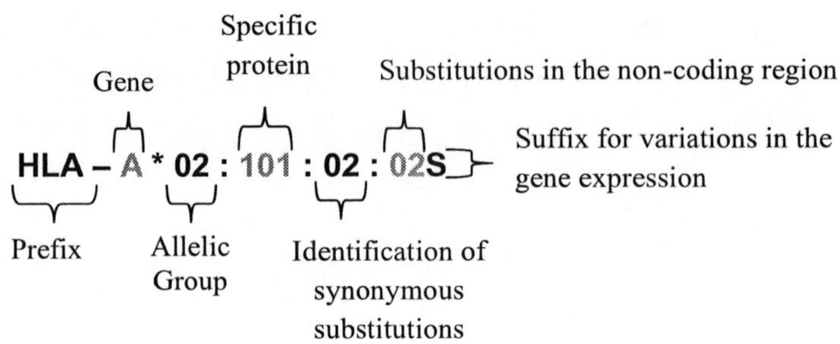

Modified from http://hla.alleles.org/nomenclature/naming.html.

This complete identification is not commonly used in many publications. It is very common to indicate a given allele using just the former numeric group (e.g. HLA-A*02 allele). However, it is important to note that this identification only indicates the allelic group, and that the second numeric group will be needed in order to identify the coding sequence of a specific protein.

THE MHC-I STRUCTURE

The MHC-I molecule is composed by two polypeptidic chains bounded non-covalently, one heavy chain (α chain) and one invariable subunit, encoded by a different *locus*, called β2-microglobulin. The amino-terminal endings (N-term) of the α chain (α1 and α2) interact with each other, forming a platform of eight β-sheets, which supports two parallel α-helixes. This structure is called the MHC-I "cleft", a space with size enough to lodge peptides from eight to eleven amino acids long. The full loaded MHC-I molecule is, in fact, an heterotrimer consisted by two chains (α and β2-m) and the endogenous peptide (epitope) bounded to its cleft (Figure 2) [9]. This heterotrimer is referred as peptide:MHC complex, or pMHC.

HLA AND INFECTIOUS DISEASE

Infection is a major selective pressure being an important cause of mortality and morbidity [11-12]. Genes involved with immune response are the most diverse in the human genome and the classical HLA genes have stood out as the leading candidates for infectious disease protection and susceptibility. Currently, there are many reports of positive associations between specific HLA alleles and major infection diseases, such as HIV/AIDS, hepatitis, leprosy, tuberculosis, malaria, leishmaniasis and schistosomiasis [11]. In this chapter we will focus on MHC class I and viral infection, briefly reviewing recent finds that have indicated the protective effect of some HLA alleles against two major viral infections: Hepatitis C Virus and Human Immunodeficiency virus.

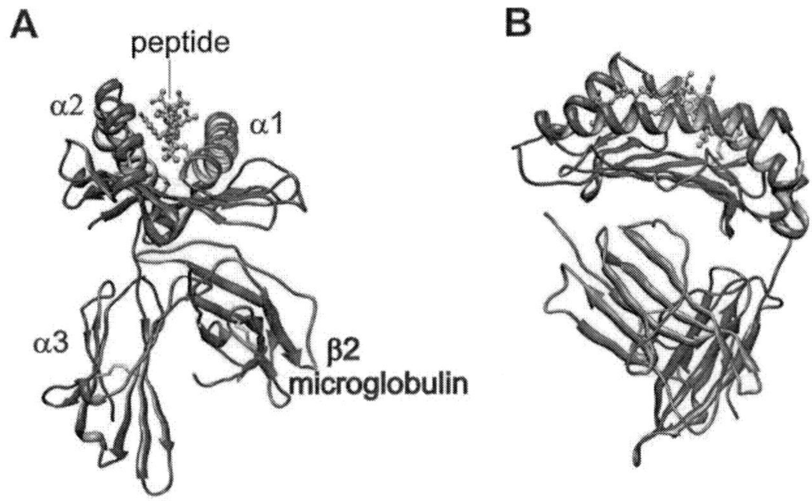

Figure 2. Peptide:MHC-I (pMHC) complex. (A) Front view and (B) side view. The images were generated using UCSF Chimera package from the Resource for Biocomputing, Visualization, and Informatics at the University of California, San Francisco (*supported by NIH P41 RR-01081*) [10].

The Hepatitis C Virus (HCV) represents a serious problem of global health, affecting about 3% of the human population [13-14]. In most cases (about 70%) the infection results in viral persistence in the host organism, being the leading cause of chronic liver disease, cirrhosis, and hepatocellular carcinoma. The remaining individuals, less than 30% of the cases, spontaneously resolve the infection, usually acquiring a protective immunity against future exposure to the pathogen [15]. Cellular immune response, especially when intensely triggered during the early stages of disease, seems to play a critical role in the response to HCV, being associated with virus control and clearance.

Several studies have shown the contribution of host genetic factors in determining the clinical phenotype of the disease. Confirming the central role of the cellular immune response, most of them indicate the involvement of genes from the MHC region [11]. In this context, stands out the work published by McKiernan et al., which showed an increased frequency of the allelic groups HLA-A*03, HLA-B*27 and HLA-Cw01 in individuals with viral clearance when compared to individuals with chronic infection [16]. This study detected a major association between HCV clearance and the presence of HLA-B*27 group. Corroborating these initial findings, a group headed by German researchers was able to identify an immunodominant epitope HCV-NS5B$_{2841}$ (ARMILMTHF), restricted to the B*27 group [17]. Furthermore, this work correlated viral clearance with cytotoxic response against this specific target, evidencing the role of the HLA-B*27 allele as a selective force driving viral evolution.

More recent studies have yielded conflicting results regarding the identification of MHC alleles with major contribution to HCV infection control. This apparent disagreement can be partially explained by the low level resolution in HLA genotyping, masking the variability given by different alleles from the same HLA group, as well as by the lack of complete identification of the HCV genotypes involved in these studies. Considering these possible bias factors, Kuniholm et al. conducted a high-resolution class I genotyping of a large multiracial cohort, which included U.S. women with high HCV and HIV prevalence [18]. This work found a significant association between the HLA-B*57:01 and HLA-B*57:03 alleles and the absence of viral RNA in infected patients, corroborating initial findings that suggests the protective role of the B*57 alleles [19-20]. Nevertheless, this work did not found significant association between viremia and some alleles previously associated with viral persistence (HLA-B*18:01 and HLA-Cw*04:01) and clearance (HLA-B*27:05).

The B*57 role in HCV infection was recently complemented by Kim *et al.*, through the identification of two immunodoiminant epitopes - HCV-$E2_{541}$ (NTRPPLGNW) and HCV-$NS5_{2629}$ (KSKKTPMGF) - restricted to the HLA-B*57:01 allele [21]. In addition, it was shown that viral particles from several chronic infected individuals presented escape mutations exactly in the region that is restricted to the B*57 group.

As expected for RNA viruses, huge nucleotide variability has been described in HCV sequences. Phylogenetic analysis of these sequences allowed the classification of six HCV genotypes, which were confirmed by several independent studies [15, 22-23]. However, the nucleotide substitution accumulation caused an intense diversification of the viruses clustered in each genotype, leading to a classification in several subtypes and *quasispecies* [24]. Identification of different genotypes is clinically important for some reasons. First, because it allows dose and time adjustment for the usual treatment, which makes combined use of Peginterferon alfa-2b and Ribavirin [15, 24]. Second, because differences among the genotypes can be critical for cellular immunity outcome.

Cellular immune response has been associated with virus control and some immunodominant targets, such as the HCV-$NS3_{1073}$ epitope (C*V/I*NGVCWTV), were identified [25]. However, even a small variation in these targets can cause defective action of HCV-specific CTLs, leading to viral persistence and chronic infection [26]. In the work published in 2008, Fytili *et al.* conducted a complete analysis of the impact of mutations over the HCV-$NS3_{1073}$ epitope sequence [27]. Using both synthetic (with alanine substitutions) and natural occurring variants of this epitope, they evaluated the immunogenic variation of these peptides, in the HLA-A*02:01 context, against a wild-type-specific lymphocyte population. The authors emphasize that even conservative amino acid exchanges were able to reduce, and even abolish, the recognition by the lymphocytes. This makes it impossible to predict the impact of viral escape mutations based only in sequence analysis.

As already discussed, there are conflicting data about the real protective effect of the B*27 group against HCV infection. In a recent study, Neumann-Haefelin *et al.* discussed the variability of the immunodominant epitope HCV-$NS5B_{2841}$ [28]. This peptide is located in a very conserved region of the RNA-dependent RNA polymerase, suffering several restrictions that prevent escape mutations. Therefore, this epitope is highly conserved among particles from a given genotype, although it presents variation across the genotypes. In fact, the authors concluded that HLA-B*27 presents protective effect in patients infected with HCV serotypes from genotype 1 (most common serotype). However, this association was not seen in patients infected with genotype 3a (second most common serotype in many countries). This work also rises the hypothesis that loss of association in patients infected with genotypes other than 1 should be driven by the impact of genotype-specific mutations over the B*27 ability to present these HCV-derived peptides.

This kind of association suggesting protective effect of specific HLA alleles against viral infections have been also described for other important pathogens, such as HIV. To note, the same alleles involved in HCV protection, have also been associated with HIV control. A small group of HIV-infected individuals are able to control the viral load and avoid, or delay, progression to AIDS. These individuals are classified as Long-Term Nonprogressors (LTNP) or Elite Controllers (EC), according to the detectable levels of HIV RNA [29]. Some genetic factors were associated with this HIV control, such as HLA-B*27 and HLA-B*57 allelic groups [30-31]. The first Genome-Wide Association Study (GWAS) for an infectious disease identified (in the asymptomatic phase of HIV-1 infection) strong association between three SNPs and low levels of viral load, a predictive sign of slower disease progression [32]. These polymorphisms are located in the MHC-I region and the strongest association occurred with a genetic marker from the HLA-B*57 group. A study performed with a wide cohort of 3,622 patients non-treated with antiretrovirals (called *The International HIV Controllers Study*), also indicated the protective effect of the HLA-B*57:01, HLA-B*27:05 and HLA-B*14 alleles [33].

There are more than 4,500 MHC class I alleles, each one of them with affinity to a specific group of peptides. It is expected that, by chance, at least some of these alleles will be able to present exactly the most conserved region of a given pathogen. However, it is very intriguing that despite all variability involved, either HIV or HCV as well HLA system variability, the same HLA alleles are associated with protection against two of the greatest current challenges to vaccine development. Besides, HLA-B*27 and HLA-B*57 groups are also associated with double control of HIV and HCV in co-infected patients [21]. Notwithstanding, the similarity between protective cellular immune response against both pathogens can be associated with the stimulation of the same (or at least closer) CTL populations. Vali *et al.* recently described the presence of a cross-reactive lymphocyte population in co-infected individuals that is able to recognize both HCV-derived epitope ($NS5B_{2594}$ - ALYDVVSKL) and HIV-derived epitope (Gag_{77} - SLYNTVATL) [34]. In another study, conducted by our group, a virtual screening of 55 selected pMHC complexes suggested a possible cross-recognition between the same HIV target (SLYNTVATL) and a well-known HCV immunodominant epitope ($NS3_{1073}$ - CVNGVCWTV) in the HLA-A*02:01 context [35]. Taken together, these data suggest the sharing of several features in cellular immune response against these two pathogens. These features probably reflect structural aspects of the pMHC complexes, formed with protective alleles and immunogenic epitopes, and should be enlightened in order to be employed in future vaccine development initiatives.

IMMUNOINFORMATICS TOOLS IN THE STUDY AND ANALYSIS OF PMHC COMPLEXES

The great amount of *in vivo*/*in vitro* data has increased dramatically, and in the immunology field it could not be different. Based on that, some questions arise: how can we manage this huge bulk of data? What can we infer from it? How to organize and perform new experiments using the generated data? Trying to solve these questions (and many more) and to accelerate the research in the immunology field, a new bioinformatics branch come to light, called Immunoinformatics.

Historically, the immunoinformatics have began early in the XX century, through an elegant study about malaria epidemiology [36]. In that time, the major interest was given over useful mathematic models to study diseases transmission. The knowledgment evolved and the immunoinformatics field expanded to cover a wide-range of immunologic aspects. With the computational advances, more immunoinformatics tools have arisen to perform *in silico* studies. A new concept was created, named immunomics, which combines the classic immunology with the computational sciences, mathematics, physics, chemistry, biochemistry, genomics and proteomics, aiming to analyze and understand the immune system function in a large-scale way [37].

Nowadays it is possible to find several immunoinformatics tools with the ability to predict, with relatively good accuracy, different aspects of immune response. It is also possible to evaluate the peptide:MHC interaction through the visualization and study of its tridimensional structure. We will present some valuable immunoinformatics tools below.

Endogenous Antigen Processing Study

There are several programs that simulate the endogenous antigen processing pathway, such as: Netchop [38], TAPPred [39], SYFPEITHI [40], NetMHC [41], IEDB Analysis Resource [42] and EpiJen [43]. All these programs perform predictions that are based on advanced algorithms and *in vitro*/*in vivo* data.

Once a protein is poly-ubiquitinated inside the cell, it is directed to a multienzymatic complex called proteasome. The proteasome is responsible by the protein cleavage, generating the exact C-terminal extremity that later will be presented at cellular surface by the MHC-I. Netchop 3.0 predicts the C-terminal cleavage site by the proteasome through a combination of neural networks algorithms. The user can choose between two prediction methods: C-term 3.0 or 20S 3.0. The first one is trained over a database of 1,260 MHC-I ligands while the 20S 3.0 is trained with *in vitro* degradation data. Once the user provides the protein sequence in the FASTA format, the program will yield an output with several values, ranging from 0 to 1, for each amino acid. These values represent the cleavage probability in that site (Figure 3).

The next step in the endogenous antigen processing pathway is the transport of the peptides generated by the proteasome (8-30 amino acids long) into the endoplasmic reticulum. This transport is mediated by TAP (Transporter Associated with Antigen Processing) protein. Based on the fact that some peptides are preferentially transported by TAP, a group of researchers from India developed TAPPred tool. This program was built using a quantitative matrix based on SVM (Support Vector Machine) and it predicts the peptides transport probability into the endoplasmic reticulum by TAP. Unlike Netchop, TAPPred provides an output where the peptides are categorized with low, intermediary or high transport probability. TAPPred takes into account not only the peptide linear sequence, but also the physical-chemical group of each amino acid.

Once the peptides are inside the endoplasmic reticulum, some will be degraded by ERAP (Endoplasmic Reticulum Aminopeptidase) enzymes, while others will be able to bind, through a complex assembly mechanism involving several proteins, into the MHC-I cleft. There are two important tools, called SYFPEITHI and NetMHC 3.2 Server, that could infer the affinity of the peptide by the MHC-I molecule. The SYFPEITHI possess a wide database with more than 7,000 peptide sequences with binding characteristics by MHC-I and MHC-II molecules. In the "Find a Motif, Ligand or Epitope" section it is possible to search MHC-restricted epitopes, while in the "Epitope Prediction" section the user could provide the linear sequence of the peptide and the program will find the best MHCs for that peptide, based on the binding strength. The NetMHC is a server that predicts the binding of peptides to a number of different MHCs. Thus, the program will compute, through algorithms based on artificial neural networks and weight matrices, and supply, for each MHC allele, a prediction score of the peptide(s) that was first provided by the user.

There are also programs that are able to predict the complete endogenous antigen processing pathway, such as EpiJen and tools from IEDB (Immune Epitope Database).

After all the endogenous processing, the epitope will be presented at cellular surface by a specific MHC allele (the complex epitope:MHC is also called pMHC), where the TCR (T Cell Receptor) from lymphocytes will recognize the pMHC complex and trigger (or not) an immunologic response against that cell. A broader understanding of the pMHC complex could be achieved through structural analysis, as discussed below, where it is possible to study its topology and charges distribution, for example.

pos	AA	C	score
1	A	S	0.092333
2	W	S	0.610934
3	R	S	0.242864
4	R	S	0.074985
5	F	S	0.478356
6	K	S	0.048452
7	L	S	0.605637
8	K	S	0.426287
9	Y	S	0.741385
10	T	S	0.027332

Figure 3. Output from Netchop. The Netchop program provides a score that represents the C-terminal cleavage probability. In this example, the program predicts with approximately 60.56% of chance that a cleavage can occur between the amino acid 7 and the amino acid 8.

Structural Analysis of pMHC Complexes

The structure of pMHC complexes can be obtained through experimental methods, such as Nuclear Magnetic Resonance (NMR) and X-Ray Crystallography. Unfortunately, both methods are very expensive and time consuming. Furthermore, the variability of the biological systems far exceeds the capacity of the current experimental methods. The HLA-B *locus*, for instance, has over 2,069 alleles described [44], each one of them able to present several peptides. The knowledge of the structure of each one of these unique pMHC complexes would be of interest for immunology, but this goal becomes absolutely unfeasible considering only experimental methodologies. The Protein Data Bank (PDB), most important repository for experimentally-determined protein structures, holds currently almost eighty thousand structures [45]. However, less than 400 of these structures are related to pMHC complexes, most from human and mice alleles.

The immunoinformatics tools presented in the previous section has great importance for the MHC study. However, most of these tools are based only in the linear protein sequence, leaving behind the tridimensional structure influence over the system. Furthermore, these tools evaluate the pMHC binding in a static point of view. This problem could be attenuated through the use of structure immunoinformatics tools, such as molecular docking and molecular dynamics, which allow the study of pMHC complexes structure. The molecular docking is used to search for the best conformation between a ligand (or a set of ligands) and a protein or between two separated proteins [46]. The molecular dynamics tools are used to evaluate the molecular behavior along the time, under determined conditions, where is possible to manage the pressure, temperature and pH of the system, for example. These tools have been already successfully applied by pharmacist industry, especially in the screening of new chemical ligands to use in novel therapies [47].

The molecular docking, as well the molecular dynamics, could be adapted to assist immunologists [48]. Bordner & Abagyan (2006), for example, used Monte-Carlo methods to refine pMHC structures that were constructed through the molecular docking, identifying the best conformation between the peptide and the MHC [49]. In another assay, Khan & Ranganathan developed a method entitled pDOCK. This method is based on the calculation of interaction molecular maps (called GRID maps) and local energy minimization steps (through molecular dynamics). The pDOCK method was tested and reproduced about 149 pMHC complexes [50].

Structural bioinformatics offer a fast and low cost alternative to assess some of the missing complexes. However, to build a pMHC complex is not an easy computational problem. Most docking algorithms have better performance for ligands with up to 10 rotatable bounds, while a typical peptide (9-mer) presents between 35 and 44 rotatable bounds. There are many strategies proposed to address this issue, normally combining molecular docking with local minimization steps or molecular modeling [49, 51-53]. Our group has also developed a methodology for the construction of pMHC complexes, which is based on the identification of structural MHC allele-specific patterns and uses two rounds of molecular docking interspersed with an Energy Minimization step (*D1-EM-D2*) [54]. This approach, schematically represented in Figure 4, was previously applied to construct the CrossTope Structural Data Bank for Cross-Reactivity Assessment, which current holds over 200 pMHC structures (http://www.crosstope.com.br/). This database includes structures from four different MHC alleles, being two from murines (H2-D^b and H2-K^b) and two from humans (HLA-A*02:01 and HLA-B*27:05).

Once the structure of interest is obtained, it can be evaluated using tools that can reveal molecular aspects of the pMHC interaction, complex stability and even TCR recognition (Figure 5) [35, 49, 54-58]. Among these tools, the Molecular Dynamics (MD) is being largely applied to a wide range of studies, supplying critical information about the pMHC behavior *in vivo*, all this data have proven correlation with experimentally-observed values [59-60].

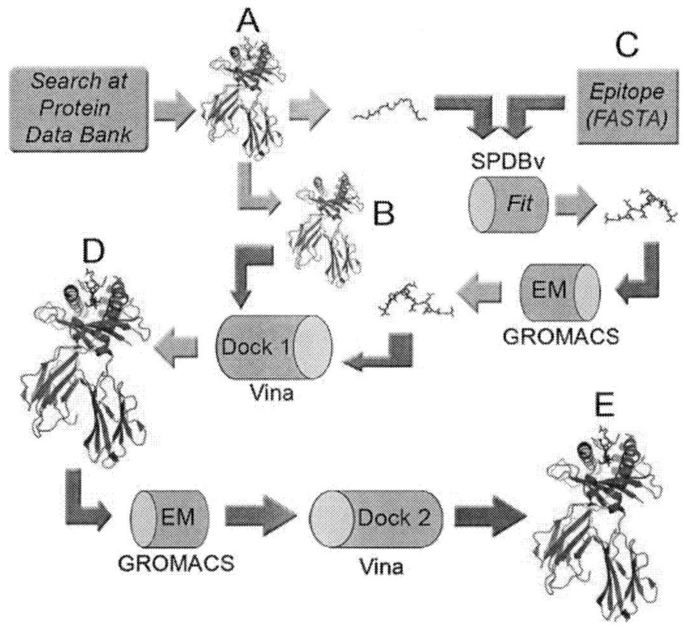

Figure 4. The *D1-EM-D2* technique for construction of new pMHC complexes. Consider the linear epitope sequence (C) which structure was not determined in the context of any MHC-I allele. A search in the PDB is performed looking for the desired MHC-I. In this example, it was found a complex represented by (A). The epitope in (A) was used as a model for the epitope in (C). The epitope in (C), after the modeling process, pass through a brief energy minimization (EM) step and, after that, is submitted to a molecular docking process (Dock 1). The best structure is retrieved, which pass through a new process of energy minimization, aiming to adjust amino acids side chains of the epitope with those of the MHC-I. A second molecular docking is performed (Dock 2) and a refined, best structure is obtained. (*Modified from Antunes et al. 2010*)

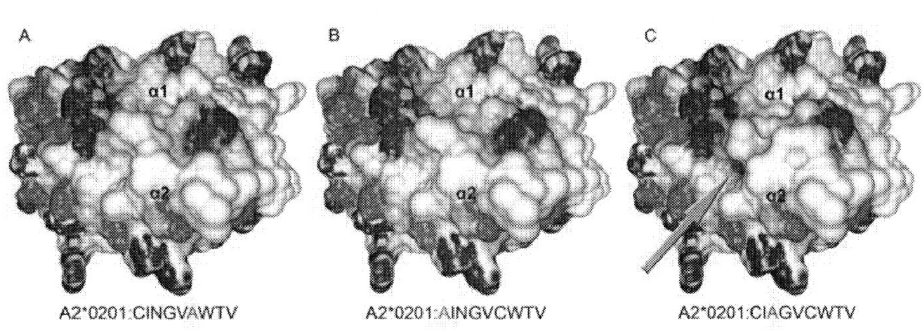

Figure 5. Topology and electrostatic potential comparison among A2*0201:HCV-**NS3**$_{1073}$ complexes. Three pMHC complexes presenting Alanine exchange variants of the HCV wild-type epitope NS3$_{1073}$(CVNGVCWTV) were constructed using a molecular docking approach [54]. TCR-interacting surfaces of these complexes, acquired with GRASP2 software, are depicted. Regions with positive (blue) and negative (red) charges are represented with a scale from -5 to +5 kiloteslas. Sequence of presented peptide is depicted below each complex with the position of the Alanine exchange depicted in red. Alpha-1 and Alpha-2 MHC domains are also indicated. TCR-interacting surfaces of complexes that stimulate high levels of IFN-γ production by CVNGVCWTV-specific CD8+ T-cells (A and B) shared both topology and electrostatic potential. One complex that stimulates low levels of IFN-γ production (C) presented differences in topology and the emergence of a positively charged region (green arrow) in the TCR-interacting surface [27, 54].

GROUNDS FOR IMMUNOGENICITY

Considering the current knowledge regarding to the MHC class I pathway, as well as the recent researches performed by our own group, we postulate the existence of three selection levels that will determine the immunogenicity of a given peptide: Processing, Stability and Reactivity. Each one of these levels can be subdivided into several processes and even alternative pathways. Processing, for instance, is related to multiple steps from the target protein polyubiquitination to the binding of a derived epitope to a given MHC allele. The major "bottlenecks" in this level of selection are the proteasome cleavage, which determines the epitope's specific C-terminal residue, the TAP transport, the N-terminal trimming and, finally, the binding to the MHC. The second level of selection refers to the dynamic capacity of the pMHC complex, passing trough protein-export step and remaining stable at the presenting cell surface. The peptide binding affinity has some influence in this level, but the heterotrimer structural integrity is not exclusively determined by this feature. Structural details of each MHC allele, such as the glycosylation of these complexes, will play a specific role over the pMHC stability. In the same way, structural aspects of the peptide will also be important, such as physical-chemical properties of the peptide side-chains, length of the main-chain (backbone) and Accessible Surface Area (ASA). Environmental changes such as pH, salt concentration, interaction with accessory molecules and the existence of other peptides in solution, can also determinate the pMHC capacity to remain stable at the surface for enough time. A peptide correctly generated through the processing steps and that is able to stay bound to the MHC cleft during the presentation at the cellular surface, will guarantee its interaction with the TCR. Its immunogenicity, however, still depends on the capability of this peptide to "react" with the TCR, in the context of the MHC allele in which it is been presented.

In the final step the pMHC complex topology and its charges distribution over the TCR-interacting area, among others aspects, will be fundamental features to determine the lymphocyte stimulation. Also, structural issues of the TCR should be considered, such as the amino acid properties over the hypervariable regions and the specific orientation of the TCR/pMHC docking. All these steps are obviously related, since key features for the processing can also have influence over the pMHC stability or reactivity. Thus, it is important to consider these three moments in the MHC-I presentation pathway. This will allow us to establish an order and scores for each methodology, integrating their results in one broader analysis, enhancing our predictions regarding to immunogenicity and cross-reactivity.

There is nowadays a vast and detailed knowledge about the molecules and mechanisms involved in Processing. However, given to methodological limitations, we still have little information regarding to immunogenicity "constitution" and the dynamics of the TCR interaction. Structural immunoinformatics studies can make an important contribution to this field of immunology, paving the way for a better understanding of the cellular immune response and enabling the manipulation of the immune system in favor of overcoming diseases that still plague mankind.

CONCLUSION

As could be seen in this chapter, the knowledge about the MHC molecule was highly improved in the last years. Initially thoughts about its restricted role in transplantation compatibility were reviewed, and the MHC now appears as a protagonist (along with TCR) in the cellular immune response against a huge variability of pathogens. Since this chapter was focused on the involvement of the MHC in viral infections clearance, more attention was given to the endogenous antigen processing pathway.

As discussed, MHC-I acts as an acceptor molecule for the peptides that reach the endoplasmic reticulum (an already tiny number of peptides, as opposed to the ideas that a given protein could be cleaved nonspecifically at any amino acid residue). Again, only some of these peptides have specific requirements for properly fit into the MHC cleft. The final step will be the transportation of the pMHC, passing through Golgi complex, to the cellular surface, where it will play its major function: "inform" to the cytotoxic T lymphocyte, through the interaction of pMHC surface with TCR loops, what kind of proteins are being produced into the cell. The resulting interaction on the immunological synapse will define the outcome of the viral infection.

Two classic viral infection examples have been discussed in this chapter, Hepatitis C virus and Human Immunodeficiency virus, stressing the importance of the proper antigen presentation to an efficiently recognition of resident viruses into the cells. The progress of the viral infection will be directly influenced by the set of HLA alleles from each individual. Currently, according to IMGT database, there are more than 4,900 HLA-I classic alleles described. This high number of allelic variants is intrinsically associated with the mutational capability of viruses. Each one of these HLA alleles has unique characteristics in its cleft residues that will or will not allow an epitope to interact and establish a stable binding. In this way, the capacity to present a given antigen will be directly proportional to the allelic HLA diversity of a population (or even to the diversity contained in a single individual).

The HLA diversity discussion raises questions about customized vaccine development. The knowledgement about HLA variability, as well about epitope conformational changes that occurs due to interactions with the HLA cleft, and its respective impact in the differential immunogenicity, reveals that could be naïve to think in worldwide useful vaccines and also makes us to reflect about current vaccines and their levels of population coverage.

It should be observed that, in all approached subjects, immunoinformatics has an important role, allowing specific questions to be answered and generalizations made. This is more evident in structural immunology, where new insights about particular issues of the MHC molecule were significantly expanded, revealing singular characteristics of the pMHC interaction surface.

It is expected that much of the information obtained through these methodologies would be applied in reverse vaccinology studies. In this way, we could envisage a new generation of vaccines, which could embrace a broader activity spectrum and, at same time, could be customized for each individual. All of this through the integration of *in vitro*, *in vivo* and *in silico* studies.

REFERENCES

[1] Horton, R; Wilming, L; Rand, V; Lovering, RC; Bruford, Ea; Khodiyar, VK, et al. Gene map of the extended human MHC. *Nature reviews Genetics,* 2004 5, 889-99.

[2] Vandiedonck, C; Knight, JC. The human Major Histocompatibility Complex as a paradigm in genomics research. *Briefings in functional genomics & proteomics,* 2009 8, 379-94.

[3] Snell, GD. Some recollections of Peter Gorer and his work on this fiftieth anniversary of his discovery of H-2. *Immunogenetics,* 1986 24, 339-40.

[4] Xie, T; Rowen, L; Aguado, B; Ahearn, ME; Madan, A; Qin, S, et al. Analysis of the gene-dense major histocompatibility complex class III region and its comparison to mouse. *Genome research,* 2003 13, 2621-36.

[5] Kelley, J; Walter, L; Trowsdale, J. Comparative genomics of major histocompatibility complexes. *Immunogenetics,* 2005 56, 683-95.

[6] ABBAS, A. *Cellular and Molecular Immunology.* 5 ed. San Francisco: Elsevier Science Limited; 2003.

[7] Piertney, SB; Oliver, MK. The evolutionary ecology of the major histocompatibility complex. *Heredity,* 2006 96, 7-21.

[8] Cao, K; Hollenbach, J; Shi, X; Shi, W; Chopek, M; Fernandez-Vina, MA. Analysis of the frequencies of HLA-A, B, and C alleles and haplotypes in the five major ethnic groups of the United States reveals high levels of diversity in these loci and contrasting distribution patterns in these populations. *Hum Immunol,* 2001 Sep 62(9), 1009-30.

[9] Hammer, GE; Kanaseki, T; Shastri, N. The final touches make perfect the peptide-MHC class I repertoire. *Immunity,* 2007 Apr 26(4), 397-406.

[10] Pettersen, EF; Goddard, TD; Huang, CC; Couch, GS; Greenblatt, DM; Meng, EC, et al. UCSF Chimera--a visualization system for exploratory research and analysis. *J Comput Chem,* 2004 Oct 25(13), 1605-12.

[11] Blackwell, JM; Jamieson, SE; Burgner, D. HLA and infectious diseases. *Clinical microbiology reviews,* 2009 22, 370-85, Table of Contents.

[12] Sabeti, PC; Reich, DE; Higgins, JM; Levine, HZ; Richter, DJ; Schaffner, SF, et al. Detecting recent positive selection in the human genome from haplotype structure. *Nature,* 2002 Oct 24 419(6909), 832-7.

[13] Walker, CM. Adaptive immunity to the hepatitis C virus. *Advances in virus research,* 2010 78, 43-86.

[14] Zeisel, MB; Fafi-Kremer, S; Robinet, E; Habersetzer, F; Baumert, TF; Stoll-Keller, F. Adaptive Immunity to Hepatitis C Virus. *Viruses,* 2009 1, 276-97.

[15] Bostan, N; Mahmood, T. An overview about hepatitis C: a devastating virus. *Critical reviews in microbiology,* 2010 36, 91-133.

[16] McKiernan, SM; Hagan, R; Curry, M; McDonald, GSa; Kelly, A; Nolan, N, et al. Distinct MHC class I and II alleles are associated with hepatitis C viral clearance, originating from a single source. *Hepatology* (Baltimore, Md), 2004 40, 108-14.

[17] Neumann-Haefelin, C; McKiernan, S; Ward, S; Viazov, S; Spangenberg, HC; Killinger, T, et al. Dominant influence of an HLA-B27 restricted CD8+ T cell response in mediating HCV clearance and evolution. *Hepatology* (Baltimore, Md), 2006 43, 563-72.

[18] Kuniholm, MH; Kovacs, A; Gao, X; Xue, X; Marti, D; Thio, CL, et al. Specific human leukocyte antigen class I and II alleles associated with hepatitis C virus viremia. *Hepatology* (Baltimore, Md), 2010 51, 1514-22.

[19] Thio, CL; Gao, X; Goedert, JJ; Vlahov, D; Nelson, KE; Hilgartner, MW, et al. HLA-Cw*04 and hepatitis C virus persistence. *J Virol,* 2002 May 76(10), 4792-7.

[20] Chuang, WC; Sarkodie, F; Brown, CJ; Owusu-Ofori, S; Brown, J; Li, C, et al. Protective effect of HLA-B57 on HCV genotype 2 infection in a West African population. *J Med Virol,* 2007 Jun 79(6), 724-33.
[21] Kim, AY; Kuntzen, T; Timm, J; Nolan, BE; Baca, Ma; Reyor, LL, et al. Spontaneous control of HCV is associated with the expression of HLA-B*57 and preservation of targeted epitopes. *Gastroenterology,* 2010 140, 686-96.e1.
[22] Simmonds, P; Bukh, J; Combet, C; Deléage, G; Enomoto, N; Feinstone, S, et al. Consensus proposals for a unified system of nomenclature of hepatitis C virus genotypes. *Hepatology* (Baltimore, Md), 2005 42, 962-73.
[23] Simmonds, P; Holmes, EC; Cha, Ta; Chan, SW; McOmish, F; Irvine, B, et al. Classification of hepatitis C virus into six major genotypes and a series of subtypes by phylogenetic analysis of the NS-5 region. *The Journal of general virology,* 1993 74 (Pt 11, 2391-9.
[24] Chayama, K; Hayes, CN. Hepatitis C virus: How genetic variability affects pathobiology of disease. *Journal of gastroenterology and hepatology,* 2011 26 Suppl 1, 83-95.
[25] Hiroishi, K; Eguchi, J; Ishii, S; Hiraide, A; Sakaki, M; Doi, H, et al. Immune response of cytotoxic T lymphocytes and possibility of vaccine development for hepatitis C virus infection. *Journal of biomedicine & biotechnology,* 2010 2010, 263810.
[26] Wedemeyer, H; He, X-S; Nascimbeni, M; Davis, AR; Greenberg, HB; Hoofnagle, JH, et al. Impaired Effector Function of Hepatitis C Virus-Specific CD8+ T Cells in Chronic Hepatitis C Virus Infection. *J Immunol,* 2002 169, 3447-58.
[27] Fytili, P; Dalekos, GN; Schlaphoff, V; Suneetha, PV; Sarrazin, C; Zauner, W, et al. Cross-genotype-reactivity of the immunodominant HCV CD8 T-cell epitope NS3-1073. *Vaccine,* 2008 Jul 23 26(31), 3818-26.
[28] Neumann-Haefelin, C; Timm, J; Schmidt, J; Kersting, N; Fitzmaurice, K; Oniangue-Ndza, C, et al. Protective effect of human leukocyte antigen B27 in hepatitis C virus infection requires the presence of a genotype-specific immunodominant CD8+ T-cell epitope. *Hepatology* (Baltimore, Md), 2010 51, 54-62.
[29] Poropatich, K; Sullivan, DJ. Human immunodeficiency virus type 1 long-term non-progressors: the viral, genetic and immunological basis for disease non-progression. *The Journal of general virology,* 2011 92, 247-68.
[30] Miura, T; Brockman, Ma; Schneidewind, A; Lobritz, M; Pereyra, F; Rathod, A, et al. HLA-B57/B*5801 human immunodeficiency virus type 1 elite controllers select for rare gag variants associated with reduced viral replication capacity and strong cytotoxic T-lymphocyte [corrected] recognition. *Journal of virology,* 2009 83, 2743-55.
[31] Ammaranond, P; van Bockel, DJ; Petoumenos, K; McMurchie, M; Finlayson, R; Middleton, MG, et al. HIV immune escape at an immunodominant epitope in HLA-B*27-positive individuals predicts viral load outcome. *Journal of immunology* (Baltimore, Md : 1950), 2011 186, 479-88.
[32] Fellay, J; Shianna, KV; Ge, D; Colombo, S; Ledergerber, B; Weale, M, et al. A whole-genome association study of major determinants for host control of HIV-1. *Science,* 2007 Aug 17 317(5840), 944-7.
[33] Pereyra, F; Jia, X; McLaren, PJ; Telenti, A; de Bakker, PIW; Walker, BD, et al. The Major Genetic Determinants of HIV-1 Control Affect HLA Class I Peptide Presentation. *Science* (New York, NY), 2010 1551.
[34] Vali, B; Tohn, R; Cohen, M; Sakhdari, A; Sheth, PM; Yue, FY, et al. Characterization of cross-reactive CD8+ T-cell recognition of HLA-A2-restricted HIV-Gag: SLYNTVATL and HCV-NS5b: ALYDVVSKL epitopes in individuals infected with

Human Immunodeficiency and Hepatitis C Viruses. *Journal of virology,* 2010, JVI.01743-10-.

[35] Antunes, DA; Rigo, MM; Silva, JP; Cibulski, SP; Sinigaglia, M; Chies, JAB, et al. Structural in silico analysis of cross-genotype-reactivity among naturally occurring HCV NS3-1073-variants in the context of HLA-A*02:01 allele. *Molecular immunology*, 2011.

[36] Ross, R. An application of the theory of probabilities to the study of a priori pathometry. Part I. Proc R Soc Lond Ser A, 1916 92, 204-30.

[37] Tong, JC; Ren, EC. Immunoinformatics: Current trends and future directions. *Drug Discov Today,* 2009 Jul 14(13-14), 684-9.

[38] Nielsen, M; Lundegaard, C; Lund, O; Kesmir, C. The role of the proteasome in generating cytotoxic T-cell epitopes: insights obtained from improved predictions of proteasomal cleavage. *Immunogenetics,* 2005 Apr 57(1-2), 33-41.

[39] Bhasin, M; Raghava, GP. Analysis and prediction of affinity of TAP binding peptides using cascade SVM. *Protein Sci,* 2004 Mar 13(3), 596-607.

[40] Rammensee, H; Bachmann, J; Emmerich, NP; Bachor, OA; Stevanovic, S. SYFPEITHI: database for MHC ligands and peptide motifs. *Immunogenetics,* 1999 Nov 50(3-4), 213-9.

[41] Lundegaard, C; Lamberth, K; Harndahl, M; Buus, S; Lund, O; Nielsen, M. NetMHC-3.0: accurate web accessible predictions of human, mouse and monkey MHC class I affinities for peptides of length 8-11. *Nucleic Acids Res,* 2008 Jul 1 36(Web Server issue), W509-12.

[42] Peters, B; Sidney, J; Bourne, P; Bui, HH; Buus, S; Doh, G, et al. The immune epitope database and analysis resource: from vision to blueprint. *PLoS Biol,* 2005 Mar 3(3), e91.

[43] Doytchinova, IA; Guan, P; Flower, DR. EpiJen: a server for multistep T cell epitope prediction. *BMC Bioinformatics,* 2006 7, 131.

[44] Robinson, J; Waller, MJ; Parham, P; Bodmer, JG; Marsh, SG. IMGT/HLA Database--a sequence database for the human major histocompatibility complex. *Nucleic Acids Res,* 2001 Jan 1 29(1), 210-3.

[45] Berman, HM; Westbrook, J; Feng, Z; Gilliland, G; Bhat, TN; Weissig, H, et al. The Protein Data Bank. *Nucleic Acids Res,* 2000 28, 235-42.

[46] Huang, SY; Zou, X. Advances and challenges in protein-ligand docking. *Int J Mol Sci,* 2010 11(8), 3016-34.

[47] Cui, Y. Using molecular simulations to probe pharmaceutical materials. *J Pharm Sci,* 2011 Jun 100(6), 2000-19.

[48] Sieker, F; May, A; Zacharias, M. Predicting affinity and specificity of antigenic peptide binding to major histocompatibility class I molecules. *Curr Protein Pept Sci,* 2009 Jun 10(3), 286-96.

[49] Bordner, AJ; Abagyan, R. Ab initio prediction of peptide-MHC binding geometry for diverse class I MHC allotypes. *Proteins,* 2006 May 15 63(3), 512-26.

[50] Khan, JM; Ranganathan, S. pDOCK: a new technique for rapid and accurate docking of peptide ligands to Major Histocompatibility Complexes. *Immunome Res,* 2010 6 Suppl 1, S2.

[51] Lafuente, EM; Reche, Pa. Prediction of MHC-peptide binding: a systematic and comprehensive overview. *Current pharmaceutical design,* 2009 15, 3209-20.

[52] Lundegaard, C; Lund, O; Buus, S; Nielsen, M. Major histocompatibility complex class I binding predictions as a tool in epitope discovery. *Immunology,* 2010 130, 309-18.

[53] Khan, JM; Ranganathan, S. pDOCK: a new technique for rapid and accurate docking of peptide ligands to Major Histocompatibility Complexes. *Immunome research,* 2010 6 Suppl 1, S2.

[54] Antunes, DA; Vieira, GF; Rigo, MM; Cibulski, SP; Sinigaglia, M; Chies, JA. Structural allele-specific patterns adopted by epitopes in the MHC-I cleft and reconstruction of MHC:peptide complexes to cross-reactivity assessment. *PLoS ONE,* 2010 5(4), e10353.

[55] Rigo, M; Antunes, D; Vieira, G; Chies, J. MHC: Peptide Analysis: Implications on the Immunogenicity of Hantaviruses' N protein. Springer Berlin / Heidelberg; 2009. p. 160-3.

[56] Kumar, N; Mohanty, D. Structure-based identification of MHC binding peptides: Benchmarking of prediction accuracy. *Molecular bioSystems,* 2010 6, 2508-20.

[57] Knapp, B; Omasits, U; Schreiner, W. Side chain substitution benchmark for peptide / *MHC interaction.* 2008, 977-82.

[58] Vivona, S; Gardy, JL; Ramachandran, S; Brinkman, FSL; Raghava, GPS; Flower, DR, et al. Computer-aided biotechnology: from immuno-informatics to reverse vaccinology. *Trends in biotechnology*, 2008 26, 190-200.

[59] Flower, DR; Phadwal, K; Macdonald, IK; Coveney, PV; Davies, MN; Wan, S. T-cell epitope prediction and immune complex simulation using molecular dynamics: state of the art and persisting challenges. *Immunome Research,* 2010 6, S4.

[60] Li, Y; Yang, Y; He, P; Yang, Q. QM/MM study of epitope peptides binding to HLA-A*0201: the roles of anchor residues and water. *Chemical biology & drug design,* 2009 74, 611-8.

In: Major Histocompatibility Complex
Editor: Natalya V. Semiletova

ISBN: 978-1-61942-999-4

Chapter 7

HLA-G: Biology, Functions and Roles in Disease

Wei-Hua Yan [*] ***and Aifen Lin***

Medical Research Center, Taizhou Hospital of Zhejiang Province, Wenzhou Medical College, 150 Xi'men Street, Linhai, Zhejiang, People's Republic of China

Abstract

Human leukocyte antigen G (HLA-G) is a non-classic major histocompatibility complex (MHC) class I molecule that functions as an immune suppressive molecule. HLA-G has direct inhibitory effects on natural killer cells (NK), dendritic cells (DC), T cells by binding to its receptors expressed on these immune cells, and has long-term indirect tolerogenic effects by inducing regulator T cells (Treg) and DCs. HLA-G has been reported to be involved in various physio-pathological conditions such as reproduction, transplantation, autoimmunity, infectious and malignant diseases. Given its tolerant properties, HLA-G expression in the fetal maternal interface during pregnancy and in transplant grafts are of beneficial significance for allogenic fetus and grafts acceptance. On the other hand, induced HLA-G expression in virus infected cells and malignant cells are of harmful outcome for the infection and tumor patients. In the context of clinical aspects, expression of HLA-G in malignant diseases including hematological and solid tumors, infectious diseases and transplantation has been extensively investigated and its relevance to clinico-parameters and potential significance in diagnosis, prognosis and immune target therapy has been postulated. In this chapter, we summarized the biology, functions and relevance of HLA-G in disease.

Introduction

The human major histocompatibility complex (MHC) is located on the short arm of chromosome 6. It spans ~3.6 Mb and encodes about 140 functional antigens. The best described and investigated are the classical human leukocyte antigen (*HLA*) *class I* (*HLA Ia*)

---

[*] Corresponding author. Tel: +86-576-85199347; Fax: +86-576-85199876; E-mail: yanwhcom@yahoo.com.

and *II* genes (*HLA-A*, *-B*, *-C*, *-DR*, *-DQ* and *-DP*). [1] However, since the late 1980s, the existence of another interesting group of non-classical *HLA class I* genes *(HLA Ib)* has become evident. The HLA *class Ib* antigens, including HLA-E, -F and -G, share some characteristics with the HLA Ia antigens, but also differ from them in a range of ways. [2] There seems to be growing evidence to support the viewpoint that HLA class Ib molecules, HLA-G in particularly, may play a role in the suppression of immune responses and contribute to long-term immune escape or tolerance. [3,4,5]

HLA-G gene was cloned in 1987 and maps on the short arm of chromosome 6 in the p21.31 region which is close to *HLA-A*, which has a gene structure consisting of eight exons and seven introns which is about 86% similarities with the consensus sequence of the *HLA-A*, *HLA-B* and *HLA-C* genes. [6] HLA-G differs from other classical HLA class I molecules with regard to its limited polymorphism, [7] slow turnover, [8] restricted tissue distribution, [9] limited peptide diversity, [10] a short cytoplasmic tail and immunosuppressive properties, [6, 11] and its primary transcripts could be generated seven isoforms. [12]

The relevance of HLA-G in human physiological and pathological contexts has been intensively investigated. The tolerogenic properties of HLA-G might have beneficial effects in reproduction, transplantation, autoimmunity, and inflammatory diseases by limiting immune reactions, whereas they might be deleterious in cancer and in viral infections by allowing escape of tumor or virus-infected cells. [5]

Gene and Molecular Structure of HLA-G

Unlike the high polymorphic classical HLA class I genes, HLA-G gene features low level of allelic polymorphisms with only 44 *HLA-G* alleles being acknowledged to date by the World Health Organization (WHO) Nomenclature Committee for Factors of the HLA System (http://www. anthonynolan.org.uk/HIG/).

The HLA-G gene shows similarity to the classical HLA loci, exhibiting 8 exons and 7 introns, coding the heavy chain of the molecule. Exon 1 encodes the peptide signal; exon 2, 3 and 4 encodes the extracellular α1, α2 and α3 domains, respectively; and exon 5 and 6 encodes the transmembrane and the cytoplasmic domain of the heavy chain. [13] Compared to classical class I molecules, HLA-G has a shortened cytoplasmic domain because of the presence of a premature stop codon in exon 6. Exon 7 is always absent from the mature mRNA and, due to the stop codon in exon 6, exon 8 is not translated. [14]

HLA-G primary transcripts could be translated to seven HLA-G isoforms including four membrane-bound (HLA-G1, -G2, -G3, and -G4) and three soluble isoforms (HLA-G5, -G6, and -G7). [12] Among these alleles, *HLA-G**0101, *0102, *0103, *0104, *0106, *0107, *0108, *0109, *0110, *0111, *0112, *0114, *0115 and *0116 could encode 14 distinct functional proteins with all isoforms. Another allele, the *G**0105N, could encode a modified HLA-G proteins due to its containing a cytosine deletion at position 1597 (first base of codon 130 or the last base of codon 129) in exon 3 resulting in a consecutive frame shift mutation and leading to a downstream stop signal (TGA) in codon 189 (exon 4). [16] Consequently, this allele is expected to disrupt the expression of HLA-G1,-G4 and -G5 isoforms containing the extracellular α2 domain, but does encode both membrane-bound and soluble functional HLA-G proteins, such as HLA-G2 and HLA-G3 and HLA-G6 and HLA-G7 proteins. [17]

The other null allele, *G**01:13N (*G**0103N), presents a C → T transition at the first base of codon 54 in exon 2 (α1 domain), yielding the formation of a premature stop codon (TAG), which prevents the production of all membrane-bound and soluble isoforms or produces presumably nonfunctional proteins. [18]

The extracellular part of the HLA-G molecule consists of the α1, α2, and α3 domains encoded by the exon 2, 3 and exon 4, respectively. HLA-G1 is a full length protein that contains α1, α2, and α3 extracellular domains linked to the transmembrane domain encoded by exon 5 and to a shortened cytoplasmic tail due to a premature stop codon in exon 6. HLA-G2, -G3, and -G4 transcripts that, lacks the exon 3, exon 3 and 4, or exon 4, respectively, generate truncated isoforms that contains only the extracellular domain α1 for HLA -G3, the domains α1 and α3 for HLA-G2, and the domains α1 and α2 for HLA-G4, joined to the transmembrane region. [19, 20] Soluble HLA-G (sHLA-G) proteins are generated by using of an intron 2 or 4 retaining mRNA. [21] The soluble full length HLA-G5 molecule retains identical leader, α1, α2, α3 domains, but includes intron 4 sequences, yielding to a HLA-G5 specific open reading frame that encodes 21 amino-acids linked to the α3 domain and excludes the transmembrane domain. A similar messenger retaining intron 4, HLA-G2, was also described suggesting the presence of a truncated HLA-G6 isoform that lacks the α2 domain of the protein. Due to the presence of a stop codon within intron 2, HLA-G7 transcript retains the capacity to be translated as soluble truncated HLA-G proteins bearing the α1 domain linked to two specific amino acids encoded by intron 2. [12] The structure of HLA-G1 and HLA-G5 is similar to that of classical HLA class I molecules: a heavy chain of three globular domains non-covalently associated with β_2-microglobulin (β_2m) which is encoded by a gene at chromosome 15, and the α1 and α2 domains form the peptide-binding cleft. However, all HLA-G isoforms contain the α1 domain. [14]

Besides the monomer of HLA-G molecules, the polymerization of HLA-G was first hypothesized after HLA-G2 sequence analysis but first observed for HLA-G1 which was then crystallized. [14,22,23] By a 1.9-A structure of a monomeric HLA-G complexe with a natural endogenous peptide ligand from histone H2A (RIIPRHLQL), data showed that the structure of monomer HLA-G1 is class I-like as a heterotrimer of heavy chain associated with the β_2m and peptide, while have a more hydrophobic for the α3 domain. [24] HLA-G1 homodimers have been shown to be expressed at the surface of normal trophoblasts *in vitro*, and at the surface of human extravillous trophoblast cells *in vivo*. HLA-G5 homodimers have also been described *in vitro*; Moreover, HLA-G1 and HLA-G5 β_2m -free heavy chains can also form homodimers. [25, 26, 27] Evidence showed that dimerization of HLA-G occurs through the creation of disulphide bonds between 2 unique cysteine residues at positions 42 (Cys42-Cys42 bonds) in the α1 domain and 147 (Cys42-Cys147 bonds) of HLA-G heavy chains in the α2 domain. [22, 28] HLA-G1 homodimers are joined head-to-tail by Cys42-Cys42 disulphide bonds and the polymerization process displayed no significant main backbone structure change from that of the monomers. However, HLA-G1 homodimers have an oblique orientation that exposes the immunoglobulin-like transcripts (ILT)-2- and ILT-4-binding sites of the α3 domain upwards, making them more accessible to the receptors, and enhancing ILT-mediated intracellular signaling. [23]

HLA-G RECEPTORS

A amount of studies have supported the role of HLA-G as a tolerogenic molecule, playing an important role in the suppression of the immune response through binding to immune inhibitory receptors expressed on various immune cells. [29] Three HLA-G-recognizing immunoglobulin-like receptors (KIRs) have been identified to interact with HLA-G including ILT-2/CD85j/(leukocyte immunoglobulin-like receptors (LILR)B1, ILT-4/CD85d/LILRB2, and KIR2DL4/CD158d. [30,31, 32] KIR2DL4 and ILT-2 expression could be detected on NK cells, while ILT-2 on T and B cells, ILT-2 and ILT-4 on monocytes/macrophages and DCs. [29] Furthermore, CD8 molecule was also found to be interacts with the α3 domain of HLA-G, which could lead to the apoptosis in CD8+ T lymphocytes and in CD8+ NK cells, which lack the T cell receptor. [33]

According to the nomenclature, KIRs have either two (2D) or three (3D) immunoglobulin (Ig)-like domains and different cytoplasmic tail length. KIRs with long cytoplasmic tails (KIR2DL, KIR3DL) contain immunoreceptor tyrosine-based inhibition motifs (ITIMs) and predicted to be inhibitory receptors, and the activating receptors are those with short cytoplasmic tails lacking ITIM and associate with the immunoreceptor tyrosinebased activation motif (ITAM) containing adapter DAP12 via a positively charged arginine or lysine residue in their transmembrane domain. [34] Among KIR family, KIR2DL4 is of unique composition, featured with both inhibitory (with a single ITIM in cytoplasmic domain) and activating (with an arginine in the transmembrane domain) functional structure, which has been described as the specific receptor for HLA-G. [35] Because of its unique features, the role of the interaction of KIR2DL4 with HLA-G in the modulation of the immune response remains much debate. Activation of resting human NK cells by KIR2DL4 stimulates the secretion of cytokines, but not cytotoxicity. Also, it reported that cross-linking of KIR2DL4 with a specific antibody or the incubation with transfectants expressing HLA-G dimers upregulates several pro-inflammatory cytokines. [36, 37, 38] For the sHLA-G, which could be endocytosed by KIR2DL4 and induces a unique proinflammatory and proangiogenic response in NK cells including an increased expression of genes encoding cytokines such as IL-1, IL-6, tumor necrosis factor-α (TNF-α), and IL-23 and chemokines including IL-8, macrophage inflammatory protein-3α (MIP-3α), MIP-1, MIP-1α, CCL3, CCL3L1, CCL15, CCL20, CCL24 and CXCL3. [39] For the signaling pathway involved in the HLA-G and KIR2DL4 interaction, Rajagopalan et al. recently demonstrated that most of KIR2DL4 in resting NK cells resides in endosomes and that the receptor endocytoses sHLA-G into intracellular compartments with a novel DNA-dependent protein kinase (DNAPKcs)-Akt-NF-κB endosomal signaling pathway. [40] Though KIR2DL4 is the specific receptor, the binding site of KIR2DL4 to HLA-G remains to be explored. In terms of this, we found that residues Met [76] and Gln [79] in HLA-G α1 domain play a crucial role in KIR2DL4 and HLA-G interaction. [41]

ILT-2 and ILT-4 are inhibitory receptors, besides HLA-G, ILT-2 and ILT-4 also bind classic HLA molecules; however, HLA-G is nonetheless the ligand of highest affinity for ILT-2 and ILT-4, and ILT-2 and ILT-4 have an even higher affinity for HLA-G multimers as mentioned above. [42] ILT-2 is a receptor for HLA-G associated with □$_2$m, whereas ILT-4 also recognizes HLA-G free heavy chains. ILT-2 and ILT-4 bind to the α3 domain and β_2m of the HLA-G molecule; however, ILT4 binds with higher affinity than ILT2. The different affinity for interaction between the ILT-2 and ILT-4 with HLA-G is mainly due to the different structure basis. ILT-4 binds more to the α3 domain than to the β_2m domain, and the binding sites of these receptors are distinct. The Tyr [36] and Arg [38] residues of ILT-4 bind to the 195-197 loop of the α3 domain of HLA-G, whereas the Tyr [38] and Tyr [76] residues of ILT-2 bind to the Phe [195] of HLA-G. [31]

HLA-G Functions

HLA-G-mediated Direct Inhibition of Immune Cell Functions

Immune cell functions could be directly inhibited by HLA-G interacting with inhibitory receptors expressed on NK cells, T cells and professional antigen-presenting cells (APC), as well as endothelial cells. [43,44]The immunosuppressive induced by HLA-G and receptor interaction including inhibition of cytotoxic activity of CTL and NK cells, [45, 46] induction of the apoptosis of activated CD8+ T cells and CD8+ NK cells, [33] and inhibition of allogeneic CD4+ T cell proliferation and interference with naive CD4+ T cell priming. [47, 48] Moreover, a novel mechanism of sHLA-G in impairment of chemotaxis could be medicated by the downregulation of T cell chemokine receptor expression such as CCR2, CXCR3 and CXCR5 in CD4+ T cells, CXCR3 in CD8+ T cells, Th1 clones and in Vγ9Vδ2 T cells. In that study, authors further suggested that the downregulation of CXCR3 expression on CD4+ T cells by sHLA-G mainly through the interaction with the receptor ILT2. [49]

A recent study with an animal model provided the first *in vivo* data revealed that HLA-G expression could promote tumor expansion by affecting both innate and adaptive immunity, where interaction between HLA-G and the murine receptor PIR-B could expand blood myeloid-derived CD11b+Gr1+PIR-B+ suppressor cells, reduce of peripheral T cells and alter cytokine balance toward Th2. [50] Furthermore, HLA-G could also impair the Vγ9Vδ2 T-cell proliferation and IFN-γ production and cytotoxicity by interacting with ILT-2 inhibitory receptor. [51]

HLA-G-Mediated Indirect Inhibitory Functions

In addition to these direct effects, HLA-G can also exert its immune suppressive activity by indirect mechanisms, in particular by the induction of tolerogenic regulatory T cells (Treg) and dendritic cells (DC), which could have a long-lasting and profound inhibitory effect on immune responses, and by the process of "trogocytosis" for immune cells acquire the HLA-G molecule from other cells. [52, 53]

Naturally occurring HLA-G1+ T cells was observed in human peripheral blood under normal physiologic conditions with an average 1.6% of HLA-G+CD4+ and 3.3% of HLA-G+CD8+ T cells. HLA-G+CD4+ or HLA-G+CD8+ T cells are phenotypically characterized by the expression of cell-surface HLA-G1 and secreted HLA-G5, but lack of CD25 and FoxP3 expression. [54] HLA-G+ regulatory T cells are hypoproliferative, hyporesponsive to stimulation, and without an increased expression of the immunosuppressive cytokines such as IL-10 or transforming growth factor- β and reduced expression of IFN-γ. The suppressive function of these HLA-G+ T cells could be mediated through soluble factors that include HLA-G, which was supported by the fact that supernatants from HLA-G+ T cells could inhibit the proliferation of autologous HLA-G- T cells. [55, 56]

HLA-G-induced regulatory T cells were first observed *in vitro*, after allogeneic stimulation by HLA-G1-transfected KG1a or LCL (HLA-G1-expressing APC). In that study, HLA-G1+ APCs could inhibit the proliferation of CD4+ T cells, induce CD4+ T cell anergy, and cause the differentiation of CD4+ T cells into suppressive cells. Thus, HLA-G1+ APC could promote the generation of long-term unresponsive HLA-G-induced CD4+ T cells. [48] HLA-G-induced tolerogenic DCs are generated through the interaction between HLA-G1 or HLA-G5 dimers and their ILT receptors. ILT4 cross-linking by HLA-G1 tetramers triggers signals by recruiting tyrosine phosphatase SHP-1 and SHP-2 in DCs. Functionally, HLA-G-induced tolerogenic DCs could induce the generation of CD4+CD25+CTLA-4+ and CD8+CD28+ regulatory T cells. [57, 58] Recently, a novel subset of tolerogenic DCs termed DC-10, which secrete high levels of IL-10, express ILT4 and HLA-G, have the potent specific function to induce IL-10-producing Treg cells through ILT4/HLA-G signaling pathway. [59]

Furthermore, it was shown that activated CD4+ and CD8+ T cells, activated NK cells, and monocytes can acquire HLA-G1-containing membrane fragments from HLA-G1-expressing antigen-presenting cells (APCs) and tumor cells. [60, 61, 62] This type of cell-to-cell contact dependent acquisition of membranes and associated molecules by a cell from another was termed as "trogocytosis". [63] Acquisition of HLA-G by NK cells could alter their functions: HLA-G-positive activated NK cells stopped proliferating, stopped being cytotoxic towards HLA-G-negative targets, and behaved as suppressor cells capable of protecting target cells from NK-mediated cytolysis. This immediate functional inversion from effector cell to regulatory cell was directly due to acquired cell-surface HLA-G1 as shown by specific blocking of HLA-G1/ILT2 interactions. [60] Similarly, resting or activated CD4+ and CD8+ T cells could acquire HLA-G1 from APCs in a few minutes and could immediately reverse their function from effectors to regulatory cells. Upon acquisition of HLA-G1-containing membranes, effector CD4+ T cells stopped proliferating, stopped responding to stimulation, and behaved as regulatory T cells capable of inhibiting the reactivity of autologous T cells *in vitro*. [60] Interestingly, T cells and monocytes both could efficiently acquire the tolerogenic molecule HLA-G1 from HLA-G-expressing tumor cells by trogocytosis, but HLA-G disappears more quickly from the surface of the monocytes in contrast to the HLA-G acquired by CD4+ and CD8+ T cells, which is due to a faster membrane internalization rate in monocytes than in lymphocytes, and in most of the cases, acquisition of HLA-G by monocytes had no impact on their function. [62, 64] By "trogocytosis", a few HLA-G1-expressing tumor cells might thus protect a comparatively larger area by quickly increasing locally the number of regulatory HLA-G1-positive cells without time-consuming and potentially hazardous unlocking of HLA-G expression; and spreading HLA-G1 presence to a larger area than that covered by the few HLA-G1-expressing cells; this would block the function of any effector cell in that area; and dampen the local reaction, preventing damage to tissues in the vicinity of HLA-G1-expressing cells. Consequently, HLA-G-mediated immune escape can be extended to HLA-G-negative cells by the "trogocytosis". [65]

REGULATION OF HLA-G EXPRESSION

HLA-G is not ubiquitously expressed but restricted to tissues such as in the pre-implanted embryo and at the maternal-fetal interface on extravillous invasive cytotrophoblasts and immune privileged sites like thymus, cornea, pancreas and the proximal nail matrix under non-pathological conditions. [66, 67, 68, 69, 70] In addition, HLA-G protein may be produced by human decidual stromal cells, mesenchymal stem cells, monocytes, keratinocytes and erythroblasts from primitive to definitive haematopoiesis. [71, 72, 73, 74, 75] However, aberrant ectopic induced HLA-G expression, particular the cell surface HLA-G isoform, has been observed in various pathological situations such as grafted organs, inflammatory and autoimmune diseases, viral aggressions and numerous tumours. [5] Also, an elevation of sHLA-G expression could be a common event in patients with tumor, allergy, inflammation and infectious diseases, etc. [76] Furthermore, the presence of stable HLA-G transcripts is often, but not always, correlated with HLA-G protein expression. [77] Studies have focused on understanding and unlocking HLA-G tissue-restricted expression, but mechanisms that drive HLA-G expression are neither simple nor easy to investigate. HLA-G expression can be modulated in HLA-G positive or negative cells under the influence of appropriate environmental factors which are essential for restoring HLA-G expression. It's suggested that multiple molecular mechanisms was involved in the HLA-G expression regulation such as micro-environmental cytokine profile, HLA-G itself genetic factor and gene epigenetic modification, and stress such as hypoxia, etc. It is conceivable that tumor cells exposed to hypoxia undergo additional epigenetic changes, such as DNA demethylation and histone acetylation, which lead to opened chromatin and HLA-G transcriptional activation. Additional inflammatory stimuli (via NF-κB) or the environmental cytokines or chemokines could further enhance the levels of HLA-G transcripts/proteins in tumor cells, providing them protection from the host immune system. [78, 79, 80] For example, multiple factors influences HLA-G expression was observed on the cultured human aortic and coronary artery endothelial cells that different stressors, including hypoxia/reoxygenation, interferon-γ, tumor necrosis factor-α, interleukin-10, immunosuppressive agents or progesterone, could modulate HLA-G expression. Similar finding was also found in coronary artery smooth muscle cells. [81] A better understanding of the molecular mechanism(s) influencing HLA-G expression might lead to the development of strategies to manage the HLA-G expression involved pathophysiologic conditions.

HLA-G promoter Structure

Similar to classical HLA class I genes, the 5′ upstream regulatory region (5′ URR) of HLA-G includes the CCAAT box and TATA element for basal regulation and transcriptional initiation. A second putative initiation site of HLA-G transcription has been reported 51 bp upstream of TATA (CTCACTCCC) including Enhancer A, IFN-stimulated response element and the SXY sequence. [82] The HLA-G promoter binding factors and respective target sequences include three CRE/TRE elements mediating its regulation by the cAMP response element binding protein 1 (CREB1), the interferon regulatory factor (IRF)-1, the heat shock transcription factor (HSF)-1, the RAS response element binding protein 1 (RREB-1), and a novel progesterone response element. [83, 84, 85] Furthermore, Monarch 1, a factor belonging to the CATERPILLER gene family, which is expressed primarily by myeloid-monocytic cells, is the only factor found to enhance both classical HLA-class I and HLA-G genes. [86]

Polymorphism within the HLA-G gene Promoter and the 3′ UT Region

HLA-G polymorphism was observed in the 5′ URR and in the 3′-untranslated region (3′ UTR) of the gene, which was reported to influence the HLA-G expression. The polymorphism -725C/G (rs1233334) in the HLA-G promoter region has been reported to be associated with fetal loss, and recent data indicated that the -725G allele could increase HLA-G transcriptional rates in the JEG-3 cells. [87, 88] Furthermore, a 14bp insertion/deletion polymorphism (rs16375) in exon 8 in the 3′ UTR was firstly reported in 1993, and later found that the 14bp polymorphism was associated with stability and splicing pattern of HLA-G mRNA, which could affect HLA-G protein expression or detection of sHLA-G. The presence of the 14 bp is associated with low levels of mRNA and protein expression. [89, 90] We found that plasma sHLA-G level with the +14bp/+14bp genotype was dramatically lower than that with +14bp/-14bp and -14bp/-14bp, while no dramatic difference was observed between the +14bp/-14bp and -14bp/-14bp genotype, indicating that 14bp deletion polymorphism in the HLA-G gene plays a determinant role in the sHLA-G expression. [91]

Cytokines, Growth Factors and Hormones

The mechanism of cytokines in HLA-G expression regulation depends on the type of cytokines and on the cell type. Induction of membrane-bound HLA-G expression on the myelomonocytic cell line U937 by cytokine IFN-γ, GM-CSF, IL-2 alone or in combination has been previously reported. Data showed that the level of HLA-G expression was induced by 15% with IL-2, 32% with IFN-γ, 51% with combined IL-2 and IFN-γ and 85% with GM-CSF and IFN-γ together. However, no response was reached in cell lines EBV-KAS (Epstein-Barr virus transformed B lymphoblastoid cells) and KG1a (CD341 myeloblastic leukemia). [92] The role of IL-10 in inducing HLA-G protein expression has been demonstrated in monocytes and purified trophoblast cells, and an association between IL-10 and HLA-G expression was demonstrated in cutaneous lymphoma and lung cancer, HLA-G immunoreactivity was often associated with IL-10 expression. [93, 94] Also, the IL-10 homolog produced by cytomegalovirus (CMV) can up-regulate HLA-G protein expression at the monocyte cell surface. [95]

HLA-G expression induced by IFN-γ was supported by many studies such as induction of HLA-G expression on the surface of myeloblastic leukemia cells and T-NHL cells by IFN-γ stimulation. Zhang et al. [96] investigated the effects of IFN-γ on regulation of HLA-G expression in a panel of cell lines including the T lymphoma cell line Karpas, melanoma cell line M21 and other cell lines. HLA-G transcript was increased significantly in Karpas, M21, Hela and T24 cells with the IFN-γ treatment. Interestingly, isoforms of HLA-G transcript is cell type dependent that only HLA-G3 mRNA was induced in M21, Hela and T24 cells and

HLA-G1~-G5 isoforms were observed in the Karpas cells. Other studies such as an increasing of sHLA-G production in acute lymphocytic leukemia (ALL) cells with the treatment of IFN-γ was also addressed. [97]

The hormone progesterone has an enhancement effect, in a dose- and time-dependent manner, on HLA-G gene expression through a specific progesterone response element in the HLA-G gene promoter region, and this effect could be completely inhibited by co-incubation with the progesterone antagonist RU486. It was reported when treated at 10, 100 and 1000 ng/ml progesterone, HLA-G mRNA expression in JEG-3 cells was increased by 2.36-, 10.53-, and 17.58-fold when compared to the controls, respectively. [98] It was confirmed that HLA-G expression induced by progesterone was through a specific binding site for the progesterone receptor (PR) complex. The identified progesterone response element (PRE)-like sequence is a 15-bp non-classical consensus core sequence which is located -37 bp from the ATG and overlaps the HLA-G TATA box. [85] In line with this observation, progesterone can also induce HLA-G expression in vascular endothelial and smooth muscle cells *in vitro*, and an association was observed between HLA-G expression and the estrogen as well as progesterone receptor status in breast cancer. [81, 99]

Epigenetic Modification and HLA-G Expression

DNA methylation of CpG islands is widely used in mammals, notably in genomic imprinting and X-chromosome inactivation, and aberrant methylation patterns in CpG are also a hallmark of human cancer. [100] DNA methylation and histone modification are interrelated epigenetic mechanisms known to play a key role in transcriptional control. Epigenetic mechanisms were also shown to be involved in the regulation of HLA-G gene and protein expression. [101] Evidence for HLA-G silencing by a DNA methylation process was reported first by Guillaudeux et al. [102] HLA-G negative choriocarcinoma cell line JAR. The use of demethylating agents such as 5-azacytidine and 5-aza-2'-deoxycitidine (5-Aza-dC) further demonstrated that the repression of HLA-G gene activity in cultured cell lines of various origins is reversed by demethylating treatment. Moreau et al. [103] reported that 5-Aza-dC could slightly induce HLA-G mRNA in a melanoma cell line M8 and cell surface HLA-G expression on 5-Aza-dC treated cell lines including JAR, LCL721.221 (lymphoblastoid B cell), and Raji (Burkitt's B lymphoma). However, by the treatment of histone deacetylase inhibitor trichostatin A, induction of HLA-G transcription was only observed in the M8 human melanoma cell line. Similar observation was obtained by another study, that histone deacetylation inhibitor (valproic acid) and hypoxia mimetic chemical ($CoCl_2$) could upregulate the HLA-G expression. Results showed that the highest activation of HLA-G transcription was achieved by treatment of choriocarcinoma JAR and lymphoblastoid Raji cell lines with demethylating agent 5-Aza-dC. Treatment of JAR and Raji cells with histone deacetylase inhibitors (sodium butyrate and valproic acid) also enhanced HLA-G transcription. [80]

In a panel of human leukemia cell lines, increased HLA-G mRNA expression was observed in 18 out of 20 leukemia cell lines, and HLA-G protein expression was observed in 10 out of these cell lines when treated with 5-Aza-dC. They further test the effects of 5-Aza-dC on HLA-G gene transcription in leukemia cells isolated from patients with acute myeloid leukemia (AML) or chronic B lymphocyte leukemia (B-CLL). In this study, HLA-G transcripts was increased when treated by the 5-Aza-dC and patient's leukemia cells with high amount of HLA-G mRNAs also expressed HLA-G1 protein, indicating that 5-Aza-dC treatment of human leukemia as AML or B-CLL may induce HLA-G protein synthesis in some patients. [104] Our study showed that, treated by the 5-Aza-dC, HLA-G expression in melanoma cell line OCM-1A could be restored. After treatment, HLA-G mRNA expression was dramatically increased and HLA-G protein was induced, however, transcription does not always correlate with protein expression. Data showed that induction of HLA-G mRNA expression could be detected on the 5-Aza-dC treated OCM-1A cells on day 1 and reached highest on day 4 and then decreased afterwards. [105] Restore of HLA-G expression with the demethylating agent 5-Aza-dC treatment was further observed in other subjects such as renal cancer and ovarian cancer cell lines. [106, 107]

Fluctuation of both cell surface HLA-G expression and plasma sHLA-G levels during other therapy regimens was also observed in recent studies. Highly active antiretroviral therapy (HAART) therapy could significantly induce HLA-G expression on monocytes in patients infected with human immunodeficiency virus type 1 (HIV-1). [108] Later, it's found that as one component of the HAART, NRTIs are the main contributor to the rise in HLA-G level. This was confirmed by the fact that the numbers of monocytes expressing HLA-G gradually diminished after NRTIs were discontinued. [109] In heart transplant recipients, plasma sHLA-G concentrations were measured in patients after cyclosporine administration in conjunction with everolimus or mycophenolate mofetil, where everolimus is associated with an increased sHLA-G expression. [110, 111] In line with this, an increased sHLA-G levels concurred with the therapy response was observed during the treatment with the methotrexate in rheumatoid arthritis patients. [112] To the contrary, sHLA-G was markedly decreased after the sublingual immunotherapy in patients with allergic rhinitis. [113] However, the mechanisms underlining the regulation of sHLA-G expression by these therapeutic agents remain elusive.

Furthermore, advance in HLA-G regulation revealed that hypoxia, a physiologic stress condition with a decrease in partial oxygen pressure, could induce HLA-G expression by hypoxia-inducible factor 1. The effect of hypoxic stress on the HLA-G transcription was first addressed by Chang CC et al. [77] using the iron chelator desferrioxamine (DFX) to stabilize HIF-1a in HLA-G negative melanoma cells. They found that DFX treatment induces HLA-G gene transcription in seven of 13 melanoma cell lines. The effect is dose- and time- dependent and approximatively 16-fold lower than the level of constitutive mRNA in the JEG-3 choriocarcinoma cell line. Mouillot et al. [114] confirmed these results with the M8 melanoma cell line, thus supporting hypoxia as a candidate micro-environmental factor to reverse HLA-G gene repression. The effect of hypoxia on the HLA-G mRNA up-regulation was also observed with undifferentiated cytotrophoblasts isolated from first-trimester placenta and the Burkitt's B lymphoma cell line Raji cultured with different low concentrations of oxygen. [80, 115]

Recent study also showed that extracellular ATP could impairs both soluble and membrane-bound HLA-G molecules expression in lipopolysaccharide (LPS)-activated human monocytes through the $P2X_7$ receptor in an IL-10-dependent fashion. [116] Moreover, MicroRNAs might participate in the regulation of the HLA-G gene expression through a putative microRNA binding site at its 3′ UTR region, where a C/G (+3142, rs1063320) polymorphism was shown to be responsible for differential microRNA (miR-148a, miR-19a*, miR-148b, miR-152, miR-218-2) binding affinity and translation suppression. [117]

Among these microRNAs, the miR152 has been shown to reduce HLA-G expression, which is associated with an increased NK cell-mediated lysis. [118]

HLA-G in Reproduction

Maternal-fetal interface is characterized by an unusual combination of human leukocyte antigen (HLA) expression on extravillous trophoblast (EVT) and maternal leukocytes distribution pattern in decidual tissues. Human EVT does not express high polymorphic HLA-A, -B and HLA class II molecules but expresses limited polymorphic non-classical HLA class I antigen HLA-E, -F, -G, besides low-level of HLA-C. [4] EVT intermingles with a variety of maternal leukocytes at the implantation site in deciduas, notably more than 85% leukocytes are $CD56^{bright}CD16^{dim}$ uterine natural killer (uNK) cells. uNK cells express HLA class I molecule specific receptors that are crucial in regulating cytolytic and cytokine production of the NK cells. [119] HLA-G binding to the KIRDL4 receptor presents on uterine NK cells upregulates their secretion of cytokines and angiogenic factors, which favors implantation and placental vascularization and development. [39]

Studies on the mice model *in vivo* and outlined that uNK cell-derived IFN-γ is indispensable for initiating pregnancy in that IFN-γ could induce decidual spiral artery remodeling and promote vessel wall thinning and lumen diameter dilation, which facilitate greater blood flow to the development of placenta and fetus. [120, 121] Studies addressed that membrane-bound HLA-G could promote proliferation and IFN-γ production of purified uNK cells, which might contribute to implantation and decidualization during early pregnancy. [122] Roles of HLA-G in pregnancy was supported by the correlations established between decreased expression of HLA-G and pregnancy disorders associated with fetal loss such as recurrent spontaneous abortions and preeclampsia, and in a HLA-G transgenic mice model, pregnancy was interrupted by the use of the antiprogesterone agent (RU486) which was followed by a rapid decrease in HLA-G expression. [123, 124, 125]

The relevance of HLA-G in human reproduction is further emphasized in the context of in vitro fertilization (IVF), as it was shown that embryo expression of sHLA-G molecules was fundamental to uterine implantation. [126] sHLA-G in the culture supernatant of preimplantation embryos is being investigated as a noninvasive marker for the selection of embryos with implantation potential. In a prospective randomized study (n=214) undergoing fresh intracytoplasmic sperm injection (ICSI) cycles and embryos were selected for transfer based on either Day 3 morphology score or graduated embryo scoring (GES)-scoring plus sHLA-G expression, by combining a positive sHLA-G expression with the highest GES-score on Day 3 resulted into significantly improved assisted reproduction technique (ART) outcome, indicating that the power of sHLA-G status is a very important criterion to identify prior to embryo transfer. [127] In this study, the miscarriage rate was nearly 12 times lower in GES-scoring plus sHLA-G group than morphology score group and the pregnancy results were superior when embryos were selected based on GES plus sHLA-G expression. Recently, a German multi-center study, in which 29 ART centers with 4212 embryo cultures (EC) from 2364 cycles were included, demonstrated that the proportion of sHLA-G-positive EC increases with the cleavage stages from 11% for zygotes to 21% in two- to nine-cell embryos and 30% in embryos larger than ten cells, and sHLA-G testing would improve the overall pregnancy rate from 30% to 40%. To be noted, this study indicated that the morphological scoring system is still the best strategy for the selection of embryos, however, when a choice has to be made between embryos of morphologically equal quality, the sHLA-G status of the embryo might be considered as a second parameter. [128]

HLA-G IN TRANSPLANTATION

Roles of HLA-G in transplantation was first demonstrated in heart-transplanted patients, and then confirmed in other contexts, such as transplantation of liver, lung, and kidney. [129] In their pioneering studies, Lila et al. showed that HLA-G could be detected in myocardial biopsies and serum samples of approximately 20% of the heart transplant population. [130] Patients with HLA-G positive had significantly fewer episodes of acute rejection when compared to the HLA-G negative group. Data revealed that only 11% of patients with recurrent moderate to severe rejection (rejecting group) showed HLA-G expression in biopsy specimens, while 86% of the HLA-G-positive patients who never experienced acute cellular rejection (non-rejecting group). Additionally, whereas 15 cases of graft vasculopathy were detected in HLA-G negative patients, none of the nine HLA-G positive patients experienced graft vasculopathy. [131] A recently study also indicated that the HLA-G genetic varies such as the 14-bp deletion polymorphism in the HLA-G gene was relative to a low risk for acute cellular rejection in heart transplant recipients. In that study, Patients with the -14-bp/-14-bp genotype had significantly higher serum HLA-G levels than those patients with the +14bp/-14bp and +14bp/+14bp genotypes, and the -14bp/-14bp genotype was significantly associated with fewer episodes of cellular rejection. [132]

In kidney and liver transplants, Creput et al. have shown that 14 out of 41 liver and 5 out of 9 kidney transplant biopsies expressed HLA-G. Data also revealed that, when a liver allograft is simultaneously transplanted with a kidney, the former protects the latter from acute rejection, as 32.5% of kidney recipients compared to only 6% of kidney and liver combined recipients developed acute kidney graft rejection. As to the liver grafts, HLA-G expression was shown to significantly decrease graft rejection, and no cases of acute or chronic rejection of the kidney graft was observed in patients who expressed HLA-G in their liver graft. [133, 134] In 64 lung transplant recipients, HLA-G expression was detected in bronchial epithelial cells from stable patients, but never in patients with acute rejection or with bronchiolitis obliterans syndrome, which is considered a form of chronic rejection. [135] Also, HLA-G level on monocytoid dendritic cells was observed to correlates with regulatory T-cell Foxp3 expression in liver transplant tolerance, and an increased serum sHLA-G levels was associated with operational tolerance of liver grafts and with a favorable outcomes in pediatric and young adult recipients. [136, 137]

In kidney transplantation, data showed that patients treated with cytotoxic T lymphocyte associated antigen4 (CTLA4)-Ig, a new recombinant molecule that interferes with the signal of T lymphocyte activation, was with significantly higher sHLA-G than patients treated with calcineurin inhibitors or healthy donors. They indentified that DC was one of the cellular sources of sHLA-G in CTLA4-Ig-treated patients, and CTLA4-Ig-treated DC could suppress T cell alloproliferation through sHLA-G, which could be restored by using a neutralizing anti-HLA-G antibody. Moreover, they found that plasma sHLA-G purified from CTLA4-Ig-treated patients could inhibit allogeneic T cell proliferation *in vitro*. [138] These results suggest that HLA-G expression may diminish the host immune response thereby reducing acute or chronic rejection and that HLA-G could be considered as a tolerance marker for the follow-up of transplanted patients. However, the 14-bp deletion/insertion polymorphism in the HLA-G gene was unrelated to the rejection status in kidney allograft recepients according to a recent study. [139]

HLA-G involved in the immunotolerance was also observed in other findings. Peripheral blood mononuclear cells (PBMCs) from transplanted patients that have been exposed to high levels of circulating HLA-G do not respond to allogenic stimulus, and PBMC from HLA-G+ transplanted patients have immunosuppressive properties and contain an increased proportion of CD3+CD4^{low} and CD3+CD8^{low} suppressor T cells. [140] Moreover, HLA-G5 purified from plasma of HLA-G+ transplanted patients suppresses T cell alloproliferation *in vitro*, where HLA-G5 secreted from human mesenchymal stem cells was observed to induce CD4+CD25^{high}FOXP3+ Treg cells expansion *in vitro,* and a positive correlation was found between sHLA-G and CD4+CD25+CD152+ Treg frequency in allogeneic peripheral blood haematopoietic stem cell transplanted patients, and that CD4+CD25+ CD152+ Treg is correlated with increased sHLA-G expression in *in vitro* mixed leucocyte reaction cultures, which all might contribute to tolerance in HLA-G+ transplanted patients. [141, 142]

HLA-G IN INFECTIOUS DISEASES

In viral infection, induced HLA-G expression by virus-infected cells was proposed as a mechanism that helps viruses to subvert host anti-virus defenses. [143] Roles of HLA-G expression induced by influenza A virus, human cytomegalovirus virus (HCMV), human immunodeficiency virus (HIV), hepatitis B and C virus (HBV and HCV), and rabies virus (RABV) were discussed. [144, 145, 146, 147, 148, 149]

A recent study revealed that HLA-G molecules were up-regulated after influenza virus (IAV) infection *in vitro* in lung epithelial cells A549 but at different levels depending on IAV strain, where A/Turkey/65 (H6N2) virus was the most efficient virus in induction of HLA-G protein expression. [144] Interestingly, when the HLA-G positive first trimester trophoblast cell lines Swan71 and HTR8 challenged with A/Udorn/72 influenza (H3N2) virus, the cell surface HLA-G expression remains unchanged. [150] Our results showed that cell surface HLA-G expression in peripheral T cells and monocytes was dramatically increased in patients with H1N1 virus of swine origin (H1N1v) and seasonal H1N1 virus infection, and an increased CD4+CD25+FoxP3+ Treg were observed in the H1N1v but not in the seasonal H1N1 infected patients. [151]

In HCV infection, our study showed that plasma sHLA-G is dramatically increased in chronic HCV-infected individuals; however, the elevation of sHLA-G expression is unrelated to the HCV genotype and viral RNA loads. [148] In a study including 90 acute hepatitis B patients (AHB), 131 chronic hepatitis B patients (CHB), 152 resolved hepatitis B individuals (RHB), and 129 normal controls. We recently found that sHLA-G levels in AHB, CHB, and RHB patients was much higher than that in normal controls. Significant difference for sHLA-G levels was also observed between patients with HBV infection (AHB *vs* CHB, AHB *vs* RHB and CHB *vs* RHB, all $p<0.001$). The area under ROC curve for sHLA-G levels was

1.000 for AHB, 0.993 for CHB, and 0.604 for RHB patients *versus* normal controls, respectively. Data also showed that the percentage of CD4+CD25+FoxP3+Treg and HLA-G+CD14+ monocytes was significantly increased in AHB and CHB patients than in normal controls, indicating that induction of HLA-G expression may play a role in HBV immune evasion and sHLA-G levels could be a useful biomarker in HBV infection. [152]

During HCMV infection, both cell surface and sHLA-G could be induced in macrophages, and bronchoalveolar macrophages collected from patients suffering from acute HCMV pneumonitis also express HLA-G molecules. Moreover, sHLA-G is induced in CMV-infected monocytes through the cooperative action of the two immediate-early-1 pp72 and immediate-early-2 pp86 products. [145] Schust et al. [153] addressed that unlike HLA-A and -B, both HLA-C and HLA-G expressed in a human trophoblast cell line were fully resistant to the rapid degradation associated with unique short region protein (US)2 and US11. Our study revealed that both HLA-G expression on CD14+ monocytes and plasma sHLA-G levels were markedly increased during active HCMV infection. [75]

In HIV-infected patients, HLA-G expression was upregulated in CD8+ T cells and monocytes. [154] This may partial due to the fact that, unlike HLA-A2 molecules which are internalized after HIV infection, HLA-G was found to be resistant to HIV Nef-induced downregulation and intracellular accumulation. [155] Moreover, sHLA-G levels were significantly higher in AIDS patients before treatment as compared with healthy controls and significantly decreased after 36 months of antiretroviral therapy. [109] The decrease of sHLA-G was correlated with the decrease of plasma HIV-RNA level and CD8+ T lymphocytes number and with the increase of CD4+ T lymphocytes number. Furthermore, sHLA-G levels were significantly higher in patients with opportunistic infections and Kaposi's sarcoma compared with patients with the wasting syndrome. [156]

Analysis of HLA-G expression in neurotropic viral infections showed that herpes simplex virus type 1 (HSV-1) and RABV upregulate the neuronal expression of HLA-G isoforms both in infected cells and neighboring uninfected cells. Indeed, upregulation of HLA-G gene expression was observed in a human neuronal line (NT2-N cells) after in vitro infection by a highly pathogenic strain of rabies virus or a strain of herpes virus inducing neuron latency. [157] Lefon et al. showed that both HSV-1 and RABV are capable of triggering up-regulation in active infected neurons to express HLA-G1 and produce HLA-G5 soluble isoforms. However, RABV primarily up-regulates HLA-G1, in contrast to HSV-1 which changes HLA-G3 and HLA-G5. [158]

HLA-G in Malignancies

In the context of cancer, HLA-G expression was firstly observed in melanoma. Later, it was observed in more than thirty kinds of neoplasmas including hematological malignancies and solid tumors. [101, 159] These studies indicated that HLA-G was preferentially detected in tumor tissue and rarely observed in normal or adjacent non-tumorous tissues, suggesting that HLA-G expression could play a critical role in tumor growth and progression. However, there are marked differences in the proportion of HLA-G expression in tumor lesions, as it ranges from 100% in hydatiform moles most likely because of its placental origin to negative in uveal melanoma and laryngeal carcinoma, and the clinical relevance of HLA-G expression in malignancies varied. [159, 160, 161, 162]

In acute myeloid leukemia (AML) patients, though HLA-G-positive patients had a significant higher bone marrow leukaemic blast cell percentage and lower total T-cell percentage; however, our recent study showed that HLA-G expression is unrelated to the prognosis in AML patients. [163, 164] In B-cell chronic lymphocytic leukemia (B-CLL), patients with leukemic cells expressing 23% or fewer HLA-G had a significantly longer progression-free survival time than those with more than 23% positive cells. Moreover, HLA-G could be a better independent prognostic factor for predicting disease progression than the Binet stage, serum β_2m and ζ associated protein-70 (ZAP-70). [165] In line with this, another study showed that HLA-G positive expression (>12%) was strongly correlated with the progression free survival in B-CLL patients, and HLA-G could be an independent factor predicting disease progression additional to Binet stage and patient age. [166] However, studies of B-CLL patients with a larger cohort demonstrated that both soluble and surface HLA-G expression was irrelative to patient age, sex, lymphocytosis, erythrocytes, platelets, hemoglobin, LDH, β_2m, Binet stage at diagnosis, cytogenetic abnormalities and patient survival. [167]

In solid tumors, HLA-G expression was detected in nearly two thirds of the ovarian carcinomas, and HLA-G protein was significantly related to the advanced ovarian cancer tissues and patients with HLA-G expression had a significantly worse prognosis. [168, 169, 170, 171] In breast cancer, studies revealed that 25%~71% lesions expressed HLA-G, and HLA-G expression was more frequently observed in advanced disease stage and tumor grade, and patient with HLA-G positive had a shorter disease-free survival or a lower survival rate. [99, 172, 173, 174, 175] In particularly, HLA-G expression in classical HLA class I-negative tumors is of prognostic value for clinical outcome of early breast cancer patients was also reported, indicating that HLA-G is an important factor in the prediction of outcome of breast cancer patients. [176] To the contrary, Sayed et al. [177] revealed the data that, though HLA-G expression is restricted to the malignant lesions, HLA-G expression is of no significance in the prognosis in breast cancer patients.

In hepatocellular carcinoma, HLA-G expression was found to be strongly correlated to advanced disease stage, and more frequently observed in elder patients. [178] In line with this finding, other studies revealed that lesion HLA-G expression is strongly correlated to the regulatory T cells/ CD8+ cells ratio, and HLA-G expression was independently associated with shortened overall survival and increased tumor recurrence. [179, 180] In addition to the HLA-G expression status was associated with the clinical parameters such as advanced stage of diseases, poor tumor cell differentiation and lymph nodal metastasis, HLA-G considered as an independent prognostic factor was also established in esophageal squamous cell carcinoma, [181, 182] non-small cell lung cancer (NSCLC), [183, 184] gastric carcinomas [185] and colorectal cancer. [186] Furthermore, in gastric cancer, besides the HLA-G expression, patients with high Tregs were also associated with poorer survival. [187] However, HLA-G expression was irrelevant to the clinical parameters such as hisotological type, tumor location, patient gender and age, tumor nuclear grade, disease stage and tumor TNM classification in renal cell carcinoma (RCC) patients in bladder and renal cancers. [188, 189, 190]

In endometrial carcinomas, HLA-G immunoreactivity was associated with metastatic disease and the performance of HLA-G staining to distinguish metastatic versus nonmetastatic endometrial carcinoma is acceptable as the area under the receiver-operating characteristics (ROC) curve was 0.75. [191] The researchers in that report argued that HLA-G may serve as a clinical marker for the preoperative prediction of metastatic endometrial carcinoma.

In additional to the lesion HLA-G expression, peripheral blood sHLA-G levels are frequently increased in patients with malignant melanoma, glioma, and breast and ovarian carcinoma as well as in patients with hematological malignancies. [192] Singer et al. [193] applied a sensitive enzyme-linked immunosorbent assay (ELISA) to measure sHLA-G levels in the supernatant of peritoneal ascites from ovarian and breast cancer patients and benign control subjects. In that study, levels of sHLA-G were significantly higher in malignant ascites than that with benign ascites in ovarian and breast carcinoma patients, and the area under the ROC curve was 0.95 for differentiating between malignant ascites and benign ascites. Two other research groups obtained similar results when they measured and compared sHLA-G levels in plasma specimens from breast cancer patients and healthy donors. In these studies, the areas under the ROC curves were reported to be 0.953 and 0.98, respectively. [99, 175]

In colorectal cancer patients, sHLA-G was significantly increased and ROC curve for sHLA-G revealed an area under the curve of 84.2% in distinguishing colorectal cancer from benign colorectal diseases such as normal colorectum, hyperplastic polyp, inflammatory bowel disease. Data also indicated that sHLA-G levels was superior to carcinoembryonic antigen (CEA) in differentiating colorectal cancer from benign colorectal diseases and the combination of sHLA-G and CEA showed a higher detection capacity than using the individual markers alone. [194] sHLA-G levels was also showed as a better diagnostic factor than carbohydrate antigen 125 in cervical cancer patients. [195]Moreover, sHLA-G was found exclusively elevated in NSCLC, especially in patients with squamous cell carcinoma (SCC) among patients with small-cell lung cancer (SCLC), NSCLC, lung adenocarcinoma, SCC and undifferentiated carcinoma, and sHLA-G level could be a potent predictor for prognosis in lung cancer patients. We showed that higher levels of sHLA-G were associated with poor survival in NSCLC patients. [196] In another study, high levels of sHLA-G correlated with neuroblastoma relapse were also observed. [197]

In hematological malignancies, plasma sHLA-G was significantly increased in B-CLL, B-NHL and T-NHL patients; however, no relation was observed between the sHLA-G levels and histological classification, grade, international prognostic index (IPI) score, lymphocytosis, remission delay, relapse occurring or death in NHL, and the Binet classification, CD38 expression, lymphocytosis, remission delay, relapse occurring or death in B-CLL patients, and unrelated to the β_2m and overall survival in multiple myeloma patients. [198, 199]

HLA-G Based Immunotherapy in Malignancies

Since HLA-G is specifically expressed in the majority of cases of various common types of cancer and it's correlated to unfavorable prognosis in kinds of malignancies, HLA-G becomes an attractive target for design of cancer immunotherapies. [192] *In vitro* assays revealed that suppression of the expression of HLA-G in choriocarcinoma cell JEG-3 by micro RNA or small interfering RNA was found to increased NK cell-mediated cytolysis, [118, 200] that the antibodies against ILT2 and ILT4 are able to restore the proliferating activity in T cells, [201] and that HLA-G derived peptide HLA-G146-154 could effectively induce peptide-specific CTLs cytotoxic activity against HLA-G-expressing HLA-A24+ RCC cells. [202] These findings indicated that HLA-G peptide-based anticancer immunotherapy is possible. Based on above observations, a HLA-G-based chemotherapy can be achieved by employing HLA-G or HLA-G receptor antibodies to block the interaction between HLA-G and its receptors, by small interfering RNA/small hairpin RNA to downregulate the HLA-G expression levels, or by using HLA-G derived immunogenic peptide and anti-idiotype antibodies to stimulate immune cell function. Finally, taking the adventure of malignant cell surface expressed HLA-G molecules, HLA-G antibody carrying anti-cancer drugs to reach the tumor site to play the anti-tumor effects.

Concluding Remarks and Future Perspectives

In addition to its initial role addressed in fetal-maternal tolerance, the immunosuppressive molecule HLA-G plays tolerogenic roles in transplant acceptance, infectious diseases as well as malignancy immune escaping. Other contexts such as autoimmune diseases and inflammations are also involved in. With respect to the clinical context, HLA-G are believed to exert beneficial functions in pregnancy, organ transplantation and autoimmune disease by promoting embryo implantation, accepting allografts, and turning down immune reaction against self-components. However, it becomes deleterious in cancer and viral infections by permitting evasion of malignant or virus-infected cells from antitumor or antiviral responses, respectively. Therefore, these biological functions of HLA-G may play an important role in clinical applications at the diagnostic, prognostic and therapeutic levels. According to the opposite roles of HLA-G under different physio-pathological conditions, the design of HLA-G-based immune therapy will depend on the pathology under consideration: induction of HLA-G expression and function might be useful to induce a favorable tolerogenic environment in pregnancy disorders, transplantation, or autoimmune diseases. By contrast, blockade of HLA-G expression or the interaction between the HLA-G and its receptors would promote the immune clearance of tumor cells or virus-infected cells. Finally, although HLA-G has postulated to be a useful biological marker in various contexts; however, this important application needs to be confirmed in multicenter studies including large cohorts of normal healthy controls and patients.

Conflicts of Interest

None declared.

ACKNOWLEDGMENTS

This work was supported by Zhejiang Provincial program for the cultivation of high-level innovative health talents, and by the grants from the National Natural Science Foundation of China (31170879, 81102218), Science and Technology Bureau of Zhejiang Province (2009C33147) and Zhejiang Provincial Natural Science Foundation of China (Y2101323).

REFERENCES

[1] MHC Sequencing Consortium. "Complete sequence and gene map of a human major histocompatibility complex". *Nature* 1999; 401(6756): 921-923.

[2] Heinrichs H, Orr HT. HLA non-A, B, C class I genes: their structure and expression. *Immunol Res* 1990; 9(4):265-74.

[3] O'Callaghan CA, Bell JI. Structure and function of the human MHC class Ib molecules HLA-E, HLA-F and HLA-G. *Immunol Rev* 1998; 163:129-38.

[4] Hunt JS. Stranger in a strange land. *Immunol Rev* 2006; 213:36-47.

[5] Carosella ED, Moreau P, Lemaoult J, Rouas-Freiss N. HLA-G: from biology to clinical benefits. *Trends Immunol* 2008; 29(3):125-32.

[6] Geraghty DE, Koller BH, Orr HT. A human major histocompatibility complex class I gene that encodes a protein with a shortened cytoplasmic segment. *Proc Natl Acad Sci* USA 1987; 84(24):9145-9.

[7] Matte C, Lacaille J, Zijenah L, Ward B, Roger M; ZVITAMBO Study Group. HLA-G exhibits low level of polymorphism in indigenous East Africans. *Hum Immunol* 2002; 63(6):495-501.

[8] Park B, Lee S, Kim E, Chang S, Jin M, Ahn K. The truncated cytoplasmic tail of HLA-G serves a quality-control function in post-ER compartments. *Immunity* 2001; 15(2):213-24.

[9] Carosella ED, Moreau P, Le Maoult J, Le Discorde M, Dausset J, Rouas-Freiss N. HLA-G molecules: from maternal-fetal tolerance to tissue acceptance. *Adv Immunol* 2003; 81:199-252.

[10] Diehl M, Münz C, Keilholz W, Stevanović S, Holmes N, Loke YW, Rammensee HG. Nonclassical HLA-G molecules are classical peptide presenters. *Curr Biol* 1996; 6(3):305-14.

[11] Rouas-Freiss N, Paul P, Dausset J, Carosella ED. HLA-G promotes immune tolerance. *J Biol Regul Homeost Agents* 2000; 14(2):93-8.

[12] Paul P, Cabestre FA, Ibrahim EC, Lefebvre S, Khalil-Daher I, Vazeux G, Quiles RM, Bermond F, Dausset J, Carosella ED. Identification of HLA-G7 as a new splice variant of the HLA-G mRNA and expression of soluble HLA-G5, -G6, and -G7 transcripts in human transfected cells. *Hum Immunol* 2000; 61(11):1138-49.

[13] Larsen MH, Hviid TV. Human leukocyte antigen-G polymorphism in relation to expression, function, and disease. *Hum Immunol* 2009; 70(12):1026-34.

[14] Ishitani A, Geraghty DE. Alternative splicing of HLA-G transcripts yields proteins with primary structures resembling both class I and class II antigens. *Proc Natl Acad Sci* USA 1992; 89(9):3947-51.

[15] Robinson J, Waller MJ, Fail SC, Marsh SG. The IMGT/HLA and IPD databases. *Hum Mutat* 2006; 27(12):1192-9.

[16] Suárez MB, Morales P, Castro MJ, Fernández V, Varela P, Alvarez M, Martínez-Laso J, Arnaiz-Villena A. A new HLA-G allele (HLA-G*0105N) and its distribution in the Spanish population. *Immunogenetics* 1997; 45(6):464-5.

[17] Le Discorde M, Le Danff C, Moreau P, Rouas-Freiss N, Carosella ED. HLA-G*0105N null allele encodes functional HLA-G isoforms. *Biol Reprod* 2005; 73(2):280-8.

[18] Lajoie J, Jeanneau A, Faucher MC, Moreau P, Roger M. Characterisation of five novel HLA-G alleles with coding DNA base changes. *Tissue Antigens* 2008; 72(5):502-4.

[19] Ulbrecht M, Maier S, Hofmeister V, Falk CS, Brooks AG, McMaster MT, Weiss EH. Truncated HLA-G isoforms are retained in the endoplasmic reticulum and insufficiently provide HLA-E ligands. *Hum Immunol* 2004; 65(3):200-8.

[20] Mallet V, Pröll J, Solier C, Aguerre-Girr M, DeRossi M, Loke YW, Lenfant F, Le Bouteiller P. The full length HLA-G1 and no other alternative form of HLA-G is expressed at the cell surface of transfected cells. *Hum Immunol* 2000; 61(3):212-24.

[21] Sangrouber D, Marcou C, Le Discorde M, Chang CC, Carosella ED, Moreau P. Cellular co-localization of intron-4 containing mRNA and HLA-G soluble protein in melanoma analyzed by fluorescence in situ hybridization. *J Immunol Methods* 2007; 326(1-2):54-62.

[22] Boyson JE, Erskine R, Whitman MC, Chiu M, Lau JM, Koopman LA, Valter MM, Angelisova P, Horejsi V, Strominger JL. Disulfide bond-mediated dimerization of HLA-G on the cell surface. *Proc Natl Acad Sci USA* 2002; 99(25):16180-5.

[23] Shiroishi M, Kuroki K, Ose T, Rasubala L, Shiratori I, Arase H, Tsumoto K, Kumagai I, Kohda D, Maenaka K. Efficient leukocyte Ig-like receptor signaling and crystal structure of disulfide-linked HLA-G dimer. *J Biol Chem* 2006; 281(15):10439-47.

[24] Clements CS, Kjer-Nielsen L, Kostenko L, Hoare HL, Dunstone MA, Moses E, Freed K, Brooks AG, Rossjohn J, McCluskey J. Crystal structure of HLA-G: a nonclassical MHC class I molecule expressed at the fetal-maternal interface. *Proc Natl Acad Sci* USA 2005; 102(9):3360-5.

[25] Gonen-Gross T, Achdout H, Arnon TI, Gazit R, Stern N, Horejsí V, Goldman-Wohl D, Yagel S, Mandelboim O. The CD85J/leukocyte inhibitory receptor-1 distinguishes between conformed and beta 2-microglobulin-free HLA-G molecules. *J Immunol* 2005; 175(8):4866-74.

[26] Apps R, Gardner L, Sharkey AM, Holmes N, Moffett A. A homodimeric complex of HLA-G on normal trophoblast cells modulates antigen-presenting cells via LILRB1. Eur J Immunol 2007; 37(7):1924-37.

[27] Morales PJ, Pace JL, Platt JS, Langat DK, Hunt JS. Synthesis of beta(2)-microglobulin-free, disulphide-linked HLA-G5 homodimers in human placental villous cytotrophoblast cells. *Immunology* 2007; 122(2):179-88.

[28] Gonen-Gross T, Achdout H, Gazit R, Hanna J, Mizrahi S, Markel G, Goldman-Wohl D, Yagel S, Horejsí V, Levy O, Baniyash M, Mandelboim O. Complexes of HLA-G protein on the cell surface are important for leukocyte Ig-like receptor-1 function. *J Immunol* 2003; 171(3):1343-51.

[29] Clements CS, Kjer-Nielsen L, McCluskey J, Rossjohn J. Structural studies on HLA-G: implications for ligand and receptor binding. *Hum Immunol* 2007; 68(4):220-6.

[30] Navarro F, Llano M, Bellón T, Colonna M, Geraghty DE, López-Botet M. The ILT2 (LIR1) and CD94/NKG2A NK cell receptors respectively recognize HLA-G1 and HLA-E molecules co-expressed on target cells. *Eur J Immunol* 1999; 29(1):277-83.

[31] Shiroishi M, Kuroki K, Rasubala L, Tsumoto K, Kumagai I, Kurimoto E, Kato K, Kohda D, Maenaka K. Structural basis for recognition of the nonclassical MHC molecule HLA-G by the leukocyte Ig-like receptor B2 (LILRB2/LIR2/ILT4/CD85d). *Proc Natl Acad Sci* USA 2006; 103(44):16412-7.

[32] Rajagopalan S, Long EO. A human histocompatibility leukocyte antigen (HLA)-G-specific receptor expressed on all natural killer cells. *J Exp Med* 1999; 189(7):1093-100.

[33] Contini P, Ghio M, Poggi A, Filaci G, Indiveri F, Ferrone S, Puppo F. Soluble HLA-A,-B,-C and -G molecules induce apoptosis in T and NK CD8+ cells and inhibit cytotoxic T cell activity through CD8 ligation. *Eur J Immunol* 2003; 33(1):125-34.

[34] Biassoni R, Ugolotti E, De Maria A. NK cell receptors and their interactions with MHC. *Curr Pharm Des* 2009; 15(28):3301-10.

[35] López-Botet M, Llano M, Navarro F, Bellón T. NK cell recognition of non-classical HLA class I molecules. *Semin Immunol* 2000; 12(2):109-19.

[36] Rajagopalan S, Fu J, Long EO. Cutting edge: induction of IFN-gamma production but not cytotoxicity by the killer cell Ig-like receptor KIR2DL4 (CD158d) in resting NK cells. *J Immunol* 2001; 167(4):1877-1881.

[37] Yan WH, Lin A, Chen BG, Zhou MY, Dai MZ, Chen XJ, Gan LH, Zhu M, Shi WW, Li BL. Possible roles of KIR2DL4 expression on uNK cells in human pregnancy. *Am J Reprod Immunol* 2007; 57(4):233-42.

[38] Li C, Houser BL, Nicotra ML, Strominger JL. HLA-G homodimer-induced cytokine secretion through HLA-G receptors on human decidual macrophages and natural killer cells. *Proc Natl Acad Sci* USA 2009; 106(14):5767-72.

[39] Rajagopalan S, Bryceson YT, Kuppusamy SP, Geraghty DE, van der Meer A, Joosten I, Long EO. Activation of NK cells by an endocytosed receptor for soluble HLA-G. *PLoS Biol* 2006; 4(1):e9.

[40] Rajagopalan S, Moyle MW, Joosten I, Long EO. DNA-PKcs controls an endosomal signaling pathway for a proinflammatory response by natural killer cells. *Sci Signal* 2010; 3(110):ra14.

[41] Yan WH, Fan LA. Residues Met76 and Gln79 in HLA-G alpha1 domain involve in KIR2DL4 recognition. *Cell Res* 2005; 15(3):176-82.

[42] Shiroishi M, Tsumoto K, Amano K, Shirakihara Y, Colonna M, Braud VM, Allan DS, Makadzange A, Rowland-Jones S, Willcox B, Jones EY, van der Merwe PA, Kumagai I, Maenaka K. Human inhibitory receptors Ig-like transcript 2 (ILT2) and ILT4 compete with CD8 for MHC class I binding and bind preferentially to HLA-G. *Proc Natl Acad Sci* USA 2003; 100(15):8856-61.

[43] Hofmeister V, Weiss EH. HLA-G modulates immune responses by diverse receptor interactions. *Semin Cancer Biol* 2003; 13(5):317-23.

[44] Fons P, Chabot S, Cartwright JE, Lenfant F, L'Faqihi F, Giustiniani J, Herault JP, Gueguen G, Bono F, Savi P, Aguerre-Girr M, Fournel S, Malecaze F, Bensussan A, Plouët J, Le Bouteiller P. Soluble HLA-G1 inhibits angiogenesis through an apoptotic pathway and by direct binding to CD160 receptor expressed by endothelial cells. *Blood* 2006; 108(8):2608-15.

[45] Le Gal FA, Riteau B, Sedlik C, Khalil-Daher I, Menier C, Dausset J, Guillet JG, Carosella ED, Rouas-Freiss N. HLA-G-mediated inhibition of antigen-specific cytotoxic T lymphocytes. *Int Immunol* 1999; 11(8):1351-6.

[46] Yu Y, Wang Y, Feng M. Human leukocyte antigen-G1 inhibits natural killer cytotoxicity through blocking the activating signal transduction pathway and formation of activating immunologic synapse. *Hum Immunol* 2008; 69(1):16-23.

[47] Mitsdoerffer M, Schreiner B, Kieseier BC, Neuhaus O, Dichgans J, Hartung HP, Weller M, Wiendl H. Monocyte-derived HLA-G acts as a strong inhibitor of autologous CD4 T cell activation and is upregulated by interferon-beta in vitro and in vivo: rationale for the therapy of multiple sclerosis. *J Neuroimmunol* 2005; 159(1-2):155-64.

[48] LeMaoult J, Krawice-Radanne I, Dausset J, Carosella ED. HLA-G1-expressing antigen-presenting cells induce immunosuppressive CD4+ T cells. *Proc Natl Acad Sci USA* 2004; 101(18):7064-9.

[49] Morandi F, Ferretti E, Bocca P, Prigione I, Raffaghello L, Pistoia V. A novel mechanism of soluble HLA-G mediated immune modulation: downregulation of T cell chemokine receptor expression and impairment of chemotaxis. *PLoS One* 2010; 5(7):e11763.

[50] Agaugué S, Carosella ED, Rouas-Freiss N. Role of HLA-G in tumor escape through expansion of myeloid-derived suppressor cells and cytokinic balance in favor of Th2 versus Th1/Th17. *Blood* 2011; 117(26):7021-31.

[51] Lesport E, Baudhuin J, Sousa S, Lemaoult J, Zamborlini A, Rouas-Freiss N, Carosella ED, Favier B. Inhibition of human Vγ9Vδ2 T-cell antitumoral activity through HLA-G: implications for immunotherapy of cancer. *Cell Mol Life Sci* 2011; 68(20):3385-99.

[52] Carosella ED, HoWangYin KY, Favier B, LeMaoult J. HLA-G-dependent suppressor cells: Diverse by nature, function, and significance. *Hum Immunol* 2008; 69(11):700-7.

[53] Carosella ED, Gregori S, Rouas-Freiss N, LeMaoult J, Menier C, Favier B. The role of HLA-G in immunity and hematopoiesis. *Cell Mol Life Sci* 2011; 68(3):353-68.

[54] Feger U, Tolosa E, Huang YH, Waschbisch A, Biedermann T, Melms A, Wiendl H. HLA-G expression defines a novel regulatory T-cell subset present in human peripheral blood and sites of inflammation. *Blood 2007*; 110(2):568-77.

[55] Huang YH, Zozulya AL, Weidenfeller C, Schwab N, Wiendl H. T cell suppression by naturally occurring HLA-G-expressing regulatory CD4+ T cells is IL-10-dependent and reversible. *J Leukoc Biol* 2009; 86(2):273-81.

[56] Gregori S, Magnani CF, Roncarolo MG. Role of human leukocyte antigen-G in the induction of adaptive type 1 regulatory T cells. *Hum Immunol* 2009; 70(12):966-9.

[57] Ristich V, Liang S, Zhang W, Wu J, Horuzsko A. Tolerization of dendritic cells by HLA-G. *Eur J Immunol* 2005; 35(4):1133-42.

[58] Liang S, Ristich V, Arase H, Dausset J, Carosella ED, Horuzsko A. Modulation of dendritic cell differentiation by HLA-G and ILT4 requires the IL-6--STAT3 signaling pathway.*Proc Natl Acad Sci* USA 2008; 105(24):8357-62.

[59] Gregori S, Tomasoni D, Pacciani V, Scirpoli M, Battaglia M, Magnani CF, Hauben E, Roncarolo MG. Differentiation of type 1 T regulatory cells (Tr1) by tolerogenic DC-10 requires the IL-10-dependent ILT4/HLA-G pathway. *Blood* 2010; 116(6):935-44.

[60] LeMaoult J, Caumartin J, Daouya M, Favier B, Le Rond S, Gonzalez A, Carosella ED. Immune regulation by pretenders: cell-to-cell transfers of HLA-G make effector T cells act as regulatory cells. *Blood* 2007; 109(5):2040-8.

[61] Caumartin J, Favier B, Daouya M, Guillard C, Moreau P, Carosella ED, LeMaoult J. Trogocytosis-based generation of suppressive NK cells. *EMBO J* 2007; 26(5):1423-33.

[62] HoWangYin KY, Alegre E, Daouya M, Favier B, Carosella ED, LeMaoult J. Different functional outcomes of intercellular membrane transfers to monocytes and T cells. *Cell Mol Life Sci* 2010; 67(7):1133-45.

[63] Davis DM. Intercellular transfer of cell-surface proteins is common and can affect many stages of an immune response. *Nat Rev Immunol* 2007; 7(3):238-43.

[64] Alegre E, Howangyin KY, Favier B, Baudhuin J, Lesport E, Daouya M, Gonzalez A, Carosella ED, Lemaoult J. Membrane redistributions through multi-intercellular exchanges and serial trogocytosis. *Cell Res* 2010; 20(11):1239-51.

[65] Umeshappa CS, Xiang J. Tumor-derived HLA-G1 acquisition by monocytes through trogocytosis: possible functional consequences. *Cell Mol Life Sci* 2010; 67(23):4107-8.

[66] Kovats S, Main EK, Librach C, Stubblebine M, Fisher SJ, DeMars R. A class I antigen; HLA-G; expressed in human trophoblasts. *Science* 1990; 248(4952): 220-3.

[67] Crisa L, McMaster MT, Ishii JK, Fisher SJ, Salomon DR. Identification of a thymic epithelial cell subset sharing expression of the class Ib HLA-G molecule with fetal trophoblasts. *J Exp Med* 1997; 186(2):289-98.

[68] Le Discorde M, Moreau P, Sabatier P, Legeais JM, Carosella ED. Expression of HLA-G in human cornea, an immune-privileged tissue. *Hum Immunol* 2003; 64(11):1039-44.

[69] Cirulli V, Zalatan J, McMaster M, Prinsen R, Salomon DR, Ricordi C, Torbett BE, Meda P, Crisa L. The class I HLA repertoire of pancreatic islets comprises the nonclassical class Ib antigen HLA-G. *Diabetes* 2006; 55(5):1214-22.

[70] Ito T, Ito N, Saathoff M, Stampachiacchiere B, Bettermann A, Bulfone-Paus S, Takigawa M, Nickoloff BJ, Paus R. Immunology of the human nail apparatus: the nail matrix is a site of relative immune privilege. *J Invest Dermatol* 2005; 125(6):1139-48.

[71] Menier C, Rabreau M, Challier JC, Le Discorde M, Carosella ED, Rouas-Freiss N. Erythroblasts secrete the nonclassical HLA-G molecule from primitive to definitive hematopoiesis. *Blood* 2004; 104(10):3153-60.

[72] Nasef A, Mathieu N, Chapel A, Frick J, François S, Mazurier C, Boutarfa A, Bouchet S, Gorin NC, Thierry D, Fouillard L. Immunosuppressive effects of mesenchymal stem cells: involvement of HLA-G. *Transplantation* 2007; 84(2):231-7.

[73] Blanco O, Tirado I, Muñoz-Fernández R, Abadía-Molina AC, García-Pacheco JM, Peña J, Olivares EG. Human decidual stromal cells express HLA-G: Effects of cytokines and decidualization. *Hum Reprod* 2008; 23(1):144-52.

[74] Ulbrecht M, Rehberger B, Strobel I, Messer G, Kind P, Degitz K, Bieber T, Weiss EH. HLA-G: expression in human keratinocytes in vitro and in human skin in vivo. *Eur J Immunol* 1994; 24(1):176-80.

[75] Yan WH, Lin A, Chen BG, Chen SY. Induction of both membrane-bound and soluble HLA-G expression in active human cytomegalovirus infection. *J Infect Dis* 2009; 200(5):820-6.

[76] Fainardi E, Castellazzi M, Stignani M, Morandi F, Sana G, Gonzalez R, Pistoia V, Baricordi OR, Sokal E, Peña J. Emerging topics and new perspectives on HLA-G. *Cell Mol Life Sci* 2011; 68(3):433-51.

[77] Chang CC, Ferrone S. HLA-G in melanoma: can the current controversies be solved? *Semin Cancer Biol* 2003; 13(5):361-9.

[78] Donadi EA, Castelli EC, Arnaiz-Villena A, Roger M, Rey D, Moreau P. Implications of the polymorphism of HLA-G on its function, regulation, evolution and disease association. *Cell Mol Life Sci* 2011; 68(3):369-95.

[79] Moreau P, Flajollet S, Carosella ED. Non-classical transcriptional regulation of HLA-G: an update. *J Cell Mol Med* 2009; 13(9B):2973-89.

[80] Polakova K, Bandzuchova E, Tirpakova J, Kuba D, Russ G. Modulation of HLA-G expression. *Neoplasma* 2007; 54(6):455-62.

[81] Sheshgiri R, Rao V, Tumiati LC, Xiao R, Prodger JL, Badiwala M, Librach C, Delgado DH. Progesterone induces human leukocyte antigen-g expression in vascular endothelial and smooth muscle cells. *Circulation* 2008; 118(14 Suppl):S58-64.

[82] Solier C, Mallet V, Lenfant F, Bertrand A, Huchenq A, Le Bouteiller P. HLA-G unique promoter region: functional implications. *Immunogenetics* 2001; 53(8):617-25.

[83] Lefebvre S, Berrih-Aknin S, Adrian F, Moreau P, Poea S, Gourand L, Dausset J, Carosella ED, Paul P. A specific interferon (IFN)-stimulated response element of the distal HLA-G promoter binds IFN-regulatory factor 1 and mediates enhancement of this nonclassical class I gene by IFN-beta. *J Biol Chem* 2001; 276(9):6133-9.

[84] Gobin SJ, Biesta P, de Steenwinkel JE, Datema G, van den Elsen PJ. HLA-G transactivation by cAMP-response element-binding protein (CREB). An alternative transactivation pathway to the conserved major histocompatibility complex (MHC) class I regulatory routes. *J Biol Chem* 2002; 277(42):39525-31.

[85] Yie SM, Xiao R, Librach CL. Progesterone regulates HLA-G gene expression through a novel progesterone response element. *Hum Reprod* 2006; 21(10):2538-44.

[86] Williams KL, Taxman DJ, Linhoff MW, Reed W, Ting JP. Cutting edge: Monarch-1: a pyrin/nucleotide-binding domain/leucine-rich repeat protein that controls classical and nonclassical MHC class I genes. *J Immunol* 2003; 170(11):5354-8.

[87] Ober C, Aldrich CL, Chervoneva I, Billstrand C, Rahimov F, Gray HL, Hyslop T. Variation in the HLA-G promoter region influences miscarriage rates. Am J Hum Genet 2003; 72(6):1425-35.

[88] Ober C, Billstrand C, Kuldanek S, Tan Z. The miscarriage-associated HLA-G -725G allele influences transcription rates in JEG-3 cells. *Hum Reprod* 2006; 21(7):1743-8.

[89] Harrison GA, Humphrey KE, Jakobsen IB, Cooper DW. A 14 bp deletion polymorphism in the HLA-G gene. *Hum Mol Genet* 1993; 2(12):2200.

[90] Rousseau P, Le Discorde M, Mouillot G, Marcou C, Carosella ED, Moreau P. The 14 bp deletion-insertion polymorphism in the 3' UT region of the HLA-G gene influences HLA-G mRNA stability. *Hum Immunol* 2003; 64(11):1005-10.

[91] Chen XY, Yan WH, Lin A, Xu HH, Zhang JG, Wang XX. The 14 bp deletion polymorphisms in HLA-G gene play an important role in the expression of soluble HLA-G in plasma. *Tissue Antigens* 2008; 72(4):335-41.

[92] Amiot L, Onno M, Drénou B, Monvoisin C, Fauchet R. HLA-G class I gene expression in normal and malignant hematopoietic cells. *Hum Immunol* 1998; 59(8):524-8.

[93] Moreau P, Adrian-Cabestre F, Menier C, Guiard V, Gourand L, Dausset J, Carosella ED, Paul P. IL-10 selectively induces HLA-G expression in human trophoblasts and monocytes. *Int Immunol* 1999; 11(5):803-11.

[94] Urosevic M, Dummer R. HLA-G and IL-10 expression in human cancer--different stories with the same message. *Semin Cancer Biol* 2003; 13(5):337-42.

[95] Spencer JV, Lockridge KM, Barry PA, Lin G, Tsang M, Penfold ME, Schall TJ. Potent immunosuppressive activities of cytomegalovirus-encoded interleukin-10. *J Virol* 2002; 76(3):1285-92.

[96] Zhang C, Tian ZG, Wei HM. The expression of non-classical class I molecules (HLA-G and HLA-E) in human tumor cell lines and the regulatory effect of IFN-γ. *Chin J Clin Oncol* (Chin) 2001; 28 (4):247-253.

[97] Rebmann V, Regel J, Stolke D, Grosse-Wilde H. Secretion of sHLA-G molecules in malignancies. *Semin Cancer Biol* 2003; 13(5):371-7.

[98] Yie SM, Li LH, Li GM, Xiao R, Librach CL. Progesterone enhances HLA-G gene expression in JEG-3 choriocarcinoma cells and human cytotrophoblasts in vitro. *Hum Reprod* 2006; 21(1):46-51.

[99] He X, Dong DD, Yie SM, Yang H, Cao M, Ye SR, Li K, Liu J, Chen J. HLA-G expression in human breast cancer: implications for diagnosis and prognosis, and effect on allocytotoxic lymphocyte response after hormone treatment in vitro. *Ann Surg Oncol* 2010; 17(5):1459-69.

[100] Ellis L, Atadja PW, Johnstone RW. Epigenetics in cancer: targeting chromatin modifications. *Mol Cancer Ther* 2009; 8(6):1409-20.

[101] Yan WH. HLA-G expression in hematologic malignancies. *Expert Rev Hematol* 2010; 3(1):67-80.

[102] Guillaudeux T, Rodriguez AM, Girr M, Mallet V, Ellis SA, Sargent IL, Fauchet R, Alsat E, Le Bouteiller P. Methylation status and transcriptional expression of the MHC class I loci in human trophoblast cells from term placenta. *J Immunol* 1995; 154(7):3283-99.

[103] Moreau P, Mouillot G, Rousseau P, Marcou C, Dausset J, Carosella ED. HLA-G gene repression is reversed by demethylation. *Proc Natl Acad Sci* USA 2003; 100(3):1191-6.

[104] Poláková K, Bandzuchová E, Kuba D, Russ G. Demethylating agent 5-aza-2'-deoxycytidine activates HLA-G expression in human leukemia cell lines. *Leuk Res* 2009; 33(4):518-24.

[105] Yan WH, Lin AF, Chang CC, Ferrone S. Induction of HLA-G expression in a melanoma cell line OCM-1A following the treatment with 5-aza-2'-deoxycytidine. *Cell Res* 2005; 15(7):523-31.

[106] Dunker K, Schlaf G, Bukur J, Altermann WW, Handke D, Seliger B. Expression and regulation of non-classical HLA-G in renal cell carcinoma. *Tissue Antigens* 2008; 72(2):137-48.

[107] Menendez L, Walker LD, Matyunina LV, Totten KA, Benigno BB, McDonald JF. Epigenetic changes within the promoter region of the HLA-G gene in ovarian tumors. *Mol Cancer* 2008; 7:43.

[108] Cabello A, Rivero A, Garcia MJ, Lozano JM, Torre-Cisneros J, González R, Dueñas G, Galiani MD, Camacho A, Santamaria M, Solana R, Montero C, Kindelán JM, Peña J. HAART induces the expression of HLA-G on peripheral monocytes in HIV-1 infected individuals. *Hum Immunol* 2003; 64(11):1045-9.

[109] Murdaca G, Contini P, Setti M, Cagnati P, Lantieri F, Indiveri F, Puppo F. Behavior of non-classical soluble HLA class G antigens in human immunodeficiency virus 1-infected patients before and after HAART: comparison with classical soluble HLA-A, -B, -C antigens and potential role in immune-reconstitution. *Clin Immunol* 2009; 133(2):238-44.

[110] Luque J, Torres MI, Aumente MD, Marín J, García-Jurado G, González R, Pascual D, Guerra N, López-Rubio F, Alvarez-López MR, Arizón JM, Peña J. Soluble HLA-G in heart transplantation: their relationship to rejection episodes and immunosuppressive therapy. *Hum Immunol* 2006; 67(4-5):257-63.
[111] Sheshgiri R, Gustafsson F, Sheedy J, Rao V, Ross HJ, Delgado DH. Everolimus but not mycophenolate mofetil therapy is associated with soluble HLA-G expression in heart transplant patients. *J Heart Lung Transplant* 2009; 28(11):1193-7.
[112] Rizzo R, Rubini M, Govoni M, Padovan M, Melchiorri L, Stignani M, Carturan S, Ferretti S, Trotta F, Baricordi OR. HLA-G 14-bp polymorphism regulates the methotrexate response in rheumatoid arthritis. Pharmacogenet Genomics 2006; 16(9):615-23.
[113] Ciprandi G, Contini P, Pistorio A, Murdaca G, Puppo F. Sublingual immunotherapy reduces soluble HLA-G and HLA-A,-B,-C serum levels in patients with allergic rhinitis. *Int Immunopharmacol* 2009; 9(2):253-7.
[114] Mouillot G, Marcou C, Zidi I, Guillard C, Sangrouber D, Carosella ED, Moreau P. Hypoxia modulates HLA-G gene expression in tumor cells. Hum Immunol 2007; 68(4):277-85.
[115] Nagamatsu T, Fujii T, Yamashita T, Miki A, Kanai T, Kusumi M, Osuga Y, Kozuma S, Taketani Y. Hypoxia does not reduce HLA-G expression on extravillous cytotrophoblasts. *J Reprod Immunol* 2004; 63(2):85-95.
[116] Rizzo R, Ferrari D, Melchiorri L, Stignani M, Gulinelli S, Baricordi OR, Di Virgilio F. Extracellular ATP acting at the P2X7 receptor inhibits secretion of soluble HLA-G from human monocytes. *J Immunol* 2009; 183(7):4302-11.
[117] Tan Z, Randall G, Fan J, Camoretti-Mercado B, Brockman-Schneider R, Pan L, Solway J, Gern JE, Lemanske RF, Nicolae D, Ober C. Allele-specific targeting of microRNAs to HLA-G and risk of asthma. *Am J Hum Genet* 2007;81(4):829-34.
[118] Zhu XM, Han T, Wang XH, Li YH, Yang HG, Luo YN, Yin GW, Yao YQ. Overexpression of miR-152 leads to reduced expression of human leukocyte antigen-G and increased natural killer cell mediated cytolysis in JEG-3 cells. *Am J Obstet Gynecol* 2010; 202(6):592.e1-7.
[119] Riley JK, Yokoyama WM. NK cell tolerance and the maternal-fetal interface. *Am J Reprod Immunol* 2008; 59(5):371-87.
[120] Ashkar AA, Di Santo JP, Croy BA. Interferon gamma contributes to initiation of uterine vascular modification, decidual integrity, and uterine natural killer cell maturation during normal murine pregnancy. *J Exp Med* 2000;192(2):259-70.
[121] Croy BA, He H, Esadeg S, Wei Q, McCartney D, Zhang J, Borzychowski A, Ashkar AA, Black GP, Evans SS, Chantakru S, van den Heuvel M, Paffaro VA Jr, Yamada AT. Uterine natural killer cells: insights into their cellular and molecular biology from mouse modelling. *Reproduction* 2003; 126(2):149-60.
[122] van der Meer A, Lukassen HG, van Lierop MJ, Wijnands F, Mosselman S, Braat DD, Joosten I. Membrane-bound HLA-G activates proliferation and interferon-gamma production by uterine natural killer cells. *Mol Hum Reprod* 2004; 10(3):189-95.
[123] Johnson PM, Christmas SE, Vince GS. Immunological aspects of implantation and implantation failure. *Hum Reprod* 1999; 14 (Suppl 2):26-36
[124] Schmidt CM, Orr HT. HLA-G transgenic mice: a model for studying expression and function at the maternal/fetal interface. *Immunol Rev* 1995; 147:53-65.

[125] Arck P, Hansen PJ, Mulac Jericevic B, Piccinni MP, Szekeres-Bartho J. Progesterone during pregnancy: endocrine-immune cross talk in mammalian species and the role of stress. *Am J Reprod Immunol* 2007; 58(3):268-79.

[126] Roussev RG, Coulam CB. HLA-G and its role in implantation (review). J Assist Reprod Genet 2007; 24(7):288-95.

[127] Kotze DJ, Hansen P, Keskintepe L, Snowden E, Sher G, Kruger T. Embryo selection criteria based on morphology VERSUS the expression of a biochemical marker (sHLA-G) and a graduated embryo score: prediction of pregnancy outcome. *J Assist Reprod Genet* 2010; 27(6):309-16.

[128] Rebmann V, Switala M, Eue I, Grosse-Wilde H. Soluble HLA-G is an independent factor for the prediction of pregnancy outcome after ART: a German multi-centre study. *Hum Reprod* 2010; 25(7):1691-8.

[129] Deschaseaux F, Delgado D, Pistoia V, Giuliani M, Morandi F, Durrbach A. HLA-G in organ transplantation: towards clinical applications. *Cell Mol Life Sci* 2011; 68(3):397-404.

[130] Lila N, Carpentier A, Amrein C, Khalil-Daher I, Dausset J, Carosella ED. Implication of HLA-G molecule in heart-graft acceptance. *Lancet* 2000; 355(9221):2138.

[131] Lila N, Amrein C, Guillemain R, Chevalier P, Latremouille C, Fabiani JN, Dausset J, Carosella ED, Carpentier A. Human leukocyte antigen-G expression after heart transplantation is associated with a reduced incidence of rejection. *Circulation* 2002; 105(16):1949-54.

[132] Twito T, Joseph J, Mociornita A, Rao V, Ross H, Delgado DH. The 14-bp deletion in the HLA-G gene indicates a low risk for acute cellular rejection in heart transplant recipients. *J Heart Lung Transplant* 2011; 30(7):778-82.

[133] Créput C, Durrbach A, Menier C, Guettier C, Samuel D, Dausset J, Charpentier B, Carosella ED, Rouas-Freiss N. Human leukocyte antigen-G (HLA-G) expression in biliary epithelial cells is associated with allograft acceptance in liver-kidney transplantation. *J Hepatol* 2003; 39(4):587-94.

[134] Creput C, Le Friec G, Bahri R, Amiot L, Charpentier B, Carosella E, Rouas-Freiss N, Durrbach A. Detection of HLA-G in serum and graft biopsy associated with fewer acute rejections following combined liver-kidney transplantation: possible implications for monitoring patients. *Hum Immunol* 2003; 64(11):1033-8.

[135] Brugière O, Thabut G, Pretolani M, Krawice-Radanne I, Dill C, Herbreteau A, Poras I, Moreau P, Colombat M, Danel C, Dehoux M, Fournier M, Carosella ED, Rouas-Freiss N. Immunohistochemical study of HLA-G expression in lung transplant recipients. *Am J Transplant* 2009; 9(6):1427-38.

[136] Castellaneta A, Mazariegos GV, Nayyar N, Zeevi A, Thomson AW. HLA-G level on monocytoid dendritic cells correlates with regulatory T-cell Foxp3 expression in liver transplant tolerance. *Transplantation* 2011; 91(10):1132-40.

[137] Zarkhin V, Talisetti A, Li L, Wozniak LJ, McDiarmid SV, Cox K, Esquivel C, Sarwal MM. Expression of soluble HLA-G identifies favorable outcomes in liver transplant recipients. *Transplantation* 2010; 90(9):1000-5.

[138] Bahri R, Naji A, Menier C, Charpentier B, Carosella ED, Rouas-Freiss N, Durrbach A. Dendritic cells secrete the immunosuppressive HLA-G molecule upon CTLA4-Ig treatment: implication in human renal transplant acceptance. *J Immunol* 2009; 183(11):7054-62.

[139] Aghdaie MH, Azarpira N, Kazemi K, Geramizadeh B, Darai M, Malekhoseini SA. Frequency of HLA-G exon 8 polymorphisms and kidney allograft outcome in Iranian population. *Mol Biol Rep* 2011; 38(5):3593-7.

[140] Naji A, Le Rond S, Durrbach A, Krawice-Radanne I, Creput C, Daouya M, Caumartin J, LeMaoult J, Carosella ED, Rouas-Freiss N. CD3+CD4low and CD3+CD8low are induced by HLA-G: novel human peripheral blood suppressor T-cell subsets involved in transplant acceptance. *Blood* 2007; 110(12):3936-48.

[141] Selmani Z, Naji A, Zidi I, Favier B, Gaiffe E, Obert L, Borg C, Saas P, Tiberghien P, Rouas-Freiss N, Carosella ED, Deschaseaux F. Human leukocyte antigen-G5 secretion by human mesenchymal stem cells is required to suppress T lymphocyte and natural killer function and to induce CD4+CD25highFOXP3+ regulatory T cells. *Stem Cells* 2008; 26(1):212-22.

[142] Le Maux A, Noël G, Birebent B, Grosset JM, Vu N, De Guibert S, Bernard M, Semana G, Amiot L. Soluble human leucocyte antigen-G molecules in peripheral blood haematopoietic stem cell transplantation: a specific role to prevent acute graft-versus-host disease and a link with regulatory T cells. *Clin Exp Immunol* 2008; 152(1):50-6.

[143] Lin A, Xu H, Yan W. Modulation of HLA expression in human cytomegalovirus immune evasion. *Cell Mol Immunol* 2007; 4(2):91-8.

[144] LeBouder F, Khoufache K, Menier C, Mandouri Y, Keffous M, Lejal N, Krawice-Radanne I, Carosella ED, Rouas-Freiss N, Riteau B. Immunosuppressive HLA-G molecule is upregulated in alveolar epithelial cells after influenza A virus infection. *Hum Immunol* 2009; 70(12):1016-9.

[145] Onno M, Pangault C, Le Friec G, Guilloux V, André P, Fauchet R. Modulation of HLA-G antigens expression by human cytomegalovirus: specific induction in activated macrophages harboring human cytomegalovirus infection. *J Immunol* 2000; 164(12):6426-34.

[146] Tripathi P, Agrawal S. The role of human leukocyte antigen E and G in HIV infection. *AIDS* 2007; 21(11):1395-404.

[147] Souto FJ, Crispim JC, Ferreira SC, da Silva AS, Bassi CL, Soares CP, Zucoloto S, Rouas-Freiss N, Moreau P, Martinelli AL, Donadi EA. Liver HLA-G expression is associated with multiple clinical and histopathological forms of chronic hepatitis B virus infection. *J Viral Hepat* 2011; 18(2):102-5.

[148] Weng PJ, Fu YM, Ding SX, Xu DP, Lin A, Yan WH. Elevation of plasma soluble human leukocyte antigen-G in patients with chronic hepatitis C virus infection. *Hum Immunol* 2011; 72(5):406-11.

[149] Lafon M. Immune evasion, a critical strategy for rabies virus. *Dev Biol (Basel)* 2008; 131:413-9.

[150] Trinh QD, Izumi Y, Komine-Aizawa S, Shibata T, Shimotai Y, Kuroda K, Mizuguchi M, Ushijima H, Mor G, Hayakawa S. H3N2 influenza A virus replicates in immortalized human first trimester trophoblast cell lines and induces their rapid apoptosis. *Am J Reprod Immunol* 2009; 62(3):139-46.

[151] Chen HX, Chen BG, Shi WW, Zhen R, Xu DP, Lin A, Yan WH. Induction of cell surface human leukocyte antigen-G expression in pandemic H1N1 2009 and seasonal H1N1 influenza virus-infected patients. *Hum Immunol* 2011; 72(2):159-65.

[152] Shi WW, Lin A, Xu DP, Bao WG, Zhang JG, Chen SY, Li J, Yan WH. Plasma soluble HLA-G expression is a potential clinical biomarker in patients with hepatitis B virus infection. *Hum Immunol* 2011; 72(11):1068-73.

[153] Schust DJ, Tortorella D, Seebach J, Phan C, Ploegh HL. Trophoblast class I major histocompatibility complex (MHC) products are resistant to rapid degradation imposed by the human cytomegalovirus (HCMV) gene products US2 and US11. *J Exp Med* 1998; 188(3):497-503.

[154] Lozano JM, González R, Kindelán JM, Rouas-Freiss N, Caballos R, Dausset J, Carosella ED, Peña J. Monocytes and T lymphocytes in HIV-1-positive patients express HLA-G molecule. *AIDS* 2002; 16(3):347-51.

[155] Pizzato N, Derrien M, Lenfant F. The short cytoplasmic tail of HLA-G determines its resistance to HIV-1 Nef-mediated cell surface downregulation. *Hum Immunol* 2004; 65(11):1389-96.

[156] Murdaca G, Contini P, Setti M, Cagnati P, Spanò F, Lantieri F, Puppo F. Soluble human leukocyte antigen-G serum levels in patients with acquired immune deficiency syndrome affected by different disease-defining conditions before and after antiretroviral treatment. *Hum Immunol* 2011; 72(9):712-6.

[157] Mégret F, Prehaud C, Lafage M, Moreau P, Rouas-Freiss N, Carosella ED, Lafon M. Modulation of HLA-G and HLA-E expression in human neuronal cells after rabies virus or herpes virus simplex type 1 infections. *Hum Immunol* 2007; 68(4):294-302.

[158] Lafon M, Prehaud C, Megret F, Lafage M, Mouillot G, Roa M, Moreau P, Rouas-Freiss N, Carosella ED. Modulation of HLA-G expression in human neural cells after neurotropic viral infections. *J Virol* 2005; 79(24):15226-37.

[159] Yan WH. HLA-G expression in cancers: potential role in diagnosis, prognosis and therapy. *Endocr Metab Immune Disord Drug Targets* 2011; 11(1):76-89.

[160] Goldman-Wohl D, Ariel I, Greenfield C, Hochner-Celnikier D, Lavy Y, Yagel S. A study of human leukocyte antigen G expression in hydatidiform moles. *Am J Obstet Gynecol* 2001; 185(2):476-80.

[161] Hurks HM, Valter MM, Wilson L, Hilgert I, van den Elsen PJ, Jager MJ. Uveal melanoma: no expression of HLA-G. *Invest Ophthalmol Vis Sci* 2001; 42(13):3081-4.

[162] Pangault C, Amiot L, Caulet-Maugendre S, Brasseur F, Burtin F, Guilloux V, Drenou B, Fauchet R, Onno M. HLA-G protein expression is not induced during malignant transformation. *Tissue Antigens* 1999; 53(4 Pt 1):335-46.

[163] Yan WH, Lin A, Chen BG, Luo WD, Dai MZ, Chen XJ, Xu HH, Li BL. Unfavourable clinical implications for HLA-G expression in acute myeloid leukaemia. *J Cell Mol Med* 2008; 12(3):889-98.

[164] Guo QY, Chen BG, Ruan YY, Lin A, Yan WH. HLA-G expression is irrelevant to prognosis in patients with acute myeloid leukemia. *Leuk Res* 2011; 35(10):1350-4.

[165] Nückel H, Rebmann V, Dürig J, Dührsen U, Grosse-Wilde H. HLA-G expression is associated with an unfavorable outcome and immunodeficiency in chronic lymphocytic leukemia. *Blood* 2005; 105(4):1694-8.

[166] Erikci AA, Karagoz B, Ozyurt M, Ozturk A, Kilic S, Bilgi O. HLA-G expression in B chronic lymphocytic leukemia: a new prognostic marker? *Hematology* 2009; 14(2):101-5.

[167] Perez-Chacon G, Rosado S, Rebolleda N, Losada-Fernandez I, Vargas JA, Morado M, Jorda J, Perez-Aciego P. Prognostic irrelevance of HLA-G in B-cell chronic lymphocytic leukemia. *Int J Lab Hematol* 2009; 31(3):327-37.

[168] Davidson B, Elstrand MB, McMaster MT, Berner A, Kurman RJ, Risberg B, Trope CG, Shih IeM. HLA-G expression in effusions is a possible marker of tumor susceptibility to chemotherapy in ovarian carcinoma. *Gynecol Oncol* 2005; 96(1):42-7.

[169] Lin A, Yan WH, Xu HH, Gan MF, Cai JF, Zhu M, Zhou MY. HLA-G expression in human ovarian carcinoma counteracts NK cell function. *Ann Oncol* 2007; 18(11):1804-9.

[170] Menier C, Prevot S, Carosella ED, Rouas-Freiss N. Human leukocyte antigen-G is expressed in advanced-stage ovarian carcinoma of high-grade histology. *Hum Immunol* 2009; 70(12):1006-9.

[171] Jung YW, Kim YT, Kim SW, Kim S, Kim JH, Cho NH, Kim JW. Correlation of human leukocyte antigen-G (HLA-G) expression and disease progression in epithelial ovarian cancer. *Reprod Sci* 2009; 16(11):1103-11.

[172] Lefebvre S, Antoine M, Uzan S, McMaster M, Dausset J, Carosella ED, Paul P. Specific activation of the non-classical class I histocompatibility HLA-G antigen and expression of the ILT2 inhibitory receptor in human breast cancer. *J Pathol* 2002; 196(3):266-74.

[173] Palmisano GL, Pistillo MP, Fardin P, Capanni P, Nicolò G, Salvi S, Spina B, Pasciucco G, Ferrara GB. Analysis of HLA-G expression in breast cancer tissues. *Hum Immunol* 2002; 63(11):969-76.

[174] Kleinberg L, Flørenes VA, Skrede M, Dong HP, Nielsen S, McMaster MT, Nesland JM, Shih IeM, Davidson B. Expression of HLA-G in malignant mesothelioma and clinically aggressive breast carcinoma. *Virchows Arch* 2006; 449(1):31-9.

[175] Chen HX, Lin A, Shen CJ, Zhen R, Chen BG, Zhang X, Cao FL, Zhang JG, Yan WH. Upregulation of human leukocyte antigen-G expression and its clinical significance in ductal breast cancer. *Hum Immunol* 2010; 71(9):892-8.

[176] de Kruijf EM, Sajet A, van Nes JG, Natanov R, Putter H, Smit VT, Liefers GJ, van den Elsen PJ, van de Velde CJ, Kuppen PJ. HLA-E and HLA-G expression in classical HLA class I-negative tumors is of prognostic value for clinical outcome of early breast cancer patients. *J Immunol* 2010; 185(12):7452-9.

[177] Sayed D, Badr G, Maximous D, Mikhail NN, Abu-Tarboush F, Alhazza IM. HLA-G and its relation to proliferation index in detection and monitoring breast cancer patients. *Tissue Antigens* 2010; 75(1):40-7.

[178] Lin A, Chen HX, Zhu CC, Zhang X, Xu HH, Zhang JG, Wang Q, Zhou WJ, Yan WH. Aberrant human leucocyte antigen-G expression and its clinical relevance in hepatocellular carcinoma. *J Cell Mol Med* 2010; 14(8):2162-71.

[179] Wang Y, Ye Z, Meng XQ, Zheng SS. Expression of HLA-G in patients with hepatocellular carcinoma. *Hepatobiliary Pancreat Dis Int* 2011; 10(2):158-63.

[180] Cai MY, Xu YF, Qiu SJ, Ju MJ, Gao Q, Li YW, Zhang BH, Zhou J, Fan J. Human leukocyte antigen-G protein expression is an unfavorable prognostic predictor of hepatocellular carcinoma following curative resection. *Clin Cancer Res* 2009; 15(14):4686-93.

[181] Lin A, Zhang X, Zhou WJ, Ruan YY, Xu DP, Wang Q, Yan WH. HLA-G expression is associated with a poor prognosis in patients with esophageal squamous cell carcinoma. *Int J Cancer* 2011; 129(6):1382-90.

[182] Yie SM, Yang H, Ye SR, Li K, Dong DD, Lin XM. Expression of HLA-G is associated with prognosis in esophageal squamous cell carcinoma. *Am J Clin Pathol* 2007; 128(6):1002-9.

[183] Lin A, Zhu CC, Chen HX, Chen BF, Zhang X, Zhang JG, Wang Q, Zhou WJ, Hu W, Yang HH, Xu HH, Yan WH. Clinical relevance and functional implications for human leucocyte antigen-g expression in non-small-cell lung cancer. *J Cell Mol Med* 2010; 14(9):2318-29.

[184] Yie SM, Yang H, Ye SR, Li K, Dong DD, Lin XM. Expression of human leucocyte antigen G (HLA-G) is associated with prognosis in non-small cell lung cancer. *Lung Cancer* 2007; 58(2):267-74.

[185] Yie SM, Yang H, Ye SR, Li K, Dong DD, Lin XM. Expression of human leukocyte antigen G (HLA-G) correlates with poor prognosis in gastric carcinoma. *Ann Surg Oncol* 2007; 14(10):2721-9.

[186] Ye SR, Yang H, Li K, Dong DD, Lin XM, Yie SM. Human leukocyte antigen G expression: as a significant prognostic indicator for patients with colorectal cancer. *Mod Pathol* 2007; 20(3):375-83.

[187] Du L, Xiao X, Wang C, Zhang X, Zheng N, Wang L, Zhang X, Li W, Wang S, Dong Z. Human leukocyte antigen-G is closely associated with tumor immune escape in gastric cancer by increasing local regulatory T cells. *Cancer Sci* 2011; 102(7):1272-80.

[188] Gan LH, Huang LF, Zhang X, Lin A, Xu DP, Wang Q, Wang TJ, Yan WH. Tumor-specific upregulation of human leukocyte antigen-G expression in bladder transitional cell carcinoma. *Hum Immunol* 2010; 71(9):899-904.

[189] Li BL, Lin A, Zhang XJ, Zhang X, Zhang JG, Wang Q, Zhou WJ, Chen HX, Wang TJ, Yan WH. Characterization of HLA-G expression in renal cell carcinoma. *Tissue Antigens* 2009; 74(3):213-21.

[190] Dunker K, Schlaf G, Bukur J, Altermann WW, Handke D, Seliger B. Expression and regulation of non-classical HLA-G in renal cell carcinoma. *Tissue Antigens* 2008; 72(2):137-48.

[191] Barrier BF, Kendall BS, Sharpe-Timms KL, Kost ER. Characterization of human leukocyte antigen-G (HLA-G) expression in endometrial adenocarcinoma. *Gynecol Oncol* 2006; 103(1):25-30.

[192] Amiot L, Ferrone S, Grosse-Wilde H, Seliger B. Biology of HLA-G in cancer: a candidate molecule for therapeutic intervention? *Cell Mol Life Sci* 2011; 68(3):417-31.

[193] Singer G, Rebmann V, Chen YC, Liu HT, Ali SZ, Reinsberg J, McMaster MT, Pfeiffer K, Chan DW, Wardelmann E, Grosse-Wilde H, Cheng CC, Kurman RJ, Shih IeM. HLA-G is a potential tumor marker in malignant ascites. *Clin Cancer Res* 2003; 9(12):4460-4.

[194] Zhu CB, Wang CX, Zhang X, Zhang J, Li W. Serum sHLA-G levels: a useful indicator in distinguishing colorectal cancer from benign colorectal diseases. *Int J Cancer* 2011; 128(3):617-22.

[195] Zheng N, Wang CX, Zhang X, Du LT, Zhang J, Kan SF, Zhu CB, Dong ZG, Wang LL, Wang S, Li W. Up-regulation of HLA-G expression in cervical premalignant and malignant lesions. *Tissue Antigens* 2011; 77(3):218-24.

[196] Schütt P, Schütt B, Switala M, Bauer S, Stamatis G, Opalka B, Eberhardt W, Schuler M, Horn PA, Rebmann V. Prognostic relevance of soluble human leukocyte antigen-G and total human leukocyte antigen class I molecules in lung cancer patients. *Hum Immunol* 2010; 71(5):489-95.

[197] Morandi F, Levreri I, Bocca P, Galleni B, Raffaghello L, Ferrone S, Prigione I, Pistoia V. Human neuroblastoma cells trigger an immunosuppressive program in monocytes by stimulating soluble HLA-G release. *Cancer Res* 2007; 67(13):6433-41.

[198] Sebti Y, Le Maux A, Gros F, De Guibert S, Pangault C, Rouas-Freiss N, Bernard M, Amiot L. Expression of functional soluble human leucocyte antigen-G molecules in lymphoproliferative disorders. *Br J Haematol 2007*; 138(2):202-12.

[199] Leleu X, Le Friec G, Facon T, Amiot L, Fauchet R, Hennache B, Coiteux V, Yakoub-Agha I, Dubucquoi S, Avet-Loiseau H, Mathiot C, Bataille R, Mary JY; Intergroupe Francophone du Myélome. Total soluble HLA class I and soluble HLA-G in multiple myeloma and monoclonal gammopathy of undetermined significance. *Clin Cancer Res* 2005; 11(20):7297-303.

[200] Sun LL, Han Y, Chen JH, Yao YQ. Down-regulation of HLA-G boosted natural killer cell-mediated cytolysis in JEG-3 cells cultured in vitro. *Fertil Steril* 2008; 90(6):2398-405.

[201] Naji A, Durrbach A, Carosella ED, Rouas-Freiss N. Soluble HLA-G and HLA-G1 expressing antigen-presenting cells inhibit T-cell alloproliferation through ILT-2/ILT-4/FasL-mediated pathways. *Hum Immunol* 2007; 68(4):233-9.

[202] Komohara Y, Harada M, Ishihara Y, Suekane S, Noguchi M, Yamada A, Matsuoka K, Itoh K. HLA-G as a target molecule in specific immunotherapy against renal cell carcinoma. *Oncol Rep* 2007; 18(6):1463-8.

In: Major Histocompatibility Complex
Editor: Natalya V. Semiletova
ISBN: 978-1-61942-999-4

Chapter 8

NON CLASSICAL MAJOR HISTOCOMPATIBILITY CLASS I IN HEALTH AND DISEASE

*Ayman Antoun**
School of Cancer Sciences, University of Birmingham, B15 2TT, Birmingham, UK

ABSTRACT

Major Histocompatibility Complex (MHC) class I molecules are divided into two major groups, the classical class I (MHC class Ia), which present peptides to T-cells and have a major role in discriminating self from non-self and the non-classical (MHC class Ib) molecules. MHC class Ia and class Ib molecules are similar in their mechanisms of peptide binding and presentation to T-cells. MHC class Ia are considered the most polymorphic molecules in the immune system and direct T cells to kill cells infected with viruses or intracellular bacteria. On the other hand, MHC class Ib are mostly conservative and include several members such as Human leukocyte antigen-E (HLA-E), Human leukocyte antigen-F (HLA-F) and Human leukocyte antigen-G (HLA-G). These molecules act as a bridge between innate and acquired immunity and are characterised by a limited diversity of presented antigens which leads to constraints on the interactions of these molecules with pathogens. They are not only recognized by pathogen-specific T cells but also serve as immune-regulatory molecules by stimulating distinct non-conventional T cell subsets. In this review, we examine their expression level and their immunological functions. HLA-E is highly conserved in evolution and we have previously investigated HLA-E gene polymorphisms in three ethnic groups using a polymerase chain reaction-sequence-specific primer method in genomic DNA. We found only two positions in HLA-E to be confirmed as polymorphic (1114 and 1446). These polymorphic positions result in two isoforms proteins expressed by human individuals. The two non-synonymous alleles differ at position 107 and are known as HLA-E^R and HLA-E^G; they differ in their relative peptide affinity and interestingly HLA-E^G expression is higher than that of HLA-E^R. How HLA-E modulates the immune response through interaction with CD94/NKG2 receptors on NK and T-cells will be discussed. HLA-G was initially shown to play a major role in feto–maternal tolerance and it has now been established that HLA-G, as a tolerogenic molecule, participates in the control of the immune response. Finally, the possible role during pregnancy of HLA-F, the least

* Email: a.antoun@bham.ac.uk; Tel: 00441214143292; Fax: 00441214144486.

studied member of this family, will be discussed. An overview of the interplay of these non-classical MHC in both health and disease will be elucidated as emerging evidence that they could influence the prognosis of several malignancies.

Keywords: Major Histocompatibility Complex, non-classical MHC, HLA-E, HLA-F, HLA-G, tumor, transplantation, T-cells, NK cells, pregnancy

INTRODUCTION

Major Histocompatibility Complex Class I

Human major histocompatibility complex class I (MHC class I) encodes 2 main groups: the classic (MHC class Ia) and non-classic (MHC class Ib) molecules [1]. The gene locus for these molecules is on the short arm of chromosome 6 [2], spans ~4 Mb and encodes at least ~130 functional genes. The best described MHC are the classical class Ia and II who play an important role in organ transplantation, antigen-peptide presentation and have strong association with several autoimmune diseases [3,4].

MHC class Ia include HLA-A, HLA-B, and HLA-C in humans and H2-K, H2-D and H2-L in mice [5]. The human MHC class Ia genes encode highly polymorphic 44-KD membrane spanning heavy chains non-covalently associated with an invariant 12-KD subunit, β2-microglobulin, at the cell surface [6]. MHC class Ia are expressed constitutively on almost all cells except red blood cells, with significant genetic variations between individuals within the same population. MHC class Ia primary function is to present antigens from within cells (virus or tumor) on the cell surface to cytotoxic CD8-positive T cells to eradicate infected or transformed cells [7]. The polymorphisms in these MHC genes are concentrated at the peptide-binding site, allowing different alleles to bind diverse and partially overlapping sets of 8-10 amino acid peptides, these peptides reside in the peptide-binding groove of the heavy chain formed by the α1 and α2 domains [8].

The class II MHC, also on chromosome 6 short arm, encodes the HLA-D family (HLA-DR, HLA-DQ, HLA-DM, and HLA-DP), which are found on antigen-presenting cells and display antigen to CD4 helper T cells [9,10].

The non-classic MHC class Ib molecules are Human leukocyte antigen-E (HLA-E), Human leukocyte antigen-F (HLA-F) and Human leukocyte antigen-G (HLA-G); and are distinguished from the classical HLA class I genes by limited expression patterns and low allelic polymorphism [11,12]. This antigens limited diversity places distinct constraints on the interactions of these molecules with pathogens. Their mouse analogues include H2–M3 and Qa1 [7] and expected to have a role in the regulation of autoimmunity. HLA-G binds a relatively narrow range of peptides [13], while HLA-E form complexes with nonamer peptide derived from the signal sequence of other MHC class I, including HLA-A, -B, -C, and -G but excluding HLA-F [14]. MHC class Ib genes are considered immune “tolerization” molecules, which not only interact with NK cells but with some T lymphocyte subsets [15,16]. They play an important role in pathogen recognition, pregnancy, tumor immunosurveillance and regulation of autoimmunity [17-19].

THE NON-CLASSICAL MHC CLASS I MOLECULES

HLA-E

HLA-E gene has been mapped between the HLA-C and HLA-A loci on the short arm of the chromosome 6 [20] (Figure 1). HLA-E presents short peptide as a complex to its receptor, and the presented peptide repertoire is normally highly restricted as HLA-E bind mainly epitopes derived from the leader peptides of HLA-A, -B, -C, and –G [21] (Table 1). The expression of HLA-E is enormously dependent on the availability of peptide as the transfection of HLA-E heavy chain alone or human β2-microglobulin and HLA-E heavy chain in a single polypeptide chain, yielded no appreciable levels of cell-surface HLA-E [22]. Most of the leader peptides efficiently bind and support HLA-E cell surface expression except some HLA-B alleles and HLA-E itself [7]. Interestingly, HLA-G leader peptide is one of the most optimal binding peptides [1]. As HLA-G and HLA-E are amongst the few HLA molecules expressed in human trophoblasts, the expression of these HLA is associated with immunosuppression needed during pregnancy [23]. In times of cellular stress, the leader peptide content is replaced with a diverse repertoire of peptides derived from heat-shock proteins (HSP60) [24], infectious agents and the HLA-E/peptide complex could be sensed by αβT-cells [25]. For example, Human Cytomegalovirus (CMV) has a peptide identical to HLA-C leader peptides and is loaded onto HLA-E independently of TAP [26].

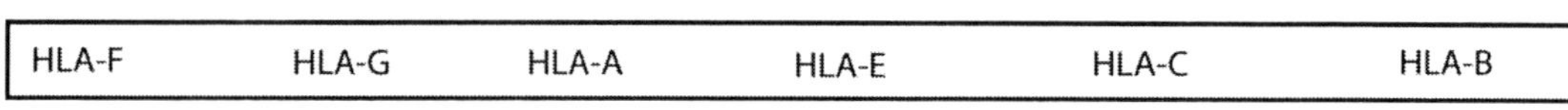

Figure 1. Schematic representation of MHC class I on chromosome 6.

The figure describes the position of the 3 human non-classical MHC class Ib in relation to each other and to classical MHC class Ia on chromosome 6. The figure is not drawn to scale.

HLA-E is expressed in a broad number of haematological cells including B and T lymphocytes, natural killer (NK) cells and macrophages [26,27]. In normal human non-lymphoid organs, HLA-E expression is mainly restricted to endothelial cells [28], where its up-regulation protects endothelial cells from NK-mediated cell lysis. HLA-E cell surface expression is up-regulated by several cytokines such as Tumour Necrosis Factor (TNFα), and interferon γ (IFN-γ) [29].

The predominant receptors for HLA-E/peptide complex are CD94/NKG2A, an inhibitory receptor, and CD94/NKG2C, an activating receptor [30] (Figure 2). CD94/NKG2 receptors are invariant transmembrane molecules expressed on NK cells and activated CD8 T cells [31]. The CD94 subunit makes contact with peptide residues and the alpha helices of HLA-E, while the NKG2 subunit contains the signal transduction domain [30]. The NKG2 receptor genes (NKG2A, NKG2C, and NKG2E) are clustered in the NK-complex locus and differ from each other only at few amino acids, which determine their affinity for CD94 and whether the specific CD94/NGK2 heterodimer acts as an inhibitory or activating receptor [7]. NKG2C is less frequently expressed on lymphocytes and associate with the activating adaptor molecule DAP12 [32], whereas the inhibitory ITIM-bearing NKG2A recruits phosphatases, like SHP-1 [33]. CD94/NKG2A has a 5- to 10-fold higher affinity for HLA-E than

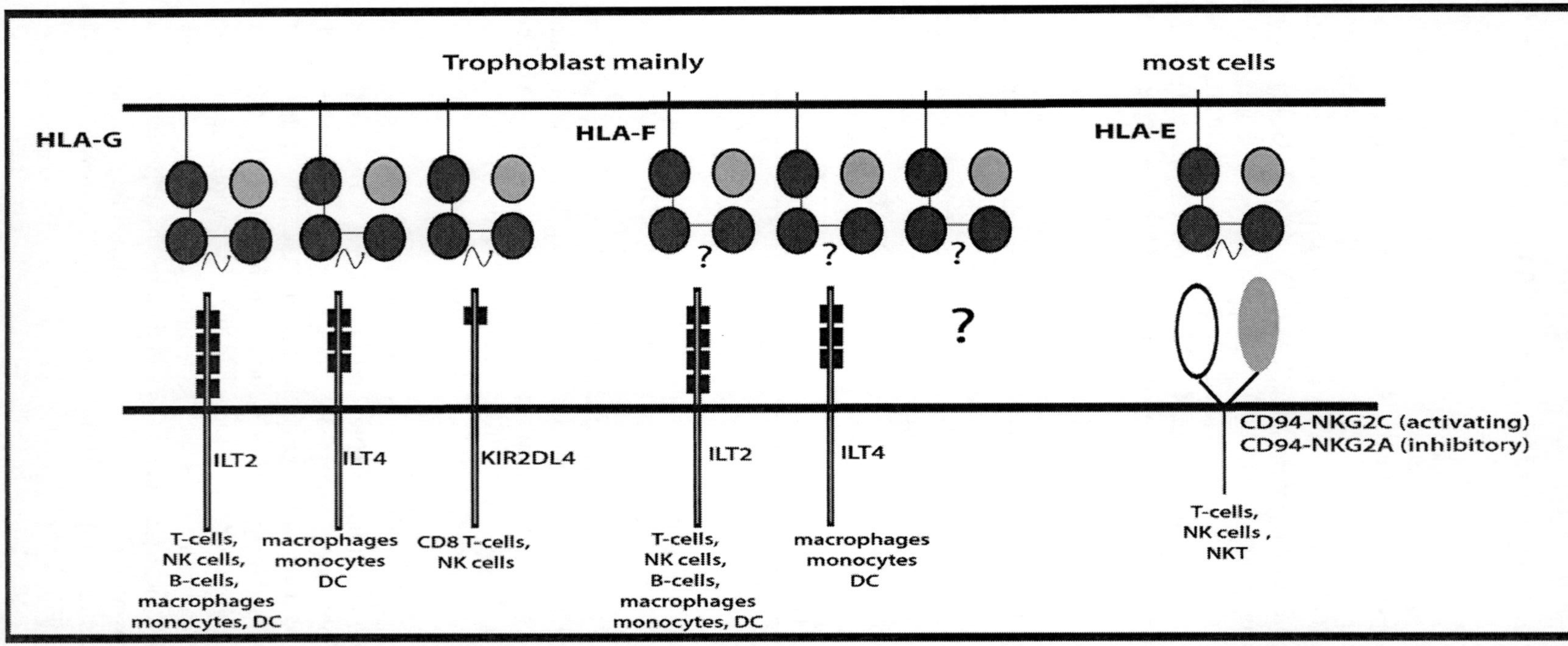

Figure 2. Human MHC class Ib and their receptors.

The figure describes the interaction of the human MHC class Ib with their respective receptors and the cells expressing these receptors. "?" denotes that no peptide was shown to bind HLA-F under favourable conditions and the possibility that another yet unidentified receptor binds HLA-F.

CD94/NKG2C [34]. The capacity of HLA class I leader peptides, including HLA-G, to modulate levels of HLA-E expression at the cell surface refines the patterns of non-classical class I expression [35].The peptide structure influences dramatically the outcome of HLA-E complex interaction with its receptors; for example, a peptide derived from the hsp60 bind HLA-E, stabilize its cell-surface expression but the resulting complex was unable to inhibit NK cell cytotoxicity [22]. HLA-E interaction with the CD94/NKG2A results in inhibition of NK and cytotoxic T cells–dependent lysis [36] (Figure 2). Furthermore, HLA-E–restricted CD8 suppressor cells are implicated in controlling the adaptive immune response to allow intracellular pathogens escaping immune detection. This is apparent in the processing defects that could lead to replacement of the signal peptides with a broad repertoire of pathogens peptides [25].

HLA-E possesses two isoforms that differ by just one single amino acid at position 107; HLA-E*0101 with arginine (E^R) and HLA-E *0103 with glycine (E^G) [14]. This position is exposed on the protein surface and does not affect the crystal structure or recognition by cytotoxic T-cells [5]. Nevertheless, the affinity of peptides for E^G is 10- to 100-fold higher than for E^R, and as a consequence, cell-surface expression of E^G usually exceeds that of E^R [5]. The frequency of both variants is equal amongst different populations [14].

The leader peptide carried by HLA-E plays an important role as evidenced in the following: the peptide derived from one of the most common HLA-C alleles (HLA-Cw7) contains a substitution of an Ala for a Thr at position 6, which, when in complex with HLA-E, directly affects recognition by CD94–NKG2 [21]. Furthermore, HLA-E in complex with the HLA-G*01 leader sequence peptide interacted with the CD94–NKG2 receptors with the highest affinity (K_D=1 μM), while HLA-Cw*07 leader sequence peptide markedly decreases the affinity of HLA-E for CD94–NKG2A (K_D=30 μM) [21]. Thus, allotypic variations in the bound leader sequences do not result in conformational changes in the HLA-E, although subtle changes in the peptide conformation could be detected within HLA-E binding groove [21]. Alterations at any of the positions of the nonamer peptide away from the canonical class I leader peptide sequence produced a significant fall in binding demonstrating that HLA-E structure is highly adapted for binding class la leader peptides [21]. HLA-E is transcribed at lower levels than MHC class Ia antigens [37]; however, high levels of HLA-E have been detected in neoplastic cells (see section on MHC class Ib and Tumour).

HLA-G

HLA-G has been mapped between the HLA-F and HLA-A loci on the short arm of chromosome 6 (Figure 1). HLA-G has tolerogenic functions especially during pregnancy [13]. It is expressed in several membrane and soluble isoforms derived from alternative splicing of the primary mRNA [38,39]. This splicing leads to seven protein isoforms (four membrane-bound: HLA-G1–HLA-G4; and three secreted: HLA-G5–HLA-G7) [38-41]. HLA-G binds a relatively narrow range of peptides probably serving as structural components rather than for antigen presentation [13,42]. Although HLA-G has eight exons, its cytoplasmic tail is only 6 amino acids long compared to 30 in the class la molecules [23]. HLA-G interacts with inhibitory receptors leukocyte immunoglobulin like receptor-1 (LIR-1 or ILT-2), leukocyte immunoglobulin like receptor-2 (LIR-2 or ILT-4), and killer immunoglobulin like receptor 2DL4 (KIR2DL4) [43] (Figure 2). ILT2 and ILT4 share 81%

sequence identity, ILT2 is expressed by lymphoid and myeloid cells, while ILT4 is solely expressed by myeloid cells and KIR2DL4 only by NK cells especially CD56bright NK cells and some CD8-T cells [44] (Table 1). The resulting HLA-G /receptor interaction influences T cell proliferation, NK cell and CD8-T cell cytotoxicity.

HLA-G molecule similar to class I molecules consists of α1, α2 and α3 domains; α1 and α2 contribute to the peptide-binding cleft [23]. The α3 domain of HLA-G, the putative binding site for ILT-2 and ILT-4, is structurally distinct from class Ia MHC molecules [6]. HLA-G regulate NK-cell activation directly through interaction with KIR2DL4, and indirectly by providing peptides that promote the HLA-E expression in the trophoblasts [1].

HLA-G displays a very restricted pattern of expression as high levels were described mainly on the foetal extravillous trophoblasts at the maternal–foetal interface and could be involved in the maternal-fetal tolerance [1]. HLA-G might present viral peptides especially CMV to the maternal immune system, so triggering lysis of infected foetal material [2]. HLA-G was also detected on the surface of human oocytes and preimplantation embryo [23] and HLA-G can be detected in serum/plasma from both women and men, especially pregnant females [45,46]. HLA-G is also expressed to a certain extent by adult thymic epithelial cells, erythroblasts, pancreatic islets and mesenchymal stem cells [47]. Ectopic induction of HLA-G expression has also been reported in solid tumors such as melanoma [48], colon carcinoma [49] and may represent an escape mechanism from anti-tumoral immune responses [45,50].

HLA-G peptide binding groove resembles that of HLA-E and the peptide repertoire of HLA-G is not as limited as HLA-E, although in the placenta, a single peptide derived from a cytokine-related protein accounts for 15% of eluted peptide [13] and only three peptides were isolated from placenta-derived HLA-G [13] (Table 1). The characterization of the HLA-G peptide repertoire led to the identification of putative anchor residues at positions 2, 3, and 9. A peptide with all three of these anchor residues stabilized cell-surface HLA-G expression on transfected cells [6]. HLA-G is found as a dimer on the cell surface and in the soluble form due to unique cysteine residues in positions 42 and 147 [51]. This dimerization increases HLA-G affinity for ILT-2 and ILT-4 [52].

HLA-G acts as a link between the innate and adaptive immunity to contribute to long-term immune escape [13,44]. HLA-G inhibits cytotoxic T- and NK cells through direct interaction with ILT2, ILT4 and KIR2DL4 [53]. Furthermore, it prevents CD4+ T cells proliferation and directs CD4+ T cells towards immunosuppression [54]. Furthermore, soluble HLA-G expression seems to induce CD8+ T-cell apoptosis through the Fas/FasL pathway [55,56].

Sequences and polymorphism in both the 5′URR and 3′UTR parts of the *HLA-G* gene has been found to be associated with differences in HLA-G expression [23]. For example, the expression of *HLA-G* mRNA isoforms containing the 14 bp sequence in exon 8 of the 3′UTR were significantly reduced when compared with forms, where the 14 bp sequence is deleted especially in first trimester trophoblast samples [38,57].

HLA-F

HLA-F, the least characterized member of the non-classical class I family, is expected to be involved in the pregnancy process. It is a 42-kDa protein, shorter than typical HLA class I due to the exclusion of exon 7 from the mature mRNA, yielding a protein with a shortened cytoplasmic domain [58].

Its expression was observed by Western blot analysis in all resting lymphocytes, all of which lacked surface expression in the resting state. Upon activation with IFN-γ, they showed an induction of surface HLA-F protein [59]. HLA-F is further expressed on lymphoid tissues such as the thymus, spleen, tonsil and fetal liver [60]. Recombinant HLA-F heavy chain was refolded with β2-microglobulin to form a stable complex even in the absence of added peptide [59]. Furthermore, MHC-I H chain was found to interact with an open conformer free of peptide HLA-F and possibly, similar to the MICA class I protein, HLA-F is expressed as a heavy chain [59].

On the other hand, HLA-F has a peptide groove with key conserved residues and dimensions similar to those of class I molecules. Although HLA-F seems to associate with a transporter associated with antigen processing (TAP) and calreticulin inside the cell; it is not yet known whether HLA-F is able to associate with peptide or other small organic molecules to present antigens and reach the cell surface [60].

HLA-F tetramers stained monocytes and CD19+ B cells, not CD56+ NK cells and CD3+ T cells. These tetramers bound ILT2 and ILT4 transfectants [60] and a direct interaction of HLA-F with these receptors was shown using Surface Plasmon Resonance. HLA-F is expressed in the cytoplasm and surface of trophoblast in the last part of pregnancy; in contrast with HLA-G that is expressed throughout pregnancy [61]. Its surface expression on decidual extravillous trophoblasts combined with its regulated expression on activated immune cells is suggestive that HLA-F is essential for the normal function of trophoblast cells in the deciduas [61]. The three class Ib molecules may act in synergy in the placenta and may functionally substitute each other [13]. In contrast to CD4+CD25+ T cells, CD4+CD25- T cells showed strong expression of surface HLA-F when activated [62].

Mouse MHC Class Ib

The mouse non-classical MHC molecules include H2–M3 and Qa1. They bind focused sets of peptides: H2–M3 binds N-formyl peptides, and Qa1 mainly bind epitopes derived from other MHC class I signal peptides or TCR variable regions in a TAP-dependent manner [63]. Qa1 constitutes the mouse homolog of HLA-E and is virtually non-polymorphic with only two dominant allelic variants: Qa-1a and Qa-1b [64]. H-2K, does not encode signal peptides for Qa-1 and thus does not contribute to Qa-1 stabilization. Qa1 molecules are expressed in the placenta, where they regulate NK cells and are expressed at high levels at the surface of activated CD4+ T cells. Qa1 molecules might also present some 'conventional' peptides to cytotoxic T-cells [65] and studies of Qa1-deficient mice confirmed the role of Qa1 in autoimmune keratitis and diabetes in mice [66].

Q9 antigen, a member of the Qa-2 family, is expressed in most tissues, including immunologically privileged sites such as the eye [67]. Qa-2 is a functional homolog of HLA-G [68]. Despite its limited polymorphism, Q9 binds a large array of peptides and has a role in anti-tumour responses [69] as Q9-restricted CTL responses capable of recognizing several tumours have been described such as ectopic expression of Q9 in the class-Ia-deficient melanoma [70].

H2-M3 has a specialized peptide-binding groove that preferentially binds N-formylated peptides of prokaryotic origin. The presentation of these epitopes to CD8+ T cells in case of Salmonella [71] and Mycobacteria infections were shown [72]. For example, polyclonal CD8+ T cells restricted by H2–M3 protect against infection with M. Tuberculosis was detected but these cells develop and peak sooner after infection than their MHC-class-Ia-restricted counterparts [5].

MHC Class Ib and Lymphocytes

NK cells are important in early responses to viruses and tumours [73]. Their activity is regulated by the balance of inhibitory and activating signals that they receive through their cell surface receptors [74]. These receptors belong to two superfamilies, the immunoglobulin-like receptors, including the killer cell immunoglobulin-like receptors and the C-type lectin superfamily, including CD94–NKG2 receptors [75]. The MHC class I–specific inhibitory receptors delivers an inhibitory signal that down-regulates several NK functions such as cytokine production and lysis of healthy autologous cells, while acting as survival receptors in NK cells [76]. On the other hand, CD94/NKG2C complex, leads to IFN-γ production, cytotoxicity, and proliferation; while the activating receptor– induced apoptosis of NK cells could play a role in eliminating potentially harmful NK cell clones [77].

Negative selection of T-cell clones in the thymus deletes strongly self-reactive T cells [78], while T cells carrying receptors with intermediate and low affinity for self-antigen are released into peripheral lymphoid tissues, which could initiate autoimmune disease. A small fraction of CD8 T-cells (CD8+ Treg) recognise Qa-1 in mouse and HLA-E in human and target autoreactive CD4+ cells [79,80]. CD8+ Treg have been implicated in the regulation of human autoimmune diseases, including inflammatory bowel disease and MS [81] and its suppressive activity was demonstrated in a murine model of multiple sclerosis (MS), experimental autoimmune encephalomyelitis (EAE) [80,82]. HLA-E restricted CD8+ Treg cloned from patients during disease exacerbation express higher levels of CD94/NKG2A than CD8 cells cloned from MS patients in remission or from healthy controls [80,83,84]. Moreover, the cytolytic activity of the CD8+ T regs from MS patients could be blocked with anti-HLA-E antibody [83,84]. Qa-1–restricted CD8 T cells were shown to be involved in the maintenance of peripheral tolerance to self-antigen and the optimization of T-cell responses to foreign antigens [85]. The Qa-1/Hsp60sp complex is only preferentially expressed at a higher level on T cells of intermediate but not high or low avidity as a biologic consequence of T-cell activation [86]. Thus, an effective approach to downregulate the intermediate avidity T-cells, expected to be responsible for auto-immune diseases, could be to reactivate the HLA-E–restricted CD8 T-cell–mediated regulatory pathway.

GroEL is the bacterial orthologue of eukaryotic HSP60. GroEL-derived epitopes are remarkably conserved among Gram-positive and Gram-negative bacteria [5] and might account for many of the HLA-E-restricted human CTLs that are specific for *M. tuberculosis* [87] and *Salmonella enterica* [88]. GroEL-specific CTLs kill both infected cells and stressed cells that express high levels of HSP60. Similarly, a GroEL-specific clone from a patient with *Yersinia enterocolitica*-induced reactive arthritis was cross-reactive with GroEL from some bacterial species [5].

Finally, "Natural HLA-G+ Treg" (thymus-derived HLA-G expressing T cells) were found to be hypo proliferative in response to stimulation via CD3 and CD28 and show a decreased production of IFN-γ and IL-10 [89].

MHC CLASS IB IN HEALTH AND DISEASE

MHC Class Ib and Pregnancy

Pregnancy is a homeostatic state whereby genetically different fetal tissues attach to the mother without triggering acute rejection [90]. Thus, changes to the immune status are needed to allow the tolerance of the genetically different fetal tissues, such as impaired cell mediated immunity [90]. During early pregnancy, trophoblasts invade into the decidua, and fuse with and open up maternal uterine arteries to facilitate an adequate blood supply to the developing fetus through interaction with decidual NK cells [1]. These extra-villous trophoblast (EVT) display an unusual pattern for HLA expression, where only HLA-E, -F and -G and HLA-C [13,91] are expressed. The absence of classical class I ensure fetal survival as they could mount a maternal immune response [1].

The main leukocytes in this site are natural-killer (NK) cells and macrophages. The uterine NK cells are distinctive in phenotype and function from cells in peripheral blood [92,93]. Approximately 90% of the decidual NK cells express high levels of CD56 and are negative for CD16 [1]. This CD56bright subset demonstrates low cytotoxicity and expresses higher levels of CD94/NKG2 compared to the CD56dim subset and are the main cytokine-producing NK cells [94]. These NK cells carry KIR and CD94/NKG2 capable of recognizing trophoblast HLA-I molecules [91] and influence the degree of trophoblast invasion. About 25% of first trimester uterine NK cells express ILT2 [53,91,95], while KIR2DL4 could module uterine NK cell function [53]. EVTs express membrane-bound HLA-G protein from early gestation to term [61]. Progesterone expressed from the trophoblast during pregnancy up-regulates HLA-G expression by human inhibitory mesenchymal stem cells [96]. Furthermore, the correlation of HLA-G expression with cleavage rate suggested an important role in human pre-embryo development [97].

HLA-E was found in all cells that expressed HLA-G, suggesting a specific role in the placenta as it may stimulate NK to secrete cytokines of specific benefit for the implanted embryo [1]. These cytokines include interferon-γ and may function in the process of vascularisation [98]. An adequate secretion of INF-γ by NK cells is necessary to increase the blood flow needed for placentation [92,93]. HLA-E expression on EVTs increases as gestation progresses from the second trimester until term [61]. HLA-E on trophoblasts binds mainly HLA-G-derived peptides and weakly HLA-C-derived peptides [99]. HLA-E/G-peptide has 10–40 times higher affinity to NKG2 receptor than HLA-E/Ia-peptide [100]. HLA-E bound peptides derived from class Ia signal peptides interact with the CD94/NKG2A NK receptor and inhibit NK cytotoxicity [99], while HLA-E bound peptide derived from HLA-G (HLA-E/Gpep) may interact with CD94/NKG2C and activate NK cells [101]. The increase in the expression of HLA-E and HLA-F from the second trimester to full term coincides with the timing of rapid growth of the fetus [13,102].

In decidua, ~10% of leukocytes are T cells [103] and the activation of these cells may be induced by recognition of fetal antigens in maternal blood [104].

Diminished or aberrant HLA-G expression seems to be associated with pregnancy complications such as implantation failure in IVF and pre-eclampsia. For example, sHLA-G levels in the serum samples of women experiencing early spontaneous abortions were significantly reduced, compared with women with intact pregnancies [105]. Furthermore, pre-eclampsia, is a disorder affecting 2–7% of all pregnancies, where the pregnant woman develops hypertension, proteinuria and often oedema. A significantly increased risk of pre-eclampsia was detected, when the fetus carries a *+14/+14 HLA-G* genotype [106]. This +14 bp sequence has been associated with greater unstability of the transcripts [107]. Moreover, women with pre-eclampsia had significantly reduced levels of sHLA-G in their serum [108]. *HLA-G* genotype homozygous for the presence of the *14 bp* sequence polymorphism was significantly associated with increased birth weight and placental weight at birth [109], which fits the mouse Qa-2 expression association with birth weight [68]. All IVF treatments with sHLA-G negative pre-implantation embryo cultures ended unsuccessfully with no signs of implantation [110] and the live birth rate in women who had HLA-G-positive embryos transferred was significantly higher than that in women who had only HLA-G-negative embryos transferred [97].

MHC Class Ib and Transplantation

The expression of soluble HLA-G (sHLA-G) in blood, heart and liver/kidney grafts has been associated with significantly better prognosis and fewer rejection episodes [111,112]. Plasma sHLA-G levels were enhanced after cyclosporine treatment for transplant rejection or tacrolimus administration in some heart transplant patients [113]. An increased sHLA-G was observed in kidney transplant patients treated with the CTLA4-Ig fusion protein, which is associated with better graft function and survival [114]. Likewise, high HLA-G5 levels in plasma of patients transplanted with peripheral blood stem cell were associated with no acute Graft versus Host Disease [115] and CD94/NKG2A was increased following allogeneic bone marrow transplantation in patients without chronic graft-versus-host disease [116].

MHC Class Ib and Tumour

Malignant cells evade the extrinsic tumour suppressor function of the immune system using mechanisms such as the expression of non-classical major histocompatibility antigens and the accumulation of regulatory T cells [117].

Ectopic expression "neoexpression" of HLA-G following neoplastic transformation is increasingly recognized as a potential contributing factor to tumor evasion of immunosurveillance [22]. For example, HLA-G and its receptors were up-regulated in breast carcinoma [118]. Moreover, HLA-G was enhanced in breast cancer cells upon estradiol/ progesterone treatment while reduced by their antagonists, tamoxifen and RU486 [16]. The expression of HLA-G on renal cell carcinoma, ovarian carcinoma and melanoma has also been reported [119]. Soluble HLA-G which could induce immunosuppressive T cells was found at elevated levels in serum and ascites from patients suffering from malignant melanoma, myeloma, glioma, breast and ovarian carcinoma and lymphoproliferative disorders [120]. HLA–G has also been implicated in the disease severity of cutaneous T-cell lymphomas [121].

HLA-E was overexpressed in lymphomas, colon cancer and melanomas [120]. In addition, individuals harbouring a polymorphism in the HLA-E gene are at an increased risk for nasopharyngeal carcinoma [122].

HLA-F was found to be overrepresented in EBV-transformed lymphoblastoid cell lines, in monocyte cell lines and in cell lines of transitional cell carcinomas of the bladder, glioblastoma and liver cancer [120] and a genome-wide association study identified association between variations in HLA-F and nasopharyngeal carcinoma [123].

MHC Class Ib and Immunological Diseases

The *HLA-G*010102* is in linkage disequilibrium with a haplotype associated with a range of immunopathological diseases, such as type I diabetes, systemic lupus erythematosus (SLE), dermatitis herpetiformis and myastenia gravis [4]. HLA-G was identified as a possible asthma-susceptibility gene [124,125] and a deletion in the 3' untranslated region of HLA-G has been associated with Pemphigus [126]. HLA-G5 play an important role in erythropoiesis as it inhibits the proliferation of normal erythoid cells through G1 cell cycle arrest [127]. An acquired activating mutation in the gene encoding JAK2, which is a downstream mediator of HLA-G was found in patients suffering from polycythemia vera (PV) [16]. Thus, HLA-G5 could reduce the increased erythroid cell proliferation, which is the critical clinical manifestation of polycythemia vera [16].

sHLA-E, almost undetected in normal sera, was dramatically increased with disease activity in patients with antineutrophil cytoplasmic antibody–associated systemic vasculitis [28].

MHC Class Ib and Viral Infections

CMV is a β-herpesvirus resulting in life-long persistent asymptomatic infection, which may cause severe morbidity in immune-compromised individuals [128]. CMV infection is the most common viral complication following hematopoietic stem cell transplantation [129] and solid organ transplantation. CMV evades the immune system through several mechanisms: CMV proteins, US2 and US11 bind to nascent HLA class I chains resulting in their shuttle from the ER to the cytosol [130]. US3 binds to HLA class I molecules and retains them in the ER [130]. As a consequence, conventional HLA class Ia-restricted CTLs may be inefficient in counteracting CMV infection [37]. UL-40 up-regulates HLA-E expression [130] through supplying peptides to HLA-E, resulting in surface expression of HLA-E at even higher concentrations than in uninfected cells [130]. On the other hand, HLA-E-restricted CD8+ T cells could represent an additional type of effector cells playing a role in defense against a virus [37]. HLA-G-restricted T cells specifically recognizing and killing HCMV-infected astrocytoma cells have been generated in transgenic mice [131]. An increase of NKG2C positive NK cells after CMV infection [132] was found, which could be an adaptation favouring protection against infectious agents.

Human Immunodeficiency virus (HIV) interferes with the MHC expression to avoid HIV-specific CTL responses [133]. Immuno-protection could also be achieved by increased expression of HLA-G and HLA-E during HIV infection [133] and significant associations of certain HLA-G and HLA-E alleles with protection from HIV infection were discovered [134-137].

Chronic hepatitis C was shown to be associated with increased intra-hepatic HLA-E expression and Hepatitis C virus supplies a peptide to HLA-E making a complex readily recognized by CD8+ T cells [37]. The frequency of HLA-E-restricted responses was higher in patients homozygous for the HLAE*0101 allele [138]. Finally, CD94/NKG2A was up-regulated on CD8+ T cells during viral activation [139].

Table 1. Human MHC class Ib molecules, their receptors and the peptides presented by these molecules

	Receptor	Type of signal	Cells carrying receptor	Self-Peptide	Non-self peptides
HLA-E	CD94/NKG2A*	Inhibitory	NK and activating CD8 T-cells	class I Leader peptide except HLA-E and HLA-F	CMV UL-40 Salmonella GroEL Mycobacterium Tumours
	CD94/NKG2C	Activating			
HLA-G	ILT2	Inhibitory	Lymphoid and Myeloid	a peptide from a cytokine-related protein ~ 15% of eluted peptide [13] and three peptides isolated from placenta [13]	
	ILT4	Inhibitory	Myeloid only		
	KIR2DL4	Inhibitory	NK cells (CD56bright) and some CD8-T cells		
HLA-F	ILT2, ILT4	Inhibitory	As above	N.I.	N.I.

N.I. not yet identified.

* CD94/NKG2A has 5- to 10-fold higher affinity for HLA-E than CD94/NKG2C [34].

CONCLUSIONS

Non classical MHC class I molecules are emerging immunological factors involved in the immune regulation process. They differ from the classical MHC class I in the extent of the presented peptide repertoire and limited polymorphism in these molecules. Their important functions especially for HLA-G are clearly illustrated during pregnancy. They are expected to work in synergism in pregnancy as they are all expressed specifically and at different levels. Furthermore, there is increasing evidence that these molecules are associated with several diseases including malignancies and auto-immune diseases.

REFERENCES

[1] Ishitani A, Sageshima N, Hatake K. The involvement of HLA-E and -F in pregnancy. *J Reprod Immunol*. 2006;69:101-113.

[2] O'Callaghan CA, Bell JI. Structure and function of the human MHC class Ib molecules HLA-E, HLA-F and HLA-G. *Immunol Rev*. 1998;163:129-138.

[3] Doherty PC, Zinkernagel RM. A biological role for the major histocompatibility antigens. *Lancet*. 1975;1:1406-1409.

[4] Svejgaard A, Platz P, Ryder LP. HLA and disease 1982--a survey. *Immunol Rev*. 1983;70:193-218.

[5] Rodgers JR, Cook RG. MHC class Ib molecules bridge innate and acquired immunity. *Nat Rev Immunol*. 2005;5:459-471.

[6] Clements CS, Kjer-Nielsen L, McCluskey J, Rossjohn J. Structural studies on HLA-G: implications for ligand and receptor binding. *Hum Immunol*. 2007;68:220-226.

[7] van Hall T, Oliveira CC, Joosten SA, Ottenhoff TH. The other Janus face of Qa-1 and HLA-E: diverse peptide repertoires in times of stress. *Microbes Infect*;12:910-918.

[8] Antoniou AN, Powis SJ. Pathogen evasion strategies for the major histocompatibility complex class I assembly pathway. *Immunology*. 2008;124:1-12.

[9] Li Y, Depontieu FR, Sidney J, et al. Structural basis for the presentation of tumor-associated MHC class II-restricted phosphopeptides to CD4+ T cells. *J Mol Biol*;399:596-603.

[10] Depontieu FR, Qian J, Zarling AL, et al. Identification of tumor-associated, MHC class II-restricted phosphopeptides as targets for immunotherapy. *Proc Natl Acad Sci U S A*. 2009;106:12073-12078.

[11] Geraghty DE, Wei XH, Orr HT, Koller BH. Human leukocyte antigen F (HLA-F). An expressed HLA gene composed of a class I coding sequence linked to a novel transcribed repetitive element. *J Exp Med*. 1990;171:1-18.

[12] Koller BH, Geraghty DE, Shimizu Y, DeMars R, Orr HT. HLA-E. A novel HLA class I gene expressed in resting T lymphocytes. *J Immunol*. 1988;141:897-904.

[13] Ishitani A, Sageshima N, Lee N, et al. Protein expression and peptide binding suggest unique and interacting functional roles for HLA-E, F, and G in maternal-placental immune recognition. *J Immunol*. 2003;171:1376-1384.

[14] Antoun A, Jobson S, Cook M, Moss P, Briggs D. Ethnic variability in human leukocyte antigen-E haplotypes. *Tissue Antigens*. 2009;73:39-45.

[15] Carosella ED, HoWangYin KY, Favier B, LeMaoult J. HLA-G-dependent suppressor cells: Diverse by nature, function, and significance. *Hum Immunol*. 2008;69:700-707.

[16] Carosella ED, Gregori S, Rouas-Freiss N, LeMaoult J, Menier C, Favier B. The role of HLA-G in immunity and hematopoiesis. *Cell Mol Life Sci*;68:353-368.

[17] Yie SM, Hu Z. Human leukocyte antigen-G (HLA-G) as a marker for diagnosis, prognosis and tumor immune escape in human malignancies. *Histol Histopathol*;26:409-420.

[18] Favier B, LeMaoult J, Carosella ED. Functions of HLA-G in the immune system. *Tissue Antigens*. 2007;69 Suppl 1:150-152.

[19] Favier B, LeMaoult J, Rouas-Freiss N, Moreau P, Menier C, Carosella ED. Research on HLA-G: an update. *Tissue Antigens*. 2007;69:207-211.

[20] Sullivan LC, Clements CS, Rossjohn J, Brooks AG. The major histocompatibility complex class Ib molecule HLA-E at the interface between innate and adaptive immunity. *Tissue Antigens*. 2008.

[21] Hoare HL, Sullivan LC, Clements CS, et al. Subtle changes in peptide conformation profoundly affect recognition of the non-classical MHC class I molecule HLA-E by the CD94-NKG2 natural killer cell receptors. *J Mol Biol*. 2008;377:1297-1303.

[22] Crew MD. Play it in E or G: utilization of HLA-E and -G in xenotransplantation. *Xenotransplantation*. 2007;14:198-207.

[23] Hviid TV. HLA-G in human reproduction: aspects of genetics, function and pregnancy complications. *Hum Reprod Update*. 2006;12:209-232.

[24] Michaelsson J, Teixeira de Matos C, Achour A, Lanier LL, Karre K, Soderstrom K. A signal peptide derived from hsp60 binds HLA-E and interferes with CD94/NKG2A recognition. *J Exp Med*. 2002;196:1403-1414.

[25] Jiang H, Canfield SM, Gallagher MP, et al. HLA-E-restricted regulatory CD8(+) T cells are involved in development and control of human autoimmune type 1 diabetes. *J Clin Invest*;120:3641-3650.

[26] Tomasec P, Braud VM, Rickards C, et al. Surface expression of HLA-E, an inhibitor of natural killer cells, enhanced by human cytomegalovirus gpUL40. *Science*. 2000;287:1031.

[27] Moretta L, Romagnani C, Pietra G, Moretta A, Mingari MC. NK-CTLs, a novel HLA-E-restricted T-cell subset. *Trends Immunol*. 2003;24:136-143.

[28] Coupel S, Moreau A, Hamidou M, Horejsi V, Soulillou JP, Charreau B. Expression and release of soluble HLA-E is an immunoregulatory feature of endothelial cell activation. *Blood*. 2007;109:2806-2814.

[29] Barrett DM, Gustafson KS, Wang J, Wang SZ, Ginder GD. A GATA factor mediates cell type-restricted induction of HLA-E gene transcription by gamma interferon. *Mol Cell Biol*. 2004;24:6194-6204.

[30] Braud VM, Allan DS, O'Callaghan CA, et al. HLA-E binds to natural killer cell receptors CD94/NKG2A, B and C. *Nature*. 1998;391:795-799.

[31] Petrie EJ, Clements CS, Lin J, et al. CD94-NKG2A recognition of human leukocyte antigen (HLA)-E bound to an HLA class I leader sequence. *J Exp Med*. 2008;205:725-735.

[32] Lanier LL, Corliss B, Wu J, Phillips JH. Association of DAP12 with activating CD94/NKG2C NK cell receptors. *Immunity*. 1998;8:693-701.

[33] Angelini DF, Zambello R, Galandrini R, et al. NKG2A inhibits NKG2C effector functions of gammadelta T cells: implications in health and disease. *J Leukoc Biol*;89:75-84.

[34] Kaiser BK, Pizarro JC, Kerns J, Strong RK. Structural basis for NKG2A/CD94 recognition of HLA-E. *Proc Natl Acad Sci U S A*. 2008;105:6696-6701.

[35] Paul P, Rouas-Freiss N, Moreau P, et al. HLA-G, -E, -F preworkshop: tools and protocols for analysis of non-classical class I genes transcription and protein expression. *Hum Immunol*. 2000;61:1177-1195.

[36] O'Callaghan CA. Molecular basis of human natural killer cell recognition of HLA-E (human leucocyte antigen-E) and its relevance to clearance of pathogen-infected and tumour cells. *Clin Sci (Lond)*. 2000;99:9-17.

[37] Pietra G, Romagnani C, Manzini C, Moretta L, Mingari MC. The emerging role of HLA-E-restricted CD8+ T lymphocytes in the adaptive immune response to pathogens and tumors. *J Biomed Biotechnol*;2010:907092.
[38] Fujii T, Ishitani A, Geraghty DE. A soluble form of the HLA-G antigen is encoded by a messenger ribonucleic acid containing intron 4. *J Immunol*. 1994;153:5516-5524.
[39] Hviid TV, Moller C, Sorensen S, Morling N. Co-dominant expression of the HLA-G gene and various forms of alternatively spliced HLA-G mRNA in human first trimester trophoblast. *Hum Immunol*. 1998;59:87-98.
[40] Ishitani A, Geraghty DE. Alternative splicing of HLA-G transcripts yields proteins with primary structures resembling both class I and class II antigens. *Proc Natl Acad Sci U S A*. 1992;89:3947-3951.
[41] LeMaoult J, Le Discorde M, Rouas-Freiss N, et al. Biology and functions of human leukocyte antigen-G in health and sickness. *Tissue Antigens*. 2003;62:273-284.
[42] Lee N, Malacko AR, Ishitani A, et al. The membrane-bound and soluble forms of HLA-G bind identical sets of endogenous peptides but differ with respect to TAP association. *Immunity*. 1995;3:591-600.
[43] Urosevic M, Dummer R. HLA-G and IL-10 expression in human cancer--different stories with the same message. *Semin Cancer Biol*. 2003;13:337-342.
[44] LeMaoult J, Zafaranloo K, Le Danff C, Carosella ED. HLA-G up-regulates ILT2, ILT3, ILT4, and KIR2DL4 in antigen presenting cells, NK cells, and T cells. *FASEB J*. 2005;19:662-664.
[45] Rebmann V, Regel J, Stolke D, Grosse-Wilde H. Secretion of sHLA-G molecules in malignancies. *Semin Cancer Biol*. 2003;13:371-377.
[46] Hviid TV, Rizzo R, Christiansen OB, Melchiorri L, Lindhard A, Baricordi OR. HLA-G and IL-10 in serum in relation to HLA-G genotype and polymorphisms. *Immunogenetics*. 2004;56:135-141.
[47] Le Bouteiller P, Blaschitz A. The functionality of HLA-G is emerging. *Immunol Rev*. 1999;167:233-244.
[48] Paul P, Rouas-Freiss N, Khalil-Daher I, et al. HLA-G expression in melanoma: a way for tumor cells to escape from immunosurveillance. *Proc Natl Acad Sci U S A*. 1998;95:4510-4515.
[49] Fukushima Y, Oshika Y, Nakamura M, et al. Increased expression of human histocompatibility leukocyte antigen-G in colorectal cancer cells. *Int J Mol Med*. 1998;2:349-351.
[50] Crisa L, McMaster MT, Ishii JK, Fisher SJ, Salomon DR. Identification of a thymic epithelial cell subset sharing expression of the class Ib HLA-G molecule with fetal trophoblasts. *J Exp Med*. 1997;186:289-298.
[51] Boyson JE, Erskine R, Whitman MC, et al. Disulfide bond-mediated dimerization of HLA-G on the cell surface. *Proc Natl Acad Sci U S A*. 2002;99:16180-16185.
[52] Carosella ED, Favier B, Rouas-Freiss N, Moreau P, Lemaoult J. Beyond the increasing complexity of the immunomodulatory HLA-G molecule. *Blood*. 2008;111:4862-4870.
[53] Rajagopalan S, Long EO. A human histocompatibility leukocyte antigen (HLA)-G-specific receptor expressed on all natural killer cells. *J Exp Med*. 1999;189:1093-1100.
[54] LeMaoult J, Krawice-Radanne I, Dausset J, Carosella ED. HLA-G1-expressing antigen-presenting cells induce immunosuppressive CD4+ T cells. *Proc Natl Acad Sci U S A*. 2004;101:7064-7069.

[55] Fournel S, Aguerre-Girr M, Huc X, et al. Cutting edge: soluble HLA-G1 triggers CD95/CD95 ligand-mediated apoptosis in activated CD8+ cells by interacting with CD8. *J Immunol*. 2000;164:6100-6104.

[56] Contini P, Ghio M, Poggi A, et al. Soluble HLA-A,-B,-C and -G molecules induce apoptosis in T and NK CD8+ cells and inhibit cytotoxic T cell activity through CD8 ligation. *Eur J Immunol*. 2003;33:125-134.

[57] Hiby SE, King A, Sharkey A, Loke YW. Molecular studies of trophoblast HLA-G: polymorphism, isoforms, imprinting and expression in preimplantation embryo. *Tissue Antigens*. 1999;53:1-13.

[58] He X, Xu L, Liu Y, Zeng Y. Identification of a novel HLA-F allele - HLA-F*010102. *Tissue Antigens*. 2004;63:181-183.

[59] Wainwright SD, Biro PA, Holmes CH. HLA-F is a predominantly empty, intracellular, TAP-associated MHC class Ib protein with a restricted expression pattern. *J Immunol*. 2000;164:319-328.

[60] Lepin EJ, Bastin JM, Allan DS, et al. Functional characterization of HLA-F and binding of HLA-F tetramers to ILT2 and ILT4 receptors. *Eur J Immunol*. 2000;30:3552-3561.

[61] Shobu T, Sageshima N, Tokui H, et al. The surface expression of HLA-F on decidual trophoblasts increases from mid to term gestation. *J Reprod Immunol*. 2006;72:18-32.

[62] Lee N, Ishitani A, Geraghty DE. HLA-F is a surface marker on activated lymphocytes. *Eur J Immunol*;40:2308-2318.

[63] Sullivan BA, Kraj P, Weber DA, Ignatowicz L, Jensen PE. Positive selection of a Qa-1-restricted T cell receptor with specificity for insulin. *Immunity*. 2002;17:95-105.

[64] Bouwer HG, Seaman MS, Forman J, Hinrichs DJ. MHC class Ib-restricted cells contribute to antilisterial immunity: evidence for Qa-1b as a key restricting element for Listeria-specific CTLs. *J Immunol*. 1997;159:2795-2801.

[65] Lu L, Ikizawa K, Hu D, Werneck MB, Wucherpfennig KW, Cantor H. Regulation of activated CD4+ T cells by NK cells via the Qa-1-NKG2A inhibitory pathway. *Immunity*. 2007;26:593-604.

[66] Panoutsakopoulou V, Huster KM, McCarty N, et al. Suppression of autoimmune disease after vaccination with autoreactive T cells that express Qa-1 peptide complexes. *J Clin Invest*. 2004;113:1218-1224.

[67] He X, Tabaczewski P, Ho J, Stroynowski I, Garcia KC. Promiscuous antigen presentation by the nonclassical MHC Ib Qa-2 is enabled by a shallow, hydrophobic groove and self-stabilized peptide conformation. *Structure*. 2001;9:1213-1224.

[68] Comiskey M, Goldstein CY, De Fazio SR, Mammolenti M, Newmark JA, Warner CM. Evidence that HLA-G is the functional homolog of mouse Qa-2, the Ped gene product. *Hum Immunol*. 2003;64:999-1004.

[69] Chiang EY, Stroynowski I. Protective immunity against disparate tumors is mediated by a nonpolymorphic MHC class I molecule. *J Immunol*. 2005;174:5367-5374.

[70] Chiang EY, Henson M, Stroynowski I. Correction of defects responsible for impaired Qa-2 class Ib MHC expression on melanoma cells protects mice from tumor growth. *J Immunol*. 2003;170:4515-4523.

[71] Ugrinovic S, Brooks CG, Robson J, Blacklaws BA, Hormaeche CE, Robinson JH. H2-M3 major histocompatibility complex class Ib-restricted CD8 T cells induced by

Salmonella enterica serovar Typhimurium infection recognize proteins released by Salmonella serovar Typhimurium. *Infect Immun*. 2005;73:8002-8008.

[72] Doi T, Yamada H, Yajima T, Wajjwalku W, Hara T, Yoshikai Y. H2-M3-restricted CD8+ T cells induced by peptide-pulsed dendritic cells confer protection against Mycobacterium tuberculosis. *J Immunol*. 2007;178:3806-3813.

[73] Zamai L, Ponti C, Mirandola P, et al. NK cells and cancer. *J Immunol*. 2007;178:4011-4016.

[74] Endt J, McCann FE, Almeida CR, et al. Inhibitory receptor signals suppress ligation-induced recruitment of NKG2D to GM1-rich membrane domains at the human NK cell immune synapse. *J Immunol*. 2007;178:5606-5611.

[75] Brooks AG, Boyington JC, Sun PD. Natural killer cell recognition of HLA class I molecules. *Rev Immunogenet*. 2000;2:433-448.

[76] Krzewski K, Strominger JL. The killer's kiss: the many functions of NK cell immunological synapses. *Curr Opin Cell Biol*. 2008;20:597-605.

[77] Spaggiari GM, Contini P, Dondero A, et al. Soluble HLA class I induces NK cell apoptosis upon the engagement of killer-activating HLA class I receptors through FasL-Fas interaction. *Blood*. 2002;100:4098-4107.

[78] Sprent J. Proving negative selection in the thymus. *J Immunol*. 2005;174:3841-3842.

[79] Lu L, Cantor H. Generation and regulation of CD8(+) regulatory T cells. *Cell Mol Immunol*. 2008;5:401-406.

[80] Lu L, Kim HJ, Werneck MB, Cantor H. Regulation of CD8+ regulatory T cells: Interruption of the NKG2A-Qa-1 interaction allows robust suppressive activity and resolution of autoimmune disease. *Proc Natl Acad Sci U S A*. 2008;105:19420-19425.

[81] Van Kaer L. Comeback kids: CD8(+) suppressor T cells are back in the game. *J Clin Invest*;120:3432-3434.

[82] Battistini L, Piccio L, Rossi B, et al. CD8+ T cells from patients with acute multiple sclerosis display selective increase of adhesiveness in brain venules: a critical role for P-selectin glycoprotein ligand-1. *Blood*. 2003;101:4775-4782.

[83] Correale J, Villa A. Role of CD8+ CD25+ Foxp3+ regulatory T cells in multiple sclerosis. *Ann Neurol*;67:625-638.

[84] Correale J, Villa A. Isolation and characterization of CD8+ regulatory T cells in multiple sclerosis. *J Neuroimmunol*. 2008;195:121-134.

[85] Jiang H, Chess L. Qa-1/HLA-E-restricted regulatory CD8+ T cells and self-nonself discrimination: an essay on peripheral T-cell regulation. *Hum Immunol*. 2008;69:721-727.

[86] Chen W, Zhang L, Liang B, et al. Perceiving the avidity of T cell activation can be translated into peripheral T cell regulation. *Proc Natl Acad Sci U S A*. 2007;104:20472-20477.

[87] Joosten SA, van Meijgaarden KE, van Weeren PC, et al. Mycobacterium tuberculosis peptides presented by HLA-E molecules are targets for human CD8 T-cells with cytotoxic as well as regulatory activity. *PLoS Pathog*;6:e1000782.

[88] Salerno-Goncalves R, Fernandez-Vina M, Lewinsohn DM, Sztein MB. Identification of a human HLA-E-restricted CD8+ T cell subset in volunteers immunized with Salmonella enterica serovar Typhi strain Ty21a typhoid vaccine. *J Immunol*. 2004;173:5852-5862.

[89] Huang YH, Zozulya AL, Weidenfeller C, Schwab N, Wiendl H. T cell suppression by naturally occurring HLA-G-expressing regulatory CD4+ T cells is IL-10-dependent and reversible. *J Leukoc Biol*. 2009;86:273-281.

[90] Yip L, McCluskey J, Sinclair R. Immunological aspects of pregnancy. *Clin Dermatol*. 2006;24:84-87.

[91] King A, Hiby SE, Gardner L, et al. Recognition of trophoblast HLA class I molecules by decidual NK cell receptors--a review. *Placenta*. 2000;21 Suppl A:S81-85.

[92] Moffett-King A. Natural killer cells and pregnancy. *Nat Rev Immunol*. 2002;2:656-663.

[93] Moffett-King A, Entrican G, Ellis S, Hutchinson J, Bainbridge D. Natural killer cells and reproduction. *Trends Immunol*. 2002;23:332-333.

[94] Yu J, Mao HC, Wei M, et al. CD94 surface density identifies a functional intermediary between the CD56bright and CD56dim human NK-cell subsets. *Blood*;115:274-281.

[95] King A, Allan DS, Bowen M, et al. HLA-E is expressed on trophoblast and interacts with CD94/NKG2 receptors on decidual NK cells. *Eur J Immunol*. 2000;30:1623-1631.

[96] Ivanova-Todorova E, Mourdjeva M, Kyurkchiev D, et al. HLA-G expression is up-regulated by progesterone in mesenchymal stem cells. *Am J Reprod Immunol*. 2009;62:25-33.

[97] Jurisicova A, Casper RF, MacLusky NJ, Mills GB, Librach CL. HLA-G expression during preimplantation human embryo development. *Proc Natl Acad Sci U S A*. 1996;93:161-165.

[98] Eriksson M, Meadows SK, Wira CR, Sentman CL. Unique phenotype of human uterine NK cells and their regulation by endogenous TGF-beta. *J Leukoc Biol*. 2004;76:667-675.

[99] Lee N, Llano M, Carretero M, et al. HLA-E is a major ligand for the natural killer inhibitory receptor CD94/NKG2A. *Proc Natl Acad Sci U S A*. 1998;95:5199-5204.

[100] Kaiser BK, Barahmand-Pour F, Paulsene W, Medley S, Geraghty DE, Strong RK. Interactions between NKG2x immunoreceptors and HLA-E ligands display overlapping affinities and thermodynamics. *J Immunol*. 2005;174:2878-2884.

[101] Llano M, Lee N, Navarro F, et al. HLA-E-bound peptides influence recognition by inhibitory and triggering CD94/NKG2 receptors: preferential response to an HLA-G-derived nonamer. *Eur J Immunol*. 1998;28:2854-2863.

[102] Grimsley C, Kawasaki A, Gassner C, et al. Definitive high resolution typing of HLA-E allelic polymorphisms: Identifying potential errors in existing allele data. *Tissue Antigens*. 2002;60:206-212.

[103] Trundley A, Moffett A. Human uterine leukocytes and pregnancy. *Tissue Antigens*. 2004;63:1-12.

[104] van Rood JJ, Claas F. Both self and non-inherited maternal HLA antigens influence the immune response. *Immunol Today*. 2000;21:269-273.

[105] Pfeiffer KA, Rebmann V, Passler M, et al. Soluble HLA levels in early pregnancy after in vitro fertilization. *Hum Immunol*. 2000;61:559-564.

[106] Hylenius S, Andersen AM, Melbye M, Hviid TV. Association between HLA-G genotype and risk of pre-eclampsia: a case-control study using family triads. *Mol Hum Reprod*. 2004;10:237-246.

[107] Hviid TV, Hylenius S, Rorbye C, Nielsen LG. HLA-G allelic variants are associated with differences in the HLA-G mRNA isoform profile and HLA-G mRNA levels. *Immunogenetics*. 2003;55:63-79.

[108] Yie SM, Li LH, Li YM, Librach C. HLA-G protein concentrations in maternal serum and placental tissue are decreased in preeclampsia. *Am J Obstet Gynecol.* 2004;191:525-529.

[109] Hviid TV. HLA-G genotype is associated with fetoplacental growth. *Hum Immunol.* 2004;65:586-593.

[110] Noci I, Fuzzi B, Rizzo R, et al. Embryonic soluble HLA-G as a marker of developmental potential in embryos. *Hum Reprod.* 2005;20:138-146.

[111] Creput C, Durrbach A, Charpentier B, Carosella ED, Rouas-Freiss N. [HLA-G: immunoregulatory molecule involved in allograft acceptance]. *Nephrologie.* 2003;24:451-456.

[112] Creput C, Le Friec G, Bahri R, et al. Detection of HLA-G in serum and graft biopsy associated with fewer acute rejections following combined liver-kidney transplantation: possible implications for monitoring patients. *Hum Immunol.* 2003;64:1033-1038.

[113] Carosella ED, Moreau P, Lemaoult J, Rouas-Freiss N. HLA-G: from biology to clinical benefits. *Trends Immunol.* 2008;29:125-132.

[114] Bahri R, Naji A, Menier C, et al. Dendritic cells secrete the immunosuppressive HLA-G molecule upon CTLA4-Ig treatment: implication in human renal transplant acceptance. *J Immunol.* 2009;183:7054-7062.

[115] Le Maux A, Noel G, Birebent B, et al. Soluble human leucocyte antigen-G molecules in peripheral blood haematopoietic stem cell transplantation: a specific role to prevent acute graft-versus-host disease and a link with regulatory T cells. *Clin Exp Immunol.* 2008;152:50-56.

[116] Tanaka M, Kanamori H, Kuwabara H, et al. [Successful second transplant from one-locus HLA-mismatched unrelated donor for graft rejection following initial transplant from another unrelated donor in a patient with chronic myelogenous leukemia]. *Rinsho Ketsueki.* 2001;42:656-658.

[117] Hayakawa S. No cancer in cancers: evolutionary trade-off between successful viviparity and tumor escape from the adaptive immune system. *Med Hypotheses.* 2006;66:888-897.

[118] He X, Dong DD, Yie SM, et al. HLA-G expression in human breast cancer: implications for diagnosis and prognosis, and effect on allocytotoxic lymphocyte response after hormone treatment in vitro. *Ann Surg Oncol*;17:1459-1469.

[119] Sheu JJ, Shih Ie M. Clinical and biological significance of HLA-G expression in ovarian cancer. *Semin Cancer Biol.* 2007;17:436-443.

[120] Wischhusen J, Waschbisch A, Wiendl H. Immune-refractory cancers and their little helpers--an extended role for immunetolerogenic MHC molecules HLA-G and HLA-E? *Semin Cancer Biol.* 2007;17:459-468.

[121] Urosevic M, Kamarashev J, Burg G, Dummer R. Primary cutaneous CD8+ and CD56+ T-cell lymphomas express HLA-G and killer-cell inhibitory ligand, ILT2. *Blood.* 2004;103:1796-1798.

[122] Hirankarn N, Kimkong I, Mutirangura A. HLA-E polymorphism in patients with nasopharyngeal carcinoma. *Tissue Antigens.* 2004;64:588-592.

[123] Tse KP, Su WH, Chang KP, et al. Genome-wide association study reveals multiple nasopharyngeal carcinoma-associated loci within the HLA region at chromosome 6p21.3. *Am J Hum Genet.* 2009;85:194-203.

[124] Rizzo R, Mapp CE, Melchiorri L, et al. Defective production of soluble HLA-G molecules by peripheral blood monocytes in patients with asthma. *J Allergy Clin Immunol.* 2005;115:508-513.

[125] Nicolae D, Cox NJ, Lester LA, et al. Fine mapping and positional candidate studies identify HLA-G as an asthma susceptibility gene on chromosome 6p21. *Am J Hum Genet.* 2005;76:349-357.

[126] Gazit E, Loewenthal R. The immunogenetics of pemphigus vulgaris. *Autoimmun Rev.* 2005;4:16-20.

[127] Menier C, Guillard C, Cassinat B, Carosella ED, Rouas-Freiss N. HLA-G turns off erythropoietin receptor signaling through JAK2 and JAK2 V617F dephosphorylation: clinical relevance in polycythemia vera. *Leukemia.* 2008;22:578-584.

[128] Larsson S, Soderberg-Naucler C, Wang FZ, Moller E. Cytomegalovirus DNA can be detected in peripheral blood mononuclear cells from all seropositive and most seronegative healthy blood donors over time. *Transfusion.* 1998;38:271-278.

[129] Widmann T, Sester U, Gartner BC, et al. Levels of CMV specific CD4 T cells are dynamic and correlate with CMV viremia after allogeneic stem cell transplantation. *PLoS One.* 2008;3:e3634.

[130] Wilkinson GW, Tomasec P, Stanton RJ, et al. Modulation of natural killer cells by human cytomegalovirus. *J Clin Virol.* 2008;41:206-212.

[131] Lenfant F, Pizzato N, Liang S, Davrinche C, Le Bouteiller P, Horuzsko A. Induction of HLA-G-restricted human cytomegalovirus pp65 (UL83)-specific cytotoxic T lymphocytes in HLA-G transgenic mice. *J Gen Virol.* 2003;84:307-317.

[132] Guma M, Budt M, Saez A, et al. Expansion of CD94/NKG2C+ NK cells in response to human cytomegalovirus-infected fibroblasts. *Blood.* 2006;107:3624-3631.

[133] Tripathi P, Agrawal S. The role of human leukocyte antigen E and G in HIV infection. *AIDS.* 2007;21:1395-1404.

[134] Lajoie J, Hargrove J, Zijenah LS, Humphrey JH, Ward BJ, Roger M. Genetic variants in nonclassical major histocompatibility complex class I human leukocyte antigen (HLA)-E and HLA-G molecules are associated with susceptibility to heterosexual acquisition of HIV-1. *J Infect Dis.* 2006;193:298-301.

[135] Martini F, Agrati C, D'Offizi G, Poccia F. HLA-E up-regulation induced by HIV infection may directly contribute to CD94-mediated impairment of NK cells. *Int J Immunopathol Pharmacol.* 2005;18:269-276.

[136] Nattermann J, Nischalke HD, Hofmeister V, et al. HIV-1 infection leads to increased HLA-E expression resulting in impaired function of natural killer cells. *Antivir Ther.* 2005;10:95-107.

[137] Segat L, Catamo E, Fabris A, et al. HLA-G*0105N allele is associated with augmented risk for HIV infection in white female patients. *AIDS*;24:1961-1964.

[138] Schulte D, Vogel M, Langhans B, et al. The HLA-E(R)/HLA-E(R) genotype affects the natural course of hepatitis C virus (HCV) infection and is associated with HLA-E-restricted recognition of an HCV-derived peptide by interferon-gamma-secreting human CD8(+) T cells. *J Infect Dis.* 2009;200:1397-1401.

[139] McMahon CW, Zajac AJ, Jamieson AM, et al. Viral and bacterial infections induce expression of multiple NK cell receptors in responding CD8(+) T cells. *J Immunol.* 2002;169:1444-1452.

In: Major Histocompatibility Complex
Editor: Natalya V. Semiletova
ISBN: 978-1-61942-999-4

Chapter 9

HLA CLASS II PRESENTATION OF HLA CLASS I BINDING ANTIGENIC 9MER PEPTIDES

Mingjun Wang[1]*, Susanne Rasmussen[2] and Mogens H. Claesson[2]

[1]Center for Cell and Gene Therapy, Baylor College of Medicine, Houston, Texas, US
[2]Laboratory of Experimental Immunology, Faculty of Health Sciences, University of Copenhagen, Panum Institute, Blegdamsvej 3, Copenhagen 2200N, Denmark

ABSTRACT

Identification of new antigenic peptides, derived from infectious agents, which bind to human leukocyte antigen (HLA) class I molecules, is of importance for the development of new effective vaccines capable of activating the cellular arm of the immune response. In a search for HLA class I restricted antigenic $CD8^+$ T cell (CTL) epitopes, a computer-based program was used to screen and predict the peptide binding affinity for the recently identified twelve HLA class I supertypes. Peptides derived from *mycobacterium tuberculosis*, vaccinia virus and influenza A protein sequences with a predicted high binding affinity were synthesized, and the binding was biochemically verified and quantified using a recombinant HLA class I molecule-based system.

Peripheral blood T cells from healthy donors, vaccinated against smallpox and tuberculosis more than 30 years ago, were used in an ELISPOT assay to test for the antigenicity of the HLA class I binding peptides. Fifty new antigenic peptide epitopes were discovered. However, T cell reactivity towards 27 of these peptides was found to be strictly HLA class II restricted in spite of their high ($\leq$ 50 nM) to medium ($\leq$ 500 nM) binding affinities to the HLA class I molecules for most of these peptides. This review discusses these and related data in the context of the possibility for alternative processing and presentation pathways of antigenic 9mer peptide.

---

* Correspondence: Dr. Mingjun Wang, Center for Cell and Gene Therapy, Baylor College of Medicine, Houston, Texas, USA. Phone: 1 832-6384249; E-mail: aydwangmj@hotmail.com

INTRODUCTION

The immune system, including the innate and adaptive as well as overlapping systems, plays a pivotal role in the defense against viral or bacterial infections, homeostasis and surveillance. T lymphocytes derived from hematopoietic stem cells in the bone marrow are crucial for adaptive immune responses, and are activated upon recognition of peptides displayed by major histocompatibility complex (MHC) class I or MHC-II molecules at the surfaces of antigen-presenting cells (APCs).

T lymphocytes express the T cell receptor (TCR) that recognizes specific peptides, which have been processed and presented in combination with an MHC molecule. There are two major subtypes of T lymphocytes: $CD8^+$ cytotoxic T cells (CTLs) and $CD4^+$ helper T cells. CTLs recognize antigen-derived peptides in the context of MHC class I molecules, while $CD4^+$ helper T cells recognize antigen-derived peptides associated with MHC class II molecules. These two subsets of T cells are said to be restricted by MHC-I and MHC-II molecules, respectively.

It is known that CTLs play a major role in killing tumor cells [1, 2] and controlling viral or bacterial infections [3-7]. Thus, Identification of new antigenic peptides, derived from infectious agents or tumor antigens, which bind to human MHC-I (HLA-I) molecules, is important for developing new effective vaccines capable of activating the cellular arm of the immune responses. To date, however, only CTL epitopes restricted by a limited number of HLA molecules have been identified.

The concept of 'Reverse immunology' is based on immuno-bioinformatics and is maturing rapidly. It has been widely used for the *in silico* identification of T-cell epitopes from tumor antigens and the proteomes of infectious micro-organisms [8-19]. The technology has now reached the stage where genome-, pathogen- and HLA-wide scanning for HLA-I binding antigenic epitopes become feasible at a scale and speed that makes it possible to exploit the genome information as fast as it can be generated.

In a search for HLA class I restricted antigenic $CD8^+$ T cell (CTL) epitopes, a computer-based program was used to screen and predict binding affinities for the twelve HLA class I supertypes [20] to peptides derived from *Mycobacterium tuberculosis* [11], vaccinia virus [12, 15] and influenza A protein sequences [13, 14]. Fifty new antigenic peptide epitopes were discovered. However, immunity towards the majority of these peptides was found to be strictly HLA class II restricted in spite of their high ($\leq$ 50 nM) to medium binding affinities ($\leq$ 500 nM) to HLA class I molecules for most of the peptides. This review discusses these and related data in the context of the possibility for alternative processing and presentation pathways of HLA class II restricted antigenic 9mer peptides.

HUMAN MHC-I MOLECULE AND ASSEMBLY OF MHC CLASS I PEPTIDE COMPLEX

MHC-I is referred to as the leukocyte antigen class I (HLA-A, B and C) in humans and as the H-2 class I (K, D and L) in mice. MHC-I consists of three non-covalently associated components: a 45-kDa glycosylated heavy chain (HC); a 12 kDa light chain (β2m) and a short peptide usually with 8–10 AA. The heavy chain of MHC-I consists of about 340 amino acid

(AA) residues, including a cytoplasmic region (about 30 AA residues), a transmembrane region (about 40 AA residues), and an extracellular region composed of three immunoglobulin-like domains (α1, α2, and α3) each consisting of approximately 90 AA. The membrane-proximal α3 domain of the HC contains a binding site for the CD8 molecule [21] expressed by CTLs, which play an important role in killing virus-infected cells and transformed cells. The α1 and α2 domains consist of two segmented alpha helices forming the walls and eight anti-parallel β strands forming the floor - together forming a unique peptide-binding groove, which is the site where the peptide (8–10 AA) binds to the polymorphic parts of the HC and is presented to peptide specific CTL for scrutiny. Beta 2 microglobulin (β2m) is non-covalently associated with the extracellular region of the MHC-I heavy chain by non-covalent interactions with α2, and α3 domains [22]. Beta 2m is essential for the correct folding of and peptide binding by the heavy chain and stabilizes the MHC-I antigen complex on the cell surface. Thus, β2m indirectly participates in the antigen presentation to specific T-cell receptors of CTL [23-25].

Assembly of MHC-I peptide complex occurs in the endoplasmic reticulum (ER). Initially, the MHC-I HC associates with the chaperone calnexin (CNX) initiating an early folding and a disulphide bond formation in HC. The newly synthesized MHC-I HC then associates with β2m to form heterodimer. This heterodimer is then rapidly recruited into the peptide-loading complex (PLC) consisting of a transporter associated with antigen processing (TAP), chaperones tapasin, calreticulin (CRT) and ERp57. The MHC-I HC/β2m heterodimer is now ready for peptide loading. Peptides are predominantly generated in the cytosol by the proteasome to degrade cytosolic proteins into short peptides, although a proteasome-independent peptide produced directly by insulin-degrading enzyme has been recently documented [26]. Thereafter, the peptides are transported into the ER by the TAP1 and TAP2. These peptides are further trimmed by aminopeptidase ERAAP (in mice) or ERAAP1 and ERAAP2 (in humans) to 8-10 AA, a length appropriate for MHC-I binding. Once MHC-I/HC-β2m dimers, physically associated with PLC, bind a subset of high affinity peptides, the fully assembled MHC-I peptide complexes are released from PLC and transported via the Golgi apparatus to the cell surface, where the peptides are presented by MHC-I to CTL for scrutiny (see details in reviews [27, 28]).

Human MHC-II Molecule and Antigen-presenting Pathway

MHC-II molecule consists of two chains: α and β chain (each one with two domains: α1 and α2, β1 and β2) and a peptide located in a cleft formed by the α1 and β1 domains. Classical human MHC-II molecules include HLA-DR, HLA-DQ and HLA-DP and are expressed mostly in the membrane of the professional antigen-presenting cells, where they present processed extracellular antigenic peptides to the $CD4^+$ T cells. In contrast to the antigen-binding groove of MHC class I molecules, which is closed at each end, the antigen-binding groove of MHC class II molecules is open at both ends and allows longer peptides (13–25 AA) to be loaded [29, 30]. During synthesis of MHC class II molecules in the ER, the α and β chains are produced and associate with an invariant chain, which stabilizes the MHC-II molecule and prevents it from binding of intracellular peptides or peptides from the endogenous pathway. The invariant chain directs transportation of MHC-II from the ER to the Golgi complex, followed by fusion with a late endosomes which contain endocytosed, degraded antigens. The invariant chain is then cleaved by cathepsins to form a small fragment known as CLIP, which occupies the peptide-binding groove of the MHC class II molecules. HLA-DM facilitates CLIP removal and makes the peptide-binding groove of MHC-II ready for peptide loading before the MHC-II-peptide complex migrates to the cell surfaces to be recognized by and stimulate $CD4^+$ T cells [31].

Bioinformatics Search Strategy for Peptides Derived from Influenza A Virus (H1N1), Vaccinia Virus and *Mycobacterium Tuberculosis*

As mentioned in the introduction, the technology behind 'Reverse immunology' is developing rapidly in order to identify T-cell epitopes from tumor antigens and infectious micro-organisms [8-15]. During the SARS epidemic back in 2003, the SARS genome was identified in a matter of weeks, and a complete CTL epitope scanning – just barely possible at that time – was completed a few months later [32]. Therefore, 'Reverse immunology' is a powerful tool to identify T cell epitopes in a large scale and at a fast speed.

To date, one of the major drawbacks of a peptide-based CTL vaccine strategy is that the restricting HLA genes are extremely polymorphic resulting in a vast diversity of peptide-binding HLA specificities and a low population coverage for any given peptide–HLA specificity. To increase population coverage, one might include defined epitopes for each HLA-I allele, however, this would lead to a vaccine comprising hundreds of peptides. One way to reduce this complexity is to group HLA-I molecules into so-called HLA-I supertypes, a classification that refers to a group of HLA alleles with largely overlapping peptide binding specificities [33-35]. Ideally this means that a peptide, which binds to one allele within a supertype, has a high probability of binding to other allelic members of the same supertype. For HLA-I molecules, Sette and Sidney [34] defined nine supertypes (A1, A2, A3, A24, B7, B27, B44, B58, B62) and suggested that >99.6% of persons in all ethnic groups surveyed possessed at least one allele within at least one of the nine supertypes. Thus, 9 epitopes representing each of these nine MHC-I supertypes would lead to virtually complete population coverage. Recently, Lund et al. [20] defined three more MHC class I supertypes (A26, B8 and B39). Our studies [11, 13-15] include all twelve HLA-I supertypes.

In a search for HLA class I restricted antigenic $CD8^+$ T cell (CTL) epitopes, the NetCTL prediction method (http://www.cbs.dtu.dk/services/) was used for predicting 9mer CTL epitopes derived from influenza A virus (10 viral proteins: PB1, PB2, PA, HA, NP, NA, M1, M2, NS1 and NS2) [13, 14], vaccinia virus (the orthologous proteins shared among seven strains of related orthopoxviruses) [15] and *Mycobacterium tuberculosis* (24 *M. tuberculosis* proteins: Rv0151c, Rv0152c, Rv0159c, Rv0284, Rv0288, Rv0834c, Rv0980c, Rv1037c, Rv1072, Rv1404, Rv1979c, Rv1980c, Rv2557, Rv2711, Rv3144c, Rv3343c, Rv3347c, Rv3350c, Rv3403c, Rv3507, Rv3514, Rv3532, Rv3555c, Rv3873) [11]. Prediction was performed for the12 HLA supertypes [20]: A1, A2, A3, A24, A26, B7, B8, B27, B39, B44, B58, and B62. This provides a broad coverage (> 99%) of the HLA alleles worldwide regardless of ethic groups of humans. The 9mer peptides were sorted on the NetCTL score, which is a combined score for MHC binding, TAP binding and proteasomal cleavage. A threshold for a predicted binding affinity of better than 500nM was used.

Biochemical Validation of HLA-I Binding

Initially, as the aims of our projects were to identify CTL epitopes derived from *mycobacterium tuberculosis*, vaccinia virus and influenza A protein sequences, a computer-based program described as above was used to screen and predict the peptide binding affinity for the recently identified twelve HLA class I supertypes [20]. By this approach, we predicted and synthesized a total of 681 9mer peptides derived from *Mycobacterium tuberculosis* (206 peptides) [11], vaccinia virus (177 peptides) [15] and influenza A protein sequences (298 peptides) [13, 14].

The biochemical assay for peptide–MHC-I binding was performed as previously described [36]. Briefly, denatured and purified recombinant HLA heavy chains were diluted into a renaturation buffer containing β_2m and graded concentrations of the test peptide, and were incubated at 18° for 48 hr allowing equilibrium to be reached. It was previously demonstrated that denatured HLA molecules can *de novo* fold efficiently, however, only in the presence of appropriate peptide [37]. The concentration of peptide–HLA complexes generated was measured using a Luminescent Oxygen Channeling Immunoassay and plotted against the concentration of peptide offered. Because the effective concentration of HLA (1–3 nm) used in these assays is below the equilibrium dissociation constant (K_D) of most high-affinity peptide–HLA interactions, the peptide concentration leading to half-saturation of the HLA is a reasonable approximation of the affinity of the interaction. According to this assay, the percentages of measured peptides bound to their respective HLA molecules with a $K_D \leq$ 500 nM in our studies are 79% for pox peptides [15], 59% for flu peptides [13, 14] and 76% for TB peptides [11], respectively.

Antigenicity of the Predicted Peptides and HLA Class II Presentation of HLA Class I Binding Antigenic 9mer Peptides

Peripheral blood T cells from healthy donors, vaccinated against smallpox and tuberculosis more than 30 years ago, were resuspended to a concentration of 6–8 × 10^6 cells per ml in RPMI-1640 supplemented with 5% heat-inactivated AB serum (Valley Biomedical, Winchester, USA), 2 mM l-glutamine, 100 U/ml penicillin and 100 µg/ml streptomycin. Cells were cultured in 24-well plates (Nunc, Roskilde, Denmark). Individual peptides were added to a final concentration of 20 µg/ml per well and incubated for 10 days at 37 °C, 5% CO_2 in humidified air. RhIL-2 (Proleukin; Chiron, The Netherlands) 20 U/ml was added on day 1. Cells were harvested on day 10, washed twice in RPMI-1640 and resuspended in complete medium to a final concentration of 1 × 10^6 cells/ml and were used in an ELISPOT assay to test for the antigenicity of the HLA class I binding peptides. Fifty new antigenic peptide epitopes (8 pox epitopes, 8 TB epitopes and 34 flu epitopes) were discovered (Table 1).

Surprisingly, we observed that four of eight immunogenic pox virus-derived 9-mer peptides elicit a $CD4^+$ T cell-dependent and HLA-II-restricted response with no traces of HLA-I-restricted reactivity [12]. Furthermore, the induction of the responses is only restricted to the peptides with very high binding affinities for HLA-I molecules ($K_D \leq 5$ nM), but not peptides with lower binding affinities. In our subsequent studies on identification of epitopes derived from influenza A virus [13] and *mycobacterium tuberculosis* [11], we also demonstrated that 15 flu peptides and 8 TB peptides induced responses that could be completely blocked in the presence of pan-specific anti-HLA class II (HLA-II) antibody. Peptide reactivity of peripheral blood mononuclear cells (PBMC) depleted of $CD4^+$ or $CD8^+$ T cells prior to the ELISPOT culture revealed that effectors are indeed $CD4^+$ T cells. In contrast to pox virus-derived peptides [12], we found no correlation between $CD4^+$ T cell reactivity and HLA-I binding affinity of peptides derived from influenza A virus and *M. tuberculosis*. Thus, the induction of immune responses was not limited to high-affinity HLA-I binding peptides. Rather, we found examples of peptides with intermediate or low binding affinities for its HLA-I allele. These observations should not be confused with so-called co-receptor mismatched T cells being restricted by HLA class I molecules, but dependent on CD4 binding to HLA class II molecules of the antigen-presenting cells, a phenomenon which has been observed in various experimental settings [38-43].

Table 1. T cell epitopes derived from vaccinia virus, influenza A virus and M. tuberculosis

Patho-gens	Number of predicted peptides	$CD4^+$ T cell epitopes	$CD8^+$ T cell epitopes	Not deter-mined	Total epitopes	References
Vaccinia virus	177	4	3	1	8	12 and 15
Infuenza A virus	298	15	5	14	34	13 and 14
M. tuberculosis	206	8	0	0	8	11
Total peptides	681	27	8	15	50	

Potential Mechanisms for HLA Class II Presentation of HLA Class I Binding Antigenic 9mer Peptides: Reverse Cross-presentation

It has been long thought that a strict segregation of the endogenous and exogenous processing/presentation pathways exists since there is a requirement of different protease systems for processing HLA-I binding peptide and HLA-II binding peptides, respectively, as well as the specific distribution of the MHC class I and class II loading machineries. Therefore, classically HLA-I molecules present peptides derived from intracellular antigens/proteins to $CD8^+$ T cells and HLA- II molecules present peptides derived from extracellular antigens to $CD4^+$ T cells during the adaptive immune responses. However, it has been clearly shown that exogenous antigens that have been internalized into an endocytic or phagocytic compartment can efficiently be presented by MHC class I molecules by a pathway named cross-presentation [44]. Conversely, natural MHC class II ligands might also be derivatives of cytosolic antigens [45-47], and presented by MHC–II molecules after intracellular processing [48-52]. Indeed, many studies have demonstrated that endogenous antigens can gain access to MHC class II loading compartments through a variety of intracellular pathways [53-58]. Here we name these pathways 'reverse cross presentation' as opposed to the classical cross presentation pathway and suggest that 'reverse cross presentation' may explain our main observation that HLA-I binding peptides induce HLA-II restricted $CD4^+$ T cell dependent responses. Translocation of intracellular proteins or peptides generated by the proteasome into a MHC class II loading compartment for MHC-II presentation pathway might require autophagy [59-64]. There are several possibilities for HLA-I binding peptides to be presented by MHC-II molecules. Firstly, these microorganisms-derived proteins in the cytoplasm might be delivered by either macroautophagy or chaperone-mediated autophagy to the MHC class II–containing compartment (MIIC) [60, 61, 63]. These intracellular antigens are then degraded by lysosomal hydrolysis into 9mer peptides for loading onto MHC class II molecules with the assistance of the chaperone HLA-DM. Secondly, some of the 9mer peptides produced in the cytoplasm by the proteasome might be transported into endosome/lysosome through autophagy [45] or other hitherto unknown mechanisms for presentation on MHC class II molecules. Thirdly, HLA-I binding 9mer peptides presented by MHC -II might be proteasome and TAP dependent [56, 58, 64]. In this case, peptides generated by the proteasome in the cytoplasm are transported by TAP into the lumen of ER from where the peptides together with MHC- II are transported to the Golgi, followed by fusion with a late endosomes. The invariant chain is then cleaved and these 9mer peptides are able to load onto MHC class II molecules with the assistance of the chaperone HLA-DM. Fourthly, antigen-presenting cells (e.g. macrophages) may phagocytose infected cells [65, 66] and process microbial antigens by the classical MHC-II antigen-presentation pathways into 9mer peptides for stimulating a $CD4^+$ T cell response. Fifthly, a large pool of unstable MHC-I molecules exists at the cell surface under physiological conditions *in vivo* [67]. These molecules are derived from previously stable class I heterodimers, and peptides released from such dissociated MHC-I molecules might interchange with peptides in adjacent MHC-II molecules. This latter mechanism would explain why some HLA-II restricted antigenic 9mer peptides are identified through scanning for peptides with high or intermediate affinity for HLA-I molecules. None of these five possibilities are mutually exclusive and they are all experimentally testable. The suggested routes for HLA-I binding 9mer peptides presented by MHC-II molecules are depicted in Figure 1.

Since the 9mer peptides in our studies [11-13] stimulate $CD4^+$ T cell responses, they must be presented by MHC-II molecules. Therefore, in our recent publication on TB peptides [11], we tried to predict the binding of all the 157 9mers with measured $K_D \leq 500$ nM used in the study to all DR alleles present among the donors using the publicly available MHC-II predictor NetMHCIIpan [68] (http://www.cbs.dtu.dk/services). Forty-eight peptides including the two antigenic ones LEEIGILLL and IVFATAARY were predicted to be either strong binders (SB) with predicted $K_D < 50$nm or weak binders (WB) with predicted $K_D < 500$ nm, respectively, to one or more DR alleles present among the donors. However, the two donors in our panel who reacted with LEEIGILLL and IVFATAARY did not express the predicted peptide-binding HLA-DR alleles. A recently developed biochemically-based technology [69] for assaying the binding of peptides to recombinant HLA-DR molecules was further used. Three of the eight antigenic *M. tuberculosis* peptides showed binding to three of the 14 tested

HLA-DR molecules, but none of these three HLA-DR molecules were expressed by the two peptide-reactive donors. These negative data might reflect the fact that the 14 assayed HLA-DR molecules only represent one-third of the HLA-DR subtypes expressed by the immune donors. In addition, our ELISPOT assay might favor MHC-II/peptide low-affinity interactions that might be missed in our biochemical assay. Thus, so far we have no definitive proof that the 27 CD4$^+$ T cell activating 9mer peptides discovered in our study do bind to HLA-II molecules.

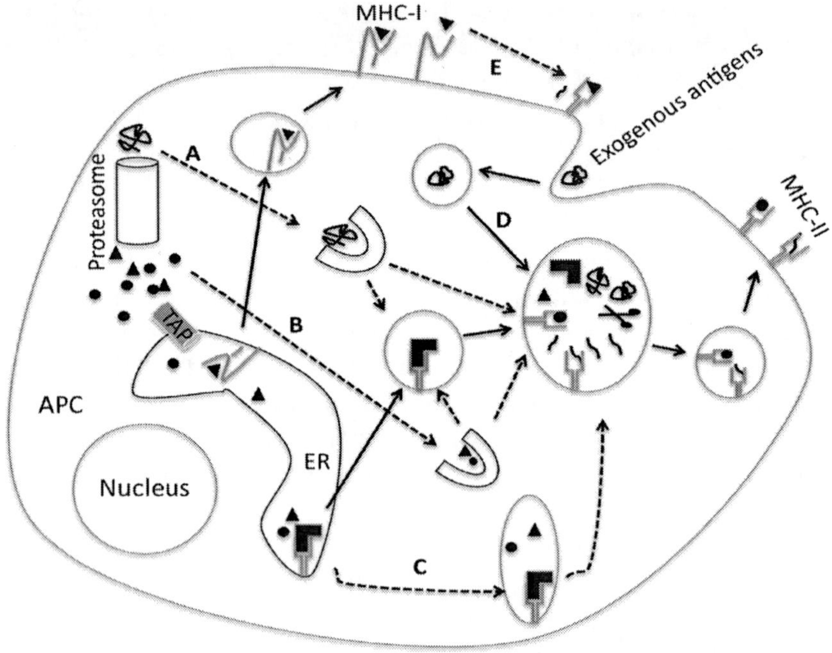

Figure 1. Reverse cross presentation of HLA-I binding peptides for HLA-II antigen presentation pathways. (A) The microorganism-derived proteins in the cytoplasm are delivered by macroautophagy or chaperone-mediated autophagy for presentation on MHC class II molecules to MHC class II–containing compartments. (B) Some of 9mer peptides produced in the cytoplasm by the proteasome are transported into endosome/lysosome through autophagy or unknown pathways for presentation on MHC class II molecules. (C) HLA-I binding 9mer peptides are generated by the proteasome in the cytoplasm are transported by TAP into the lumen of ER and together with MHC- II transported to the Golgi, followed by fusion with a late endosome. (D) antigen-presenting cells (e.g. macrophages) phagocytose the microorganisms-infected cells and process the microorganisms-derived antigen by classical MHC-II antigen-presentation pathways into 9mer peptides for stimulating a CD4$^+$ T cell response. (E) Unstable MHC-I molecules at the cell surface might release peptides with high affinity for MHC-II binding.

Conclusion

'Reverse immunology' has now reached the stage where genome-, pathogen- and HLA-wide scanning for HLA-I binding antigenic epitopes become feasible at a scale and speed that makes it possible to exploit the genome information as fast as it can be generated. Importantly, the computer-based algorithms for predicting peptides binding to an MHC-II molecule, which is of pivotal importance for understanding the immune response and its effect on host-pathogen interactions, are also becoming mature and important tools for identification of MHC-II restricted epitopes [68, 70-73]. Those tools will definitely lead to fast identification of novel peptides for use in vaccines against infectious agents as well as tumors.

By using the NetCTL prediction (http://www.cbs.dtu.dk/services/), we have discovered fifty new antigenic peptide epitopes and demonstrated that 27 of the HLA-I binding 9mer peptides derived from vaccinia virus, influenza A virus and *M. tuberculosis* induce $CD4^+$ T-cell responses. This observation suggests that certain HLA-I binding 9mer peptides might stimulate $CD4^+$ T-cell immune responses most probably restricted by HLA-II molecules. Hence, to identify the phenotype of the responding T cell, ELISPOT-based analyses of reactivity against 9mer class I binding peptides should always include either anti-CD4/CD8 blocking, $CD4^+$/$CD8^+$ T-cell subset depletion experiments or perforin- or granzyme B-based ELISPOT analyses - although $CD4^+$ T cells might occasionally express perforin/granzyme activity [74]. Alternatively, proliferation assays and flow cytometry analyses in which PBMC are stained for specific T cell surface markers should be included to obtain the true phenotype of the antigen-specific T cells.

It has been shown that $CD4^+$ T cells are required for priming as well as secondary expansion of $CD8^+$ memory T cells [75-79]. It might therefore be of critical importance to incorporate both HLA-I and -II restricted epitopes in peptide-based vaccines to obtain participation of both $CD4^+$ and $CD8^+$ T cells for generation of strong and long-lasting immunity. Nine-mer peptides, such as those discovered in our studies, which bind to both HLA-I and HLA-II molecules, may potentially activate both the T helper and CTL arms of the immune system. Our studies may have important implications for a new design of epitope-based diagnostics and vaccines, which incorporate both HLA-I and HLA-II restricted epitopes in the same peptide entity.

ACKNOWLEDGMENTS

This work was supported by National Institute of Allergy and Infectious Disease contracts HHSN266200400083C, HHSN266200400025C, EU 6FP 503231, National Institutes of Health contract HHSN266200400081C and a grant from the Lundbeck Fundation, Copenhagen, Denmark. The authors thank all the staffs from Ole Lund's Lab at the Technical University of Denmark and Soren Buus's Lab at the University of Copenhagen, Denmark for their cooperation.

REFERENCES

[1] Kanodia S, Kast WM: Peptide-based vaccines for cancer: realizing their potential. *Expert Rev Vaccines* 2008, 7(10):1533-1545.

[2] Rosenberg SA, Dudley ME: Adoptive cell therapy for the treatment of patients with metastatic melanoma. *Curr Opin Immunol* 2009, 21(2):233-240.

[3] Woodworth JS, Wu Y, Behar SM: Mycobacterium tuberculosis-specific $CD8^+$ T cells require perforin to kill target cells and provide protection in vivo. *J Immunol* 2008, 181(12):8595-8603.

[4] Woodworth JS, Behar SM: Mycobacterium tuberculosis-specific $CD8^+$ T cells and their role in immunity. *Crit Rev Immunol* 2006, 26(4):317-352.

[5] Kennedy R, Poland GA: T-Cell epitope discovery for variola and vaccinia viruses. *Rev Med Virol* 2007, 17(2):93-113.

[6] McMichael AJ, Gotch FM, Noble GR, Beare PA: Cytotoxic T-cell immunity to influenza. *N Engl J Med* 1983, 309(1):13-17.

[7] Bender BS, Croghan T, Zhang L, Small PA, Jr.: Transgenic mice lacking class I major histocompatibility complex-restricted T cells have delayed viral clearance and increased mortality after influenza virus challenge. *J Exp Med* 1992, 175(4):1143-1145.

[8] Sette A, Rappuoli R: Reverse vaccinology: developing vaccines in the era of genomics. *Immunity* 2010, 33(4):530-541.

[9] Lundegaard C, Lund O, Buus S, Nielsen M: Major histocompatibility complex class I binding predictions as a tool in epitope discovery. *Immunology* 2010, 130(3):309-318.

[10] Kessler JH, Melief CJ: Identification of T-cell epitopes for cancer immunotherapy. *Leukemia* 2007, 21(9):1859-1874.

[11] Wang M, Tang ST, Stryhn A, Justesen S, Larsen MV, Dziegiel MH, Lewinsohn DM, Buus S, Lund O, Claesson MH: Identification of MHC class II restricted T-cell-mediated reactivity against MHC class I binding Mycobacterium tuberculosis peptides. *Immunology* 2011, 132(4):482-491.

[12] Wang M, Tang ST, Lund O, Dziegiel MH, Buus S, Claesson MH: High-affinity human leucocyte antigen class I binding variola-derived peptides induce $CD4^+$ T cell responses more than 30 years post-vaccinia virus vaccination. *Clin Exp Immunol* 2009, 155(3):441-446.

[13] Wang M, Larsen MV, Nielsen M, Harndahl M, Justesen S, Dziegiel MH, Buus S, Tang ST, Lund O, Claesson MH: HLA class I binding 9mer peptides from influenza A virus induce CD4 T cell responses. *PLoS One* 2010, 5(5):e10533.

[14] Wang M, Lamberth K, Harndahl M, Roder G, Stryhn A, Larsen MV, Nielsen M, Lundegaard C, Tang ST, Dziegiel MH *et al*: CTL epitopes for influenza A including the H5N1 bird flu; genome-, pathogen-, and HLA-wide screening. *Vaccine* 2007, 25(15):2823-2831.

[15] Tang ST, Wang M, Lamberth K, Harndahl M, Dziegiel MH, Claesson MH, Buus S, Lund O: MHC-I-restricted epitopes conserved among variola and other related orthopoxviruses are recognized by T cells 30 years after vaccination. *Arch Virol* 2008, 153(10):1833-1844.

[16] Tang ST, van Meijgaarden KE, Caccamo N, Guggino G, Klein MR, van Weeren P, Kazi F, Stryhn A, Zaigler A, Sahin U *et al*: Genome-based in silico identification of new Mycobacterium tuberculosis antigens activating polyfunctional $CD8^+$ T cells in human tuberculosis. *J Immunol* 2011, 186(2):1068-1080.

[17] Anderson LD, Jr., Cook DR, Yamamoto TN, Berger C, Maloney DG, Riddell SR: Identification of MAGE-C1 (CT-7) epitopes for T-cell therapy of multiple myeloma. *Cancer Immunol Immunother* 2011, 60(7):985-997.

[18] Liu W, Zhai M, Wu Z, Qi Y, Wu Y, Dai C, Sun M, Li L, Gao Y: Identification of a novel HLA-A2-restricted cytotoxic T lymphocyte epitope from cancer-testis antigen PLAC1 in breast cancer. *Amino Acids* 2011.

[19] Zvi A, Rotem S, Bar-Haim E, Cohen O, Shafferman A: Whole-Genome Immunoinformatic Analysis of F. tularensis: Predicted CTL Epitopes Clustered in Hotspots Are Prone to Elicit a T-Cell Response. *PLoS One* 2011, 6(5):e20050.

[20] Lund O, Nielsen M, Kesmir C, Petersen AG, Lundegaard C, Worning P, Sylvester-Hvid C, Lamberth K, Roder G, Justesen S *et al*: Definition of supertypes for HLA molecules using clustering of specificity matrices. *Immunogenetics* 2004, 55(12):797-810.

[21] Salter RD, Benjamin RJ, Wesley PK, Buxton SE, Garrett TP, Clayberger C, Krensky AM, Norment AM, Littman DR, Parham P: A binding site for the T-cell co-receptor CD8 on the alpha 3 domain of HLA-A2. *Nature* 1990, 345(6270):41-46.

[22] Bjorkman PJ, Saper MA, Samraoui B, Bennett WS, Strominger JL, Wiley DC: Structure of the human class I histocompatibility antigen, HLA-A2. *Nature* 1987, 329(6139):506-512.

[23] York IA, Rock KL: Antigen processing and presentation by the class I major histocompatibility complex. *Annu Rev Immunol* 1996, 14:369-396.

[24] Vitiello A, Potter TA, Sherman LA: The role of beta 2-microglobulin in peptide binding by class I molecules. *Science* 1990, 250(4986):1423-1426.

[25] Perarnau B, Siegrist CA, Gillet A, Vincent C, Kimura S, Lemonnier FA: Beta 2-microglobulin restriction of antigen presentation. *Nature* 1990, 346(6286):751-754.

[26] Parmentier N, Stroobant V, Colau D, de Diesbach P, Morel S, Chapiro J, van Endert P, Van den Eynde BJ: Production of an antigenic peptide by insulin-degrading enzyme. *Nat Immunol* 2010, 11(5):449-454.

[27] Cresswell P, Ackerman AL, Giodini A, Peaper DR, Wearsch PA: Mechanisms of MHC class I-restricted antigen processing and cross-presentation. *Immunol Rev* 2005, 207:145-157.

[28] Kloetzel PM: Antigen processing by the proteasome. *Nat Rev Mol Cell Biol* 2001, 2(3):179-187.

[29] Chicz RM, Urban RG, Lane WS, Gorga JC, Stern LJ, Vignali DA, Strominger JL: Predominant naturally processed peptides bound to HLA-DR1 are derived from MHC-related molecules and are heterogeneous in size. *Nature* 1992, 358(6389):764-768.

[30] Rudensky A, Preston-Hurlburt P, Hong SC, Barlow A, Janeway CA, Jr.: Sequence analysis of peptides bound to MHC class II molecules. *Nature* 1991, 353(6345):622-627.

[31] Watts C: The exogenous pathway for antigen presentation on major histocompatibility complex class II and CD1 molecules. *Nat Immunol* 2004, 5(7):685-692.

[32] Sylvester-Hvid C, Nielsen M, Lamberth K, Roder G, Justesen S, Lundegaard C, Worning P, Thomadsen H, Lund O, Brunak S *et al*: SARS CTL vaccine candidates; HLA supertype-, genome-wide scanning and biochemical validation. *Tissue Antigens* 2004, 63(5):395-400.

[33] Sidney J, del Guercio MF, Southwood S, Engelhard VH, Appella E, Rammensee HG, Falk K, Rotzschke O, Takiguchi M, Kubo RT *et al*: Several HLA alleles share overlapping peptide specificities. *J Immunol* 1995, 154(1):247-259.

[34] Sette A, Sidney J: Nine major HLA class I supertypes account for the vast preponderance of HLA-A and -B polymorphism. *Immunogenetics* 1999, 50(3-4):201-212.

[35] del Guercio MF, Sidney J, Hermanson G, Perez C, Grey HM, Kubo RT, Sette A: Binding of a peptide antigen to multiple HLA alleles allows definition of an A2-like supertype. *J Immunol* 1995, 154(2):685-693.

[36] Harndahl M, Justesen S, Lamberth K, Roder G, Nielsen M, Buus S: Peptide binding to HLA class I molecules: homogenous, high-throughput screening, and affinity assays. *J Biomol Screen* 2009, 14(2):173-180.

[37] Ostergaard Pedersen L, Nissen MH, Hansen NJ, Nielsen LL, Lauenmoller SL, Blicher T, Nansen A, Sylvester-Hvid C, Thromsen AR, Buus S: Efficient assembly of recombinant major histocompatibility complex class I molecules with preformed disulfide bonds. *Eur J Immunol* 2001, 31(10):2986-2996.

[38] Boyle LH, Goodall JC, Gaston JS: Major histocompatibility complex class I-restricted alloreactive $CD4^+$ T cells. *Immunology* 2004, 112(1):54-63.

[39] Boyle LH, Goodall JC, Gaston JS: The recognition of abnormal forms of HLA-B27 by $CD4^+$ T cells. *Curr Mol Med* 2004, 4(1):51-58.

[40] Boyle LH, Goodall JC, Opat SS, Gaston JS: The recognition of HLA-B27 by human $CD4(^+)$ T lymphocytes. *J Immunol* 2001, 167(5):2619-2624.

[41] Darrow TL, Abdel-Wahab Z, Quinn-Allen MA, Seigler HF: Recognition and lysis of human melanoma by a $CD3^+$, $CD4^+$, CD8- T-cell clone restricted by HLA-A2. *Cell Immunol* 1996, 172(1):52-59.

[42] Kobayashi H, Kimura S, Aoki N, Sato K, Celis E, Katagiri M: Existence of MHC class I-restricted alloreactive $CD4^+$ T cells reacting with peptide transporter-deficient cells. *Immunogenetics* 2001, 53(8):626-633.

[43] Moore RL, Fox BS: $CD4^+$ class I-restricted T cells specific for HIV gp160 315-329. *Cell Immunol* 1994, 154(1):43-53.

[44] Ackerman AL, Cresswell P: Cellular mechanisms governing cross-presentation of exogenous antigens. *Nat Immunol* 2004, 5(7):678-684.

[45] Dengjel J, Schoor O, Fischer R, Reich M, Kraus M, Muller M, Kreymborg K, Altenberend F, Brandenburg J, Kalbacher H *et al*: Autophagy promotes MHC class II presentation of peptides from intracellular source proteins. *Proc Natl Acad Sci U S A* 2005, 102(22):7922-7927.

[46] Marrack P, Ignatowicz L, Kappler JW, Boymel J, Freed JH: Comparison of peptides bound to spleen and thymus class II. *J Exp Med* 1993, 178(6):2173-2183.

[47] Rammensee HG, Friede T, Stevanoviic S: MHC ligands and peptide motifs: first listing. *Immunogenetics* 1995, 41(4):178-228.

[48] Gueguen M, Long EO: Presentation of a cytosolic antigen by major histocompatibility complex class II molecules requires a long-lived form of the antigen. *Proc Natl Acad Sci U S A* 1996, 93(25):14692-14697.

[49] Jacobson S, Sekaly RP, Bellini WJ, Johnson CL, McFarland HF, Long EO: Recognition of intracellular measles virus antigens by HLA class II restricted measles virus-specific cytotoxic T lymphocytes. *Ann N Y Acad Sci* 1988, 540:352-353.

[50] Jacobson S, Sekaly RP, Jacobson CL, McFarland HF, Long EO: HLA class II-restricted presentation of cytoplasmic measles virus antigens to cytotoxic T cells. *J Virol* 1989, 63(4):1756-1762.

[51] Jaraquemada D, Marti M, Long EO: An endogenous processing pathway in vaccinia virus-infected cells for presentation of cytoplasmic antigens to class II-restricted T cells. *J Exp Med* 1990, 172(3):947-954.

[52] Malnati MS, Marti M, LaVaute T, Jaraquemada D, Biddison W, DeMars R, Long EO: Processing pathways for presentation of cytosolic antigen to MHC class II-restricted T cells. *Nature* 1992, 357(6380):702-704.

[53] Sant AJ: Endogenous antigen presentation by MHC class II molecules. *Immunol Res* 1994, 13(4):253-267.

[54] Oxenius A, Bachmann MF, Ashton-Rickardt PG, Tonegawa S, Zinkernagel RM, Hengartner H: Presentation of endogenous viral proteins in association with major histocompatibility complex class II: on the role of intracellular compartmentalization, invariant chain and the TAP transporter system. *Eur J Immunol* 1995, 25(12):3402-3411.

[55] Lich JD, Elliott JF, Blum JS: Cytoplasmic processing is a prerequisite for presentation of an endogenous antigen by major histocompatibility complex class II proteins. *J Exp Med* 2000, 191(9):1513-1524.

[56] Tewari MK, Sinnathamby G, Rajagopal D, Eisenlohr LC: A cytosolic pathway for MHC class II-restricted antigen processing that is proteasome and TAP dependent. *Nat Immunol* 2005, 6(3):287-294.

[57] Crotzer VL, Blum JS: Cytosol to lysosome transport of intracellular antigens during immune surveillance. *Traffic* 2008, 9(1):10-16.

[58] van Luijn MM, Chamuleau ME, Ressing ME, Wiertz EJ, Ostrand-Rosenberg S, Souwer Y, Zevenbergen A, Ossenkoppele GJ, van de Loosdrecht AA, van Ham SM: Alternative Ii-independent antigen-processing pathway in leukemic blasts involves TAP-dependent peptide loading of HLA class II complexes. *Cancer Immunol Immunother* 2010, 59(12):1825-1838.

[59] Gannage M, Munz C: Autophagy in MHC class II presentation of endogenous antigens. *Curr Top Microbiol Immunol* 2009, 335:123-140.

[60] Munz C: Enhancing immunity through autophagy. *Annu Rev Immunol* 2009, 27:423-449.

[61] Munz C: Antigen processing via autophagy--not only for MHC class II presentation anymore? *Curr Opin Immunol* 2010, 22(1):89-93.

[62] Nimmerjahn F, Milosevic S, Behrends U, Jaffee EM, Pardoll DM, Bornkamm GW, Mautner J: Major histocompatibility complex class II-restricted presentation of a cytosolic antigen by autophagy. *Eur J Immunol* 2003, 33(5):1250-1259.

[63] Schmid D, Pypaert M, Munz C: Antigen-loading compartments for major histocompatibility complex class II molecules continuously receive input from autophagosomes. *Immunity* 2007, 26(1):79-92.

[64] Comber JD, Robinson TM, Siciliano NA, Snook AE, Eisenlohr LC: Functional Macroautophagy Induction by Influenza A Virus without a Contribution to Major Histocompatibility Complex Class II-Restricted Presentation. *J Virol* 2011, 85(13):6453-6463.

[65] Fujimoto I, Pan J, Takizawa T, Nakanishi Y: Virus clearance through apoptosis-dependent phagocytosis of influenza A virus-infected cells by macrophages. *J Virol* 2000, 74(7):3399-3403.

[66] Shiratsuchi A, Kaido M, Takizawa T, Nakanishi Y: Phosphatidylserine-mediated phagocytosis of influenza A virus-infected cells by mouse peritoneal macrophages. *J Virol* 2000, 74(19):9240-9244.

[67] Rock KL, Gamble S, Rothstein L, Gramm C, Benacerraf B: Dissociation of beta 2-microglobulin leads to the accumulation of a substantial pool of inactive class I MHC heavy chains on the cell surface. *Cell* 1991, 65(4):611-620.

[68] Nielsen M, Lundegaard C, Blicher T, Peters B, Sette A, Justesen S, Buus S, Lund O: Quantitative predictions of peptide binding to any HLA-DR molecule of known sequence: NetMHCIIpan. *PLoS Comput Biol* 2008, 4(7):e1000107.

[69] Justesen S, Harndahl M, Lamberth K, Nielsen LL, Buus S: Functional recombinant MHC class II molecules and high-throughput peptide-binding assays. *Immunome Res* 2009, 5:2.

[70] Nielsen M, Lundegaard C, Worning P, Hvid CS, Lamberth K, Buus S, Brunak S, Lund O: Improved prediction of MHC class I and class II epitopes using a novel Gibbs sampling approach. *Bioinformatics* 2004, 20(9):1388-1397.

[71] Nielsen M, Lund O, Buus S, Lundegaard C: MHC class II epitope predictive algorithms. *Immunology* 2010, 130(3):319-328.

[72] Nielsen M, Justesen S, Lund O, Lundegaard C, Buus S: NetMHCIIpan-2.0 - Improved pan-specific HLA-DR predictions using a novel concurrent alignment and weight optimization training procedure. *Immunome Res* 2010, 6:9.

[73] Wang P, Sidney J, Kim Y, Sette A, Lund O, Nielsen M, Peters B: Peptide binding predictions for HLA DR, DP and DQ molecules. *BMC Bioinformatics* 2010, 11:568.

[74] Lewinsohn DM, Bement TT, Xu J, Lynch DH, Grabstein KH, Reed SG, Alderson MR: Human purified protein derivative-specific $CD4^+$ T cells use both CD95-dependent and CD95-independent cytolytic mechanisms. *J Immunol* 1998, 160(5):2374-2379.

[75] Janssen EM, Droin NM, Lemmens EE, Pinkoski MJ, Bensinger SJ, Ehst BD, Griffith TS, Green DR, Schoenberger SP: $CD4^+$ T-cell help controls $CD8^+$ T-cell memory via TRAIL-mediated activation-induced cell death. *Nature* 2005, 434(7029):88-93.

[76] Janssen EM, Lemmens EE, Wolfe T, Christen U, von Herrath MG, Schoenberger SP: $CD4^+$ T cells are required for secondary expansion and memory in $CD8^+$ T lymphocytes. *Nature* 2003, 421(6925):852-856.

[77] Shedlock DJ, Shen H: Requirement for CD4 T cell help in generating functional CD8 T cell memory. *Science* 2003, 300(5617):337-339.

[78] Sun JC, Bevan MJ: Defective CD8 T cell memory following acute infection without CD4 T cell help. *Science* 2003, 300(5617):339-342.

[79] Sun JC, Williams MA, Bevan MJ: $CD4^+$ T cells are required for the maintenance, not programming, of memory $CD8^+$ T cells after acute infection. *Nat Immunol* 2004, 5(9):927-933.

In: Major Histocompatibility Complex
Editor: Natalya V. Semiletova
ISBN: 978-1-61942-999-4

Chapter 10

IMMUNOREGULATORY EFFECT OF THE SYNGENEIC SERUM CONDITIONED BY DONOR-LIKE sMHC CLASS I PROTEINS

Natalya V. Semiletova*
Division of General Surgery, Department of Surgery,
David Geffen School of Medicine at UCLA, Los Angeles, CA, US

ABSTRACT

The major histocompatibility complex antigens (MHC) can exist in several forms as membrane complex on all nucleated cells and as soluble form in physiological fluids like blood, tears, saliva, and urine. The three forms of soluble MHC (sMHC) were found in the blood serum: whole heavy chains of class I MHC; MHC molecules lacking the transmembrane and intracellular parts; and molecules merely missing a cytoplasmic tail. Solid organ transplantation stimulates MHC shedding from recipient and donor cellular membranes and it was shown that concentrations of certain forms of sMHC depend on the immunological state of the graft and clinical condition of recipient. Understanding the role of sMHC antigens in the immunoregulation and development of graft chronic rejection is one of the principal goals of organ transplantation. Therapy with donor-like sMHC class I proteins, in conjunction with the short course of CsA, prolonged cardiac graft survival and averted development of chronic rejection in the rat cardiac model of heart transplantation. The tolerant state was characterized by the deviation of alloantibody (allo-Abs) response. This study examines the immunoregulatory effect of the singeneic serum conditioned with sMHC class I proteins on the development of vascular transplant injuries in the MHC disparate cardiac allografts and emergence of protective donor allo-Abs.

Keywords: Allo-Abs, allo-specific antibodies; WF, Wistar Furth; BN, Brown Norway; CsA, cyclosporine; i.v., intravenous; MHC, major histocompatibility complex; HPF, high power field

---

* E-mail: nsemiletova@mednet.ucla.edu.

INTRODUCTION

1. Effect of Class I MHC on Organ Allograft Survival

Pre-transplant host immunomodulation in addition to intrathymic inoculation of donor-type alloantigens provides evidence that indirect donor alloantigen presentation in the thymus to immature T cells during their ontogeny may induce acquired systemic tolerance [1, 2]. It was shown that intrathymic injection of immunogenic peptides derived from the hypervariable domain of rat class I MHC, RT1.A^U sequences induced antigen-specific tolerance to cardiac allografts in MHC class I mismatched rats. Further, soluble HLA class I molecules have been shown to induce apoptosis in alloreactive cytotoxic T lymphocytes [3], suggesting that intrathymic administration of MHC class I peptides may cause deletion of developing thymocytes with high avidity/affinity T cell receptor-MHC/allopeptide interactions. However, induction of thymic tolerance to extrathymic allografts requires pre-transplant intrathymic administration of either membrane–expressed antigen [4], extracted soluble alloantigen [5], or class I allopeptides [6] into a T cell depleted immunomodulated host, several weeks prior to transplantation. Due to such requirements, thymic tolerance has not been translated to the clinical arena. Further, the majority of long-term surviving heart allografts, following thymic tolerance induction, exhibited severe chronic rejection in the presence of a T helper (Th)-2 cytokine response [7,8]. Pre-transplant peripheral administration of membrane-expressed alloantigens also slightly prolonged cardiac allograft survival [9]. Pre-transplant i.v. administration of donor-type class I H-$2K^b$ alloantigen, expressed on C3H/He (H-2^k) L cells, was more potent than similarly expressed class II H-$2IA^b$ or class I H-$2D^b$ in prolongation of H-2^b heart allografts [10, 11]. In a clinically applicable strategy of peripheral *peri-operative* intravenous administration of soluble donor-type class I and class II extracted allopeptides specifically strengthened the effect of CsA to prolong rodent heart allograft survival [12], but failed to induce long-term graft acceptance. Thus, peripheral administration of non-modified MHC antigens failed to induce indefinite allograft survival.

2. Effect of Modified Class I MHC on Organ Survival and Chronic Rejection

Although multideterminant protein antigens exhibit a hierarchy of dominant and subdominant immungenic epitopes, host responses towards native protein antigens are orchestrated by a limited number of immunogenic determinants [13]. Alteration of critical amino acid (aa) residues in such immunogenic determinants has been shown to inhibit T-cell-proliferative responses, induce T-cell anergy, and alter host immune responses toward native antigens [14]. Strong evidence suggests that murine, rodent, and human host indirect immune responses to organ allografts are focused on a restricted number of donor alloantigenic determinants that correspond to short aa peptide residues, [15] after indirect recognition of processed MHC alloantigens. Thus, administration of modified donor MHC antigens to allograft recipients may interfere with the immune response toward wild type MHC antigens expressed on grafts, thereby leading to acceptance rather than rejection of allografts.

Our group was the first to adopt a molecular strategy to identify the immunogenic epitopes of class I MHC antigens by construction of donor-like class I molecules that contain donor-type polymorphic epitopes displayed on recipient-type heavy chains. These studies revealed the presence of immunodominant determinants within the α_1-helical region (aa 58-80) of RT1.A^u, RT1.A^l, and RT1.A^a that caused accelerated cardiac allograft rejection, increased the alloreactive cytotoxic T cell frequency and T cell proliferation [16-20].

Peripheral *peri- or post-operative* portal delivery of donor immunogenic epitopes displayed on recipient self-determinants via the soluble composite [$\alpha_{1h}{}^{l/u}$]-RT1.A^a donor-like molecule, in the presence of sub-therapeutic CsA, induced donor-specific transplantation tolerance to cardiac allografts obtained from the genetically distinct RT1^l and RT1^u rat strains in RT1^a hosts and abrogated the development of chronic rejection [20-22]. Such a tolerant state was confirmed by the acceptance of second donor-type heart allografts. Our approach is based on selection of donor immunodominant epitopes that are introduced onto the backbone of recipient class I MHC sequences in an effort to deliver a tolerogenic rather than immunogenic signal through the alloantigen-specific T-cell receptor (TCR). In a similar strategy, Langowski et al. recently demonstrated that alteration of two polymorphic residues in the α_1-helical region of RT1.A^l (Arg$_{77}$ and Glu$_{80}$), produced the donor-like MHC class I [$\alpha_{1h}{}^{77,80\ L}$]-RT1A^a protein that induced tolerance to Lewis (RT1^l) heart allografts in ACI recipients [23]. These findings confirm the ability of modified class I sMHC molecules to induce chronic rejection-free donor-specific transplantation tolerance. The mechanisms and treatment of cardiac allograft vasculopathy (CAV) remain elusive despite that 75% of patients exhibit detectable intimal thickening after 1 year post-transplant. It is known that MHC class I antigens play an important role in the pathogenesis of CAV [24, 25]. Donor-like sMHC class I molecules offer the potential of not only inhibiting chronic rejection, but also inducing tolerance to heart allografts – the ultimate goal of organ transplantation. In addition, donor-like sMHC molecules synergistically interact with CsA, which is commonly utilized in clinical practice.

3. Immunoregulatory Effect of the Syngeneic Serum

A number of studies show that serum from immunomodulated experimental animals transferred into syngeneic or allogeneic recipients could affect immune system of experimental animals [26-30]. Serum collected from mice 1 hr after a single intragastric dose of ovalbumin induced the suppression of delayed-type hypersensitivity reactions when injected intraperitoneally into recipient mice [26]. Serum from UV-irradiated BALB/c mice had suppressive effect on leukocyte adherence of CBA mice *in vitro* [27]. Specific unresponsiveness to bacterial lipopolysaccharide could be passively transferred with the serum from LPS-tolerant donors into recipient mice at the time of immunization [28]. In clinical practice, it has become apparent that blood transfusion generalized effects on the patient's immune system. These effects have been postulated to underline the clinical observations that transfused patients have more frequent recurrences of malignant tumors, decreased rates of allograft rejection, spontaneous abortion, and a reduced rate of recurrence of Crohn's disease, as well as increased postoperative bacterial infections [29]. Conflicting data have been reported in clinical trials of the postoperative infection rate and outcome in tumor patients who underwent surgery and received either allogeneic or autologous blood transfusion [30].

The fine processes by which blood transfusions exert their immunomodulatory effect are still undefined. It seems likely that such an effect is based on a combination of mechanisms, including of anergy, anti-idiotypic antibody-mediated immunosuppression, imbalance of cytokines and/or cytokine receptor expression, T-cell clone deletion and/or regulatory cell activation, and the presence of soluble factors [31]. Such soluble factors were investigated but did not receive wide attention. Wang et al. showed the results of using donor serum to prevent passive transfer of hyperacute rejection. Authors found that the donor serum prevented hyperacute rejection without an antibody blocking mechanism, and that the donor MHC class I antigen was not a key player in this model [32]. In an other work, it is indicated that the passive transfer of cytotoxic alloantibodies has resulted either in hyperacute rejection or graft enhancement [33]. Several articles described the appearance of donor-specific regulatory factors in the blood of recipients treated with immunosuppressive drugs and/or donor-like sMHC class I antigens [34, 35]. MHC antigens are heterodimeric glycoproteins that, besides being expressed on the membrane of most nucleated cells, are present in serum as soluble β_2-microglobulin (β_2m)-associated (sMHC-I) and soluble β_2m-free MHC class I heavy chains. Soluble MHC class I proteins possess immunomodulating features. *In vitro* studies showed that an MHC molecule can inhibit T cell functions by receptor blockade [36], MHC molecules can be phagocytosed by antigen-presenting cells, degraded to peptides, and presented to $CD4^+$ T cells in the context of membrane MHC class II antigens [37]. Soluble MHC may also stimulate Fas ligand expression by activated $CD8^+$ T cells and induce apoptosis [38]. Donor-like sMHC class I proteins, that have donor sequences within α_1 domains on the background of a recipient sequences, have been shown as an immunomodulators as well [9, 17, 20]. Donor-like sMHC class I therapy with short course of CsA prolonged cardiac graft survival and averted development of chronic rejection through emergence of protective donor alloantibodies that caused vascular graft accommodation in allogeneic transplants [20].

This study examines the immunoregulatory effect of sMHC class I protein conditioned serum on the development of vascular transplant injuries in the MHC disparate cardiac allografts and emergence of protective donor allo-Abs.

Materials and Methods

Animals

Adult male inbred Wistar Furth (WF; RT1.A^u), Brown Norway (BN; RT1.A^n), and ACI (RT1.A^a) rats (200-250 gm) were purchased from Harlan Sprague Dawley (Indianapolis, IN) and housed in standard rat cages. Animals received humane care according to the criteria outlined in the "Guide for the Care and Use of Laboratory Animals" prepared by the National Academy of Sciences and published by the National Institutes of Health (publication no. 86-23). Study was approved by the local ethical committee for animals.

Cardiac Transplantation

Heterotopic cardiac allografts were performed by using the modified technique of Ono and Lindsey [39]. Cold ischemia time was less than 45 min. Graft survival was assessed by daily palpation; rejection was defined by cessation of heartbeat and confirmed by histological evaluation. The day on which beating was last palpable was defined as the day of rejection. Data are presented as mean survival time ± SD and were compared using Student's *t* test. *P* values <0.05 were considered statistically significant.

Passive Transfer Studies

One mL of syngeneic serum from ACI naïve rats or tolerant ACI recipients of WF hearts (120 days posttransplant) was injected intravenously (i.v.) at day of cardiac transplantation into new ACI hosts. Experimental groups: 1) untreated hosts (acute rejection, n=8), 2) hosts treated with syngeneic naïve serum (n=5), 3) ACI rats treated with syngeneic tolerant serum (n=7), 4) animals i.v. injected with 0.1 mg/rat or 1 mg/rat of IgG purified from whole serum collected from naïve ACI (n=3 for each group), 5) ACI hosts i.v. treated with either 0.1 mg or 1 mg of total IgG purified from tolerant ACI serum (n = 6 & 3, respectively). Specificity was confirmed by treatment of ACI recipients of BN hearts (third-party) with tolerant ACI serum (n=3) or by transfer of WF and BN naïve serum into ACI recipients of WF hearts (n=3 for each group). Experimental design schematically presented on Figure 1.

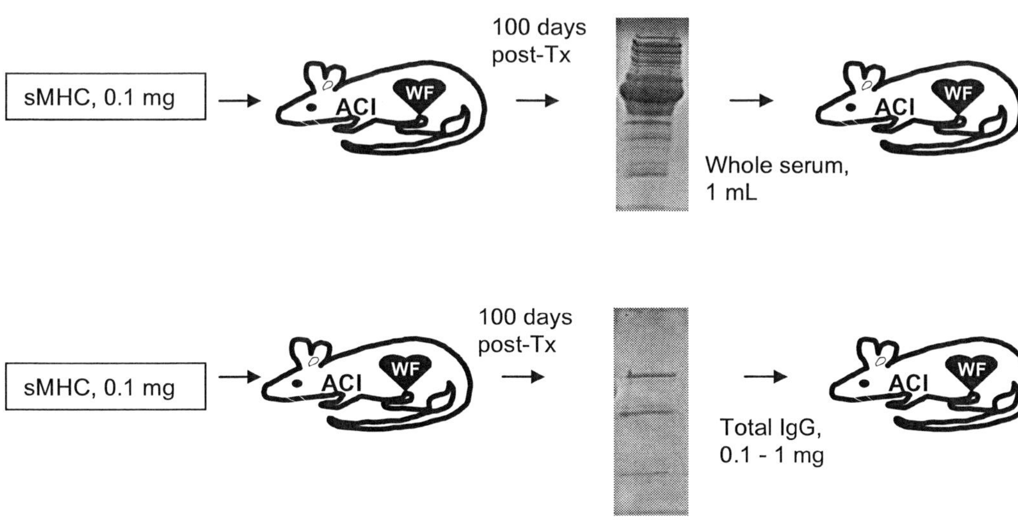

Figure 1. Experimental design. Passive transfer experiments included group of sMHC protein treated animals. Single dose of 0.1 mg of sMHC soluble protein was administered *peri-operatively* into primary ACI recipients of WF cardiac grafts in addition to a sub-therapeutic 3 day course of cyclosporine (10 mg/kg/day, days 0-2). Serums were harvested at 100 days post-transplant from recipients with alive, beating cardiac grafts. IgG fractions were prepared with Melon Gel IgG spin purification system and purity assessed on SDS-PAGE gel (>95%). Secondary ACI recipients of WF hearts were i.v. injected with 0.1 mg or 1 mg of pure IgG fractions in PBS at day of cardiac transplantation or with 1 mL of whole, unfractioned serum. Control groups were treated with IgG purified from naïve syngeneic or with whole naïve serums.

Flow Cytometry Analysis

Sera from control and long-term survived ACI recipients of WF cardiac allografts was analyzed for the presence of binding anti-RT1.A^u alloantibodies at 120 days posttransplantation as previously described [20]. A collected serum was heat inactivated (56°C/30 minutes) and stored at -80°C until the time of analysis. In brief, target LN cells ($1x10^6$) were suspended in phosphate-buffered saline (PBS Ca^{2+} & Mg^{2+} free) containing 2% fetal calf serum. Serially diluted experimental sera (1:4, 1:16 & 1:64) was added to the cells (100 μl) and incubated for 30 min at 4°C. After washing, rabbit anti-rat IgM-FITC (1:100 dilution) and mouse anti-rat IgG, IgG1, IgG2a, IgG2b and IgG2c (1:200 dilution per $1x10^6$ cells, 100 μl, PharMingen BD Biosciences, San Diego, CA) were added and cells were incubated for additional 30 min at 4°C in the dark. Thereafter cells were washed and analyzed immediately on a Becton-Dickinson Laser Flow Cytometry System (Mountain View, CA). Non-specific fluorescence was assessed by staining with the second FITC-conjugated antibody alone. Data are presented as X-Mean ± SD.

Mixed Lymphocyte Reaction (MLR)

Lymph node (LN) T cells harvested from ACI rats were used as responders toward stimulator cell populations harvested from the spleens of syngeneic ACI or donor WF or BN (third-party) rats. Responder T cells ($0.5x10^6$/well) were incubated on 96 well plate U-bottom for 5 days with $0.5x10^6$ mitomycin treated spleen stimulator cells at $37^0C/5\%$ CO_2, cultured in RPMI-1640 medium (Cellgro, Manassas, VA) supplemented with 10% heat-inactivated FCS (GibcoBRL, Gaithersburg, MD) with L-Glutamine final concentration 2mM, Sodium pyruvate 1mM, 1x Non-Essential amino acids, 10 mM HEPES, $0.5x10^{-5}$ M β-mercaptoethanol, penicillin/streptomycin 100μg/100 units, Sodium bicarbonate 1.5 g/L. Wells including stimulator cells from syngeneic ACI rats served as control for nonspecific proliferation. Proliferation was assessed by ^{3}H-thymidine incorporation (specific activity 5.0 Ci/mM; Amersham, Arlington, IL) added 1.0 μCi per well on fourth day of incubation for 24 hours. Results of triplicate cultures were expressed as the mean cpm/min±SD.

Endothelial Cell Primary Culture

The rat aortas were aseptically harvested and rinsed in cold HBSS to remove blood. Tissue was cut into short sections and digested in fresh collagenase II (0.5% w/v in HBSS, supplemented with 3mM $CaCl_2$, Invitrogen, Carlsbad, CA) solution for 1 hour at 37^0C on an orbital shaker. Cell solution and undigested tissue was pushed through a 70 μm cell strainer and washed with cold HBSS. Cells were then grown in the BIOCOAT Endothelial Cell Growth Environment (BD Biosciences, Bedford, MA) according to the manufacture's instructions. Purity of endothelial cells (EC) was verified by staining with antibodies against von Willebrand factor (BD Bioscience, Bedford, MA).

RNA Turnover Assay

To test whether serum conditioned with sMHC proteins can alter metabolic function of ECs *in vitro* we performed RNA turnover assay that utilized ^{3}H-uridine incorporation into newly synthesized RNA approach. EC cultures were incubated in full endothelial cell medium (ECM) on 6 cm collagen plates with or without rIFN-γ 500U/ml) for 72 hrs. Cell were harvested, washed and seeded into 96 well collagen coated plates in RPMI 1640 media. Wells that had only ECs with media served as baseline for RNA synthesis. Wells that contained resting or rIFN-γ activated ECs plus naïve serum from untreated syngeneic rats served as control (serum was added as 5%/well volume). Test wells had ECs plus syngeneic sMHC-conditioned serum from long-term surviving cardiac hosts (5%/well volume). Plates were pulsed with 2 μCi/well of ^{3}H-uridine and incubated for 20 hr. ECs was harvested with a semi-automated cell harvesting apparatus (Skatron, Sterling, VA) on glass-fiber filters and relative incorporation of ^{3}H-uridine was determined with a TM Analytic model Mark V scintillation counter. All experimental points were performed in quadruplicate in three separate experiments and the results averaged and presented as mean cpm/min±SD.

ELISA

Donor WF aortic EC were seeded (20x10^4/well) into 96-well plates coated with Collagen I in complete EC cultivation medium (Biocoat EC Growth Medium, DB Bioscience, Bedford, MA) and incubated for 2-3 days or until cells reach confluence. Untreated or IFN-γ treated (500 U/ml) EC were incubated on the same plate. Cells were fixed by adding 200 ml of 0.25% glutaraldehyde in PBS for 5-10 min at 4^{0}C. Cells fixed in this way could be stored at 4°C for at least 10 days without losing the ability to bind immunoglobulins. Serums from naïve and long-term graft surviving ACI recipients were diluted 1:4, 1:8 & 1:16 in PBS-AE (PBS/0.1% BSA/5 mM EDTA) and added into experimental wells (100 μL/well) in parallel with negative control (PBS-AE only) or blank wells (no EC). Plates were incubated for 60 min at room t^0 and washed 4 times with PBS-AE. Peroxidase-conjugated rabbit anti-rat IgG or IgG2c specific antibodies were added (100 μl/well, concentration 1:4000 - 1:8000) and incubated for 60 min at room t^0. Plates were washed and incubated with fresh OPDA-C/P-0.01% H_2O_2 (30 mM o-phenylene-diamine dihydrochloride (OPDA, *Sigma-Aldrich*, Taufkirchen, Germany) in 0.1 M citrate-phosphate ((C/P, pH 5) buffer with 0.01 % hydrogen peroxide) for 30 min at room t^0. Sample analysis was performed at 450 nm wave length (OD) on a plate reader (Power Waive XS, BioTek, Highland Park, VT). All experimental, negative and blank samples were seeded in triplicates. Four independent experiments were performed. Total rat immunoglobulin isotypes were detected in whole serum of naïve and long-term surviving cardiac recipients with Rat Immunoglobulin Isotyping ELISA Kit (BD Pharmingen, Bedford, MA) according to specified protocol.

Serum IgG Purification

Rat IgG from whole serum was separated with Melon Gel IgG Spin Purification System (Thermo Scientific/Pierce Rockford, IL). Non-antibody serum proteins were removed by applying 10 μL of undiluted serum on 100 μl of settled gel. Column was incubated for 5 min at room t^0 with en-over-end mixing. Purified antibody was collected after 1 min centrifugation at 6,000 x g. Quality of purification was analyzed on SDS-PAGE gel. Purity of IgG fraction was close to 95%.

Western Blotting, DNA Fragmentation (TUNEL) and RT-PCR

Total proteins were purified from snap-frozen cardiac tissue with a mammalian cell lysis kit (Sigma, St. Luis, MO) and analyzed by Western blotting against NF-κB rabbit polyclonal antibodies (StressGen, Victoria, Canada). Detection was performed with goat anti-rabbit-HRP antibodies (Pierce, Rockford, IL). TUNEL assay was performed on paraffin sections according to specification from the Klenow-FragEL DNA fragmentation detection kit (Oncogene, Boston, MA). Total RNA was extracted from homogenized frozen tissue samples and concentration determined by spectrophotometer. Total of 5 μg of RNA was reverse-transcribed using oligo (dT) primers and superscript reverse transcriptase according to the manufacturer's instructions (Invitrogen, Carlsbad, CA). Oligonucleotide primer pairs for the 5' and 3' rat NF-κB were selected based on published sequence for complete NF-κB cDNA [40]. PCR products were analyzed in ethidium bromide-stained 2% agarose gel and photographed. The PCR results were scanned, and the densities of gene-specific bands were analyzed using Kodak Digital Science 1D Analysis Software (Version 2.0). All samples were normalized against respective β-actin and results presented as Sum Intensity $\pm$ SD.

Immunohistology

Tissue paraffin sections were incubated with appropriate primary antibody against rat IgG, IgM and NF-kB (BD Biosciences, San Diego, CA). Bound primary antibody was detected using biotinylated rabbit anti-mouse IgG or goat-anti rabbit IgG and streptavidin peroxidase-conjugated complexes obtained from Vector Laboratories (Carpinteria, CA). The control sections were performed by replacing the primary mAb with dilution buffer, normal mouse serum, or normal rabbit serum. Sections were evaluated blindly by counting labeled cells in triplicates within 5 high-power fields (HPF)/section.

Statistical Analysis

Data are presented as mean ± SD. Comparison between groups was done by independent sample t-tests. Probability values (p) of less than 0.05 were considered significant. Statistical analysis was performed with the Microsoft Excel statistical software.

Results

1. Donor-like sMHC Class I Protein Therapy Upregulates Expression of Th2 Dependent Anti-donor Class I Antibodies without Increase of Total amount of Serum Immunoglobulins (Igs)

We have previously demonstrated that treatment with [α_{1h} $^{1/u}$]-RT1.A^a donor-like sMHC proteins, which contains donor-recipient class I MHC sequences, induced indefinite allograft survival and modulated alloantibody responses in ACI (RT1.A^a) recipients of WF (RT1.A^u) hearts [41]. First we tested whether sMHC therapy increased total amount of IgGs in the blood of long-term surviving cardiac recipients. The immunoglobulin isotyping analysis demonstrated no increase in the levels for total IgG1, IgG2a, IgG2b and IgG2c in the serums obtained from long-term ACI cardiac hosts after sMHC therapy compared to control syngeneic serum from untreated rats (Figure 2, A). However, sMHC-conditioning of cardiac recipients resulted in elevated IgG, but not IgM type anti-MHC specific alloantibodies when compared to serums obtained from long-term cardiac hosts after high-dose CsA therapy. Subclass analysis revealed higher titers of allo-IgG1 and allo-IgG2c in sMHC-conditioned hosts (Figure 2, B). Graft vascular endothelial cells (ECs) are first targets for host allo-antibodies and most affected during the development of graft vascular chronic rejection. We have examined whether sMHC-induced sera exhibits altered effector (serum) - target (EC) adhesion qualities by detecting changes in ability of activated WF-donor EC cultures to bind allo-antibodies after incubation with sMHC-conditioned serum. Marked increase in allo-IgG2c binding to activated donor ECs was detected through several serial dilutions. No sufficient difference was found for IgM or IgG binding to IFN-γ activated ECs (Figure 2 C).

2. Prolongation of Survival of Fully Mismatched Cardiac Allografts with Donor-like sMHC Class I Protein Modulated Sera

Singeneic ACI sMHC-modulated sera was obtained from long-term primary ACI recipients of WF hearts with donor-like sMHC protein 100 days post-transpant (Figure 1). To test the role of donor-like sMHC protein-modulated sera on allograft survival, secondary ACI recipients were treated either with 1 mL of unfractioned, whole serum (i.v.) at the day of cardiac engraftment or ACI hosts received a single whole body dose of γ-irradiation (130 Rad) in addition to i.v. serum injection on the day of transplantation. Cardiac recipients treated with ACI syngeneic serum that had high-titer of allo-IgG demonstrated 20% rate of graft survival beyond 100 days (12x2, 15x2, 48, 54, 55, 100x2 d; n=9) unlike hosts that were administered naive serums. Allo-Abs high-titer serum failed to prolong graft life in syngeneic recipients transplanted with third-party cardiac grafts (BN-ACI, MST 16$\pm$3, n=3 vs WF-ACI, MST 46.1$\pm$36.5). Untreated ACI recipients rejected WF cardiac allografts within 7.5$\pm$1.4 days. (Table 1).

Irradiation alone prolonged survival of WF (RT1^u) hearts in ACI (RT1^a) hosts to a mean survival time (MST) of 26.4$\pm$2.1 days ($p<0.001$). The combination of γ-irradiation and syngeneic naive sera resulted in prolongation of graft survival with MST of 25.25$\pm$2.2 days, which was not significantly different from irradiation alone. In sharp contrast, ACI irradiated secondary WF-engrafted hosts that were treated with sMHC-conditioned high-titer allo-IgG sera uniformly showed long-term survival of WF hearts for more then 120 days. The specificity of the response was shown by the inability of sMHC-conditioned high-titer allo-IgG sera to prolong the survival of third-party Brown Norway (BN, $RT1^n$) hearts in secondary ACI rats (MST 17.3±3.7, *P* NS). Surprisingly, ACI syngeneic serum harvested from long-term surviving cardiac hosts treated with high-dose CsA which contained minimal all-antibody levels combined with small dose whole body irradiation demonstrated mild immunosuppressive effect and prolonged WF heart survival time in average up to 51 days (Table 2).

3. Vascular Endothelial Antibody Binding and DNA Fragmentation in Long-term Surviving Cardiac Grafts after Therapy with High-titer allo-IgG Serums

Immunohistological assessment of WF allografts at 120 days in secondary sera-treated recipients, where chronic rejection and neointimal proliferation were averted, showed mild IgM and strong IgG antibody binding to vascular endothelial cells. In marked contrast, hearts of naive animals that were used as negative controls demonstrated no immunoglobulin staining or visible deposits on the vascular endothelial cells (Figure 3, A). DNA fragmentation was utilized to access level of cell apoptosis in the graft tissue. As shown in figure 3 B, the amount of positive apoptotic elements in chronically rejected grafts following CsA therapy was similar to acute rejecting controls (45±8.1 and 75±6, per 5/HPF, respectively). In marked contrast, cardiac allografts in secondary recipients treated with sMHC-conditioned sera where chronic rejection was abrogated, demonstrated a decreased number of apoptotic cells (13.4±2), similar to naïve, untreated control (7.5±1.2, *P* NS).

Table 1. Long-term cardiac allograft survival in ACI recipients treated with serum conditioned by sMHC proteins

Donor Strain	Number per group	Treatment[I]	Graft Survival, days	Mean ± SD
WF	8	N/A	6x2, 7x3, 8, 9, 10	7.5±1.4
WF	3	naïve ACI serum	35, 27, 28	30 ± 4.4
WF	3	naïve WF serum	13, 14, 15	14 ± 1
WF	3	naïve BN serum	14, 15, 16	15±1
BN	3	sMHC-conditioned serum	12, 18, 19	16.3±3.8
WF	9	sMHC-conditioned serum	12x2, 15x2, 48, 54, 55, 100, 104	46.1±36.5

[I] ACI secondary recipients were injected on the day of transplantation with i.v. injection of 1 mL of serum obtained from naïve, untreated rats or from primary long-term (100 days) ACI recipients of WF hearts treated with sMHC proteins (0.1 mg/rat).

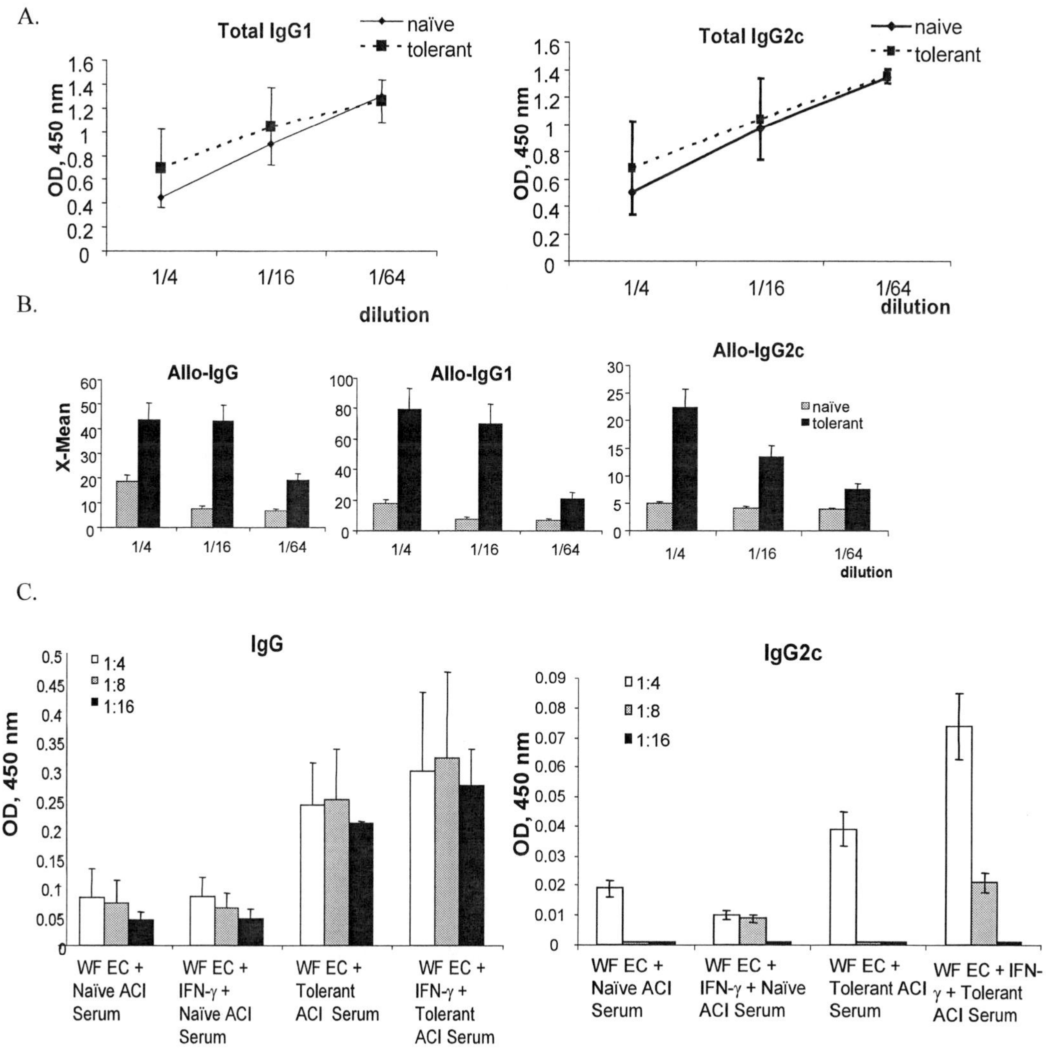

Figure 2. A. sMHC therapy does not increase the total amount of IgGs in the blood of long-term surviving cardiac recipients. Total rat immunoglobulin isotypes were detected in whole serum of naïve or long-term surviving cardiac recipients with Rat Immunoglobulin Isotyping ELISA Kit. Data present three independent experiments; each group includes 5 animals and data presented as 450 nm OD mean $\pm$ SD. All data points were done in triplicates. B. Allo-Abs production in primary hosts. Sera were collected at 100 days from ACI recipients of WF hearts, which were treated with low-dose CsA (10 mg/kg/day, 3days) and $[\alpha_{1h}^{u/l}]$-RT1.A^a donor-like class I MHC (0.1 mg, p.v., day 0); and compared to naïve serum from untreated ACI rats. Presence of allo-Abs against WF antigens in the serum of ACI recipients was analyzed by Flow cytometry (dilutions 1:4; 1:16; 1:64). Allo-IgM, IgG, IgG1, IgG2a, IgGb and IgGc were tested. Data presented as X-Mean $\pm$ SD, each bar represents 3 independent experiments. C. sMHC-induced sera exhibits altered effector (serum) - target (EC) adhesion qualities. IgG subtypes ELISA binding test to resting or IFN-γ activated WF ECs was performed with 1:4, 1:8 & 1:16 dilutions of experimental or control serums. Marked increase in IgG2c binding to activated donor ECs was detected through several serial dilutions.

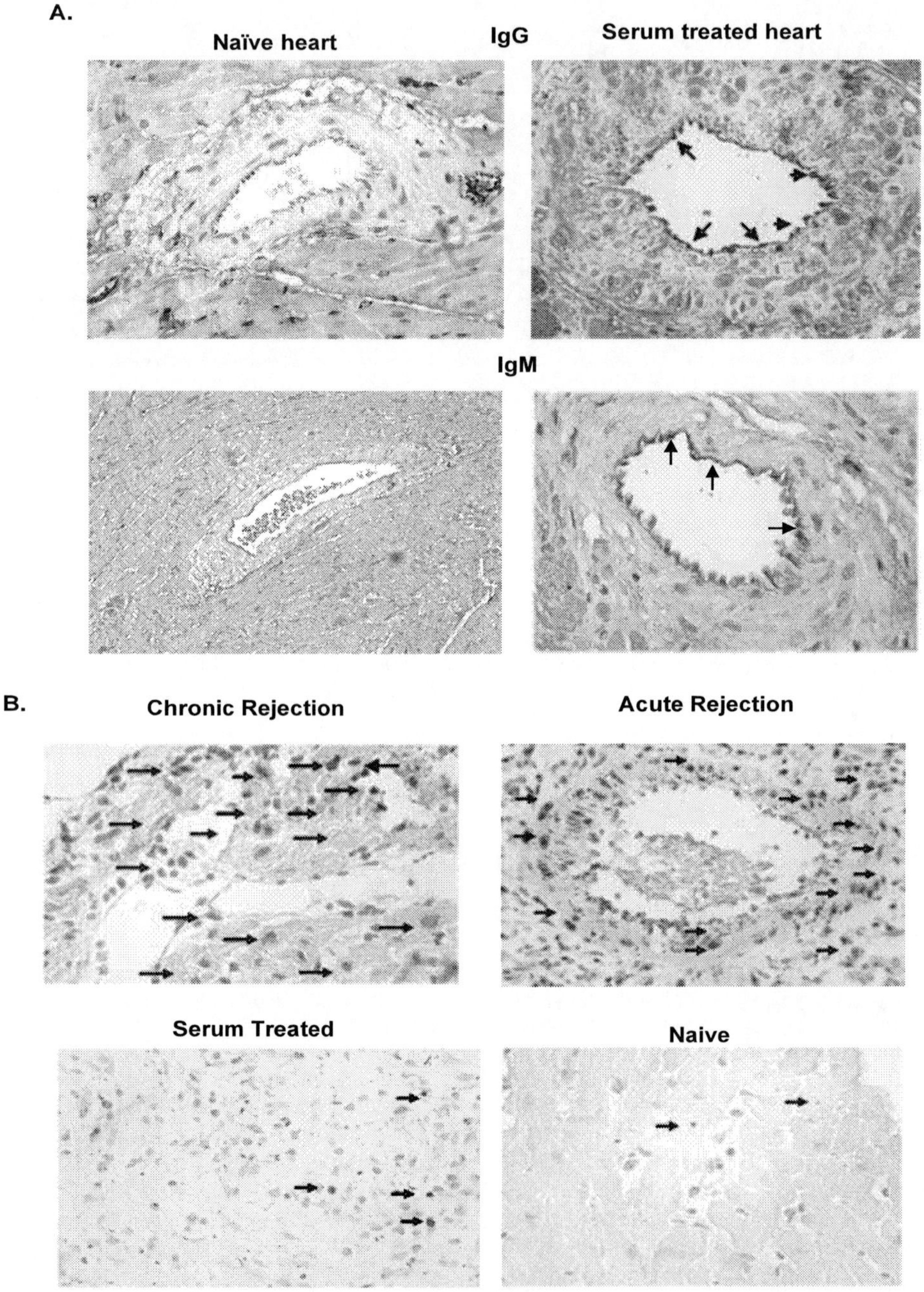

Figure 3. A. Immunohistological analysis for IgG and IgM immunoglobulin deposits in WF heart allografts of ACI recipients at day 100 posttransplant. Cardiac grafts from syngeneic ACI recipients and cardiac allografts in ACI recipients treated with sMHC-conditioned serum demonstrate evidence of vascular endothelial antibody binding but no signs of chronic rejection. There were three to five animals per group. B. DNA fragmentation (TUNEL). DNA fragmentation analysis was performed on WF allografts that exhibited chronic rejection in ACI hosts following high-dose CsA therapy, allografts in sera-treated ACI secondary hosts, WF grafts that were acutely rejected by ACI recipients with no treatment and on naïve, untreated ACI hearts. Acutely rejecting cardiac allografts and naive hearts served as positive and negative controls, respectively. Arrows demonstrate apoptotic cells within graft myocardium. A representative of 3 different experiments is shown.

Table 2. Long-term cardiac allograft survival in secondary ACI recipients

Donor Strain	Number per group	Treatment[1]	Graft Survival, days	Mean ± SD
WF	5	γ-irradiation	24, 25, 26, 28, 29	26.4±2.1
WF	4	γ-irradiation + naïve ACI serum	23, 24, 28, 26	25.25 ± 2.2
WF	10	γ-irradiation + low-titer allo-IgG serum	38, 39, 43, 46 48, 50, 57, 62, 65, 70	51.8±11.2
WF	13	γ-irradiation + high-titer allo-IgG serum	80x2, >120x11	>120
BN	3	γ-irradiation + high-titer allo-IgG serum	14, 18, 19	17.3±3.7

[1] Lightly γ-irradiated ACI secondary recipients (130 Rad) were treated on the day of transplantation with i.v. injection of 1 mL of serum obtained from naïve ACI rats or from primary long-term (100 days) ACI recipients of WF heart allografts. Low-titer and high-titer allo-IgG serums were obtained by treating primary ACI hosts either with high-dose CsA (10 mg/kg/day, 3 days, p.o.) or with donor-like sMHC protein (1 mg/rat).

4. Effect of sMHC-conditioned Serum on EC Metabolism and T Cell Responses

In vitro studies on whether a sMHC-conditioned serum that has high titers of allo-IgGs can alter metabolic functions of ECs assessed on the level of RNA synthesis demonstrated that allogeneic serum (ACI) conditioned with sMHC class I proteins directly inhibits metabolic activity of IFN-γ activated donor (WF) ECs without significant changes in metabolic activity in non-activated EC cultures. Interestingly, an experiment with naïve serum that does not have allo-IgG antibodies and was obtained from untreated ACI rats revealed suppressing effect of naïve serum on IFN-γ activated EC cultures also. In contrast, serum from ACI recipients that rejected WF cardiac grafts in acute manner significantly stimulated RNA synthesis in WF EC cultures both IFN-γ activated and non-stimulated (data not shown). ECs that were incubated with fetal bovine serum (FBS, 5%) added to media served as positive control for a normal EC metabolic activity *in vitro*. WF EC cells that were incubated in serum-free media were used as baseline to detect a minimal RNA synthesis activity (Fig 4, A).

Mixed lymphocyte reaction (MLR) was performed on LN T cells from naïve ACI rats (responders) stimulated with syngeneic (ACI), donor (WF) or third-party (BN) splenocytes in the presence of naïve (no allo-IgG) or sMHC-conditioned (allo-IgG) serums. sMHC-conditioned but not naïve serum significantly blocked ACI T cell proliferative responses against WF donor antigens. Unexpectedly, sMHC-conditioned serum non-specifically suppressed proliferative response in the wells that had third-party (BN) and syngeneic (ACI) antigens as well (Figure 4 B).

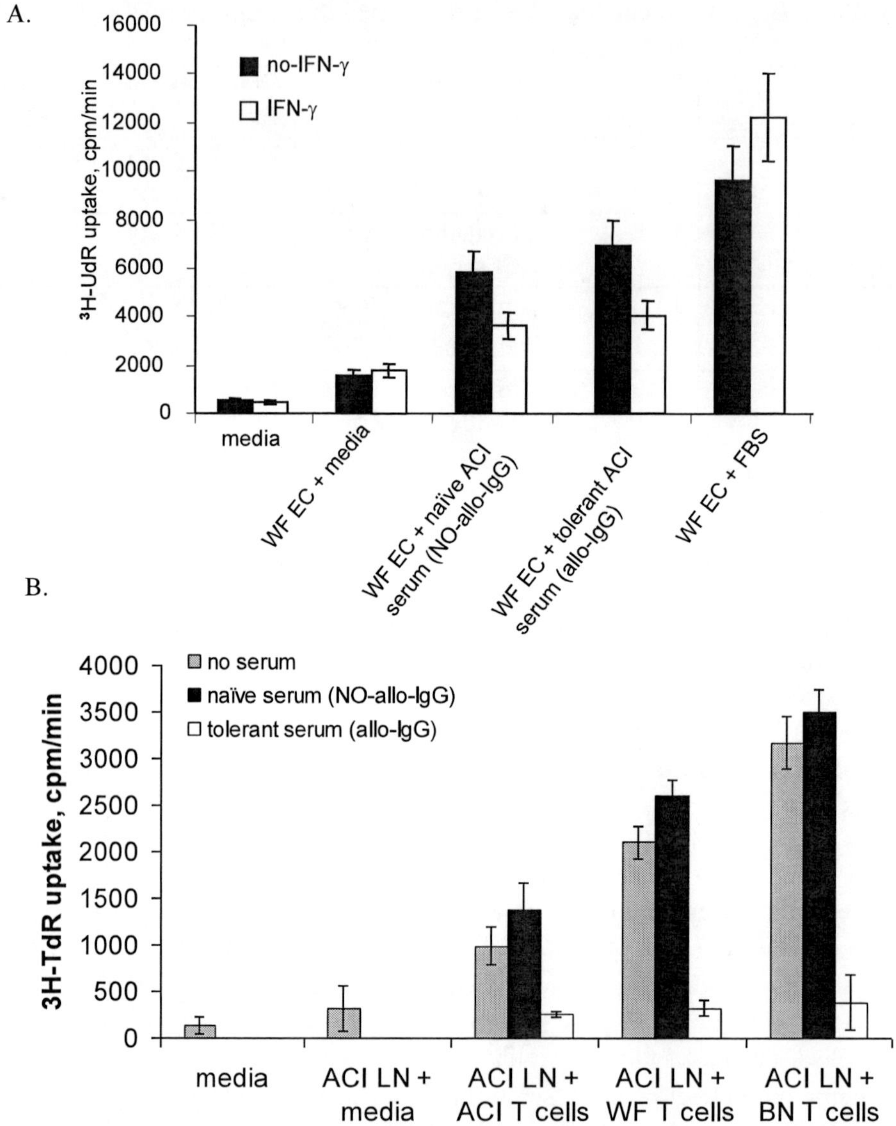

Figure 4. A. Serum conditioned with sMHC proteins can alter metabolic function of ECs. RNA turnover assay uses ^{3}H-uridine incorporation into newly synthesized RNA as indicator of cell metabolic activity. Three day ECs cultures incubated with or without rIFN-γ (500U/ml) and pulsed with 2 μCi/well of ^{3}H-uridine for 20 hrs were used in RNA turnover assay to demonstrated effect of sMHC-conditioned serum. B. *In vitro* suppression of T cell responses. Mixed lymphocyte reaction (MLR) was performed on LN T cells from naïve ACI rats (responders) and stimulated with syngeneic ACI or donor WF or third-party BN spleen cells. MRL cultures were incubated either with no syngeneic serum or with naïve serum (no allo-IgG) or with sMHC-conditioned serum. sMHC-conditioned but not naïve serum significantly blocked ACI recipient T cell proliferative responses to WF T cell donor stimulation. Data represent three independent experiments and presented as cpm/min $\pm$ SD, all cultures were done in triplicates.

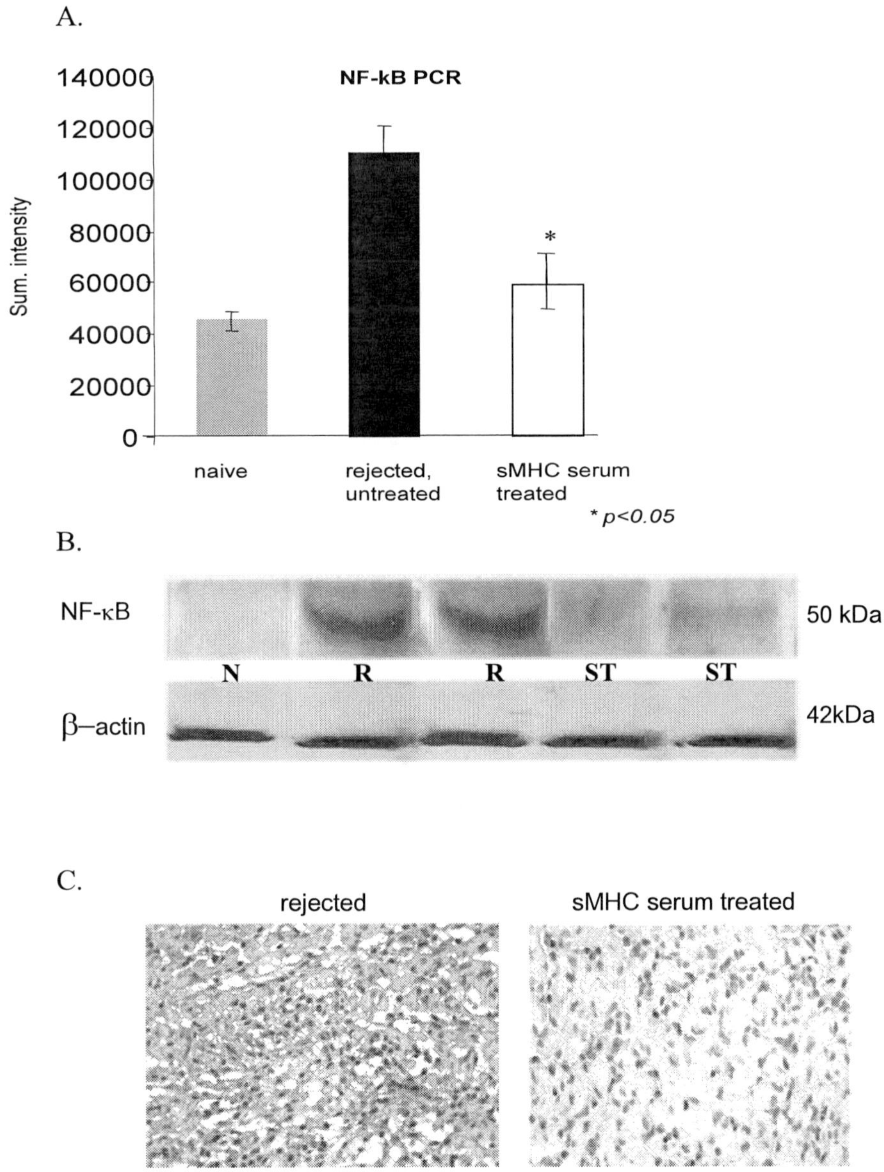

Figure 5. Level of NF-κB activation in the graft could contribute into development of transplant chronic rejection. A. PCR analysis of NF-κB gene expression in naïve WF hearts, acutely rejecting WF hearts and long-term surviving WF transplants treated with sMHC-conditioned serum. Long-term surviving grafts demonstrated reduced level of NF-κB gene expression. NF-κB gene expression was quantified by RT-PCR method with subsequent normalization to housekeeping gene and presented as summarized intensity. B. Western-blot for expression of NF-κB protein in the grafts. Protein expression repeats PCR pattern. C. Immunohistology of acutely rejecting cardiac tissue and sMHC-serum treated heart. sMHC-serum treated transplants demonstrated significantly less NF-κB positive cells then rejecting heart.

5. Prolongation of Cardiac Graft Survival after sMHC-conditioned Serum Treatment Could be Partially Dependent on the Level of NF-κB Activation

It is well known that NF-κB transcription factors are involved in many processes that are important for B cell development, differentiation and IgM/IgG immunoglobulin switch [42]. The cardiac recipients treated with sMHC-conditioned serum demonstrated impaired allo-antibody production, moreover, detected allo-antibodies were mostly IgG2b type (data not shown) that known to be Th2 dependent, we suggested that it would be logical to test level of NF-κB gene and protein expression in the cardiac graft tissue. NF-κB gene expression was quantified by RT-PCR method with subsequent normalization to housekeeping gene and presented as summarized intensity (Figure 5, A). mRNA from long-term surviving grafts had significantly less copies of NF-κB gene than samples from acutely rejecting recipients (positive control). Furthermore, detection of p50 subunit of NF-κB that reduces IgM and IgG synthesis in B cells [42] showed strongly diminished content of this protein in cardiac tissue of long-term surviving hosts treated with sMHC-conditioned serum compared to acutely rejecting hearts (Figure 5, B). Immunohistological analysis clearly demonstrated presence of the numerous NF-κB positive cells in acutely rejecting grafts on the background of significantly necrotic tissue while long-term serum treated hearts represented much less positive cells on a very good morphological surrounding (Figure 5, C).

6. Effect of IgG Serum Fractions on Cardiac Allograft Survival

To elucidate the role of serum humoral factors on prolongation of transplant survival, we prepared immunoglobulin fractions (IgG/PBS) from sMHC-conditioned rat serum with Melon Gel IgG spin purification system (purity assessed on SDS-PAGE gel was >95%). The new cohorts of syngeneic cardiac test recipients were i.v. treated with 0.1 and 1 mg of IgGs at day of cardiac transplantation. We analyzed allogeneic cardiac grafts for the survival and development of chronic rejection. Control groups were treated with IgG purified from naïve syngeneic serum. Hearts in the control group treated with 0.1 mg of IgG were acutely rejected after 15 days post-transplant (MST 15.0±0, n=3) and ten-fold dose increase had not effect on prolongation of graft survival. All transplants in the experimental groups were acutely rejected also (Table 3). However, combination of 0.1 mg of IgG and whole body γ-irradiation (130 Rad) resulted in sufficient prolongation of graft life up to 73 days in average (MST 73.8±51, n=7).

CONCLUSION

The aim of the present study was to determine whether soluble donor-like MHC class I proteins can induce donor-specific regulatory factors in the blood of long-term surviving allogeneic cardiac graft recipients. Our findings show that MHC class I donor-like molecules administrated peri-transplant through the portal vein in the presence of subtherapeutic CsA induced donor-specific regulatory factors in the blood of allogeneic cardiac recipients. These factors could be passively transferred to the new syngeneic cardiac transplant recipients. Such factors affect recipient immune system toward donor specific tolerance. In our experiments, only ACI rats transferred with sMHC-conditioned serum from long-term graft surviving recipients demonstrated prolongation of allo-graft survival. ACI recipients that received naïve ACI syngeneic or third party serums rejected their cardiac transplants within 4 weeks post-transplantation in compare to 17 weeks in long-term surviving group.

Table 3. Long-term cardiac allograft survival in secondary ACI recipients treated with serum IgG fractions

Donor Strain	Number per group	Treatment[1]	Graft Survival, days	Mean ± SD
WF	3	0.1 mg	10, 11, 14	11.1±2
WF	3	1 mg	16x3	16±0
WF	7	γ-irradiation + 0.1 mg	20x3, 97, 120x3	73.8±51

[1] ACI recipients of WF hearts were i.v. injected on the day of transplantation with IgG fractions purified from whole serums obtained from long-term surviving ACI cardiac recipients treated with sMHC proteins.

The ability of sera to induce rejection or enhancement of allograft survival has been well established [43]. However, the underlying mechanisms for such seemingly opposing effects in transplantation are not well defined. Our data indicate that IgG antibodies (Abs) detected in the sera were responsible for allograft protection. Transfer of class I modulated sera, which contained high IgG titers, induced long-term graft survival and abrogated chronic rejection. In sharp contrast, graft protection was not afforded in secondary hosts after transfer of sera from CsA-treated recipients that exhibit minimal antibody levels.

Immunomodulating effect of sMHC-conditioned serum on immune system of ACI rats resulted in abrogation of chronic rejection in allogeneic cardiac transplants. In previous work we have showed that donor-like MHC class I proteins regulate immune system of recipients through the development of vascular accommodation [15]. Accommodation in our model was characterized by vascular endothelial Abs binding and reduced apoptosis in long-term sMHC-treated allografts. Analysis of serum from long-term sMHC-treated recipients demonstrated up-regulation of IgG, IgG1 and IgG2c alloantibodies that reached its peak by 44 days post-transplant and then stayed stable up to 120 days post-transplantation [20]. In the present study, transfer of syngeneic serum that has donor allo-Abs did not prevent IgM/IgG switch in recipients with allogeneic cardiac transplants moreover we detected attenuated IgG and no visible IgM allo-Abs in the blood of long-term survived passively transferred WF cardiac recipients. Further analysis showed strong dichotomization of IgG allo-Abs toward Th2 dependent types [44]. We found significant increase for IgG2b and attenuated level of IgG1. Unlike sMHC protein treated recipients, cardiac hosts that were injected with one mL of sMHC-conditioned serum demonstrated impaired allo-Ab production, statistically significant changes were detected for IgG2b only. Elevated level of these immunoglobulins was higher than in control group and in some samples was comparable to samples from acute rejecting cardiac recipients. Such selective inhibition of immunoglobulin expression cannot be explained by a simple passive transfer of blocking serum antibody including anti-MHC antibody or by modification of T-helper subsets. We cannot explain such prolonged effect of serum transfer by a simple passive increase of anti-idiotypic antibody against anti-MHC or soluble MHC antigens.

Antibodies administered to animals together with their specific antigen (Ag) are known to feedback regulate the Ab response to this Ag [45]. The regulatory effects are potent, as small doses of syngeneic Ab can result in 99% suppression or a 1000-fold enhancement. The best described negative feedback regulation is the ability of all IgG subclasses to completely suppress and IgM to enhance the response to erythrocytes [46]. Although IgG suppresses the Ab response to erythrocytes, it can enhance responses to soluble proteins [45]. The IgG1-, IgG2a-, and IgG2b-mediated enhancement takes place in the absence of complement [47, 48] but seem to require activating FcγR [49] and probably act by increasing of Ag presentation to Th cells. Such activation was dependent on $CD23^+$ B cells. Taken together, these data indicate that administered sera which contains high titer of allo-Abs initiates a complex antigen presentation sequel to activate naive T cells *in vivo*, and thus suggest a critical role for B cells [50]. Such complex serum-induced Ag presentation, where the final outcome may be determined by the type of activated T cell, may explain the different effects of enhancement or rejection of allografts following sera transfer. It may also explain the different Ab profile obtained in our secondary recipients with high levels of the Th2-dependant IgG2b when compared to the primary hosts that displayed up-regulation of IgG1 and IgG2c alloantibodies. Another very interesting observation connects the anti-inflammatory activity of IgGs with the form of Fc fragment sialylation. There are data indicating that passive immunization with IgG Abs can switch from a pro-inflamatory to an anti-inflamatory species by changing the extent of sialylation of the N-linked glycan on the Fc domain [51].

The roles that different immunoglobulins play in graft rejection/survival have not been clearly defined. Some authors have reported that the binding of IgG2c to vascular endothelium of hamster xenograft was associated with long-term survival of the grafts while rejection was probably due to IgG1, or IgG2a or IgG2b isotypes. Others have suggested only purified IgG2b and IgG2c are capable of inducing xenograft rejection in a compliment-dependent manner in hamsters [52]. In our model of tolerance development we found that the transfer of sMHC-conditioned serum with allo-reactive Abs leads to a positive regulation of T-dependent IgG2b production after IgM/IgG isotype switch, and immunohistology staining of long-term surviving cardiac grafts after sMHC-conditioned serum treatment showed noticeable IgG and IgM deposits on graft vascular endothelium. Nevertheless, the exact mechanisms by which chronic rejection is inhibited and prolongation of graft survival is achieved can be only elucidated by analysis of the type of binding antibody and dissection of its effects on endothelial cell function. The identification of the critical antibodies and corresponding targets may pave the way for development of antibody therapy that inhibits chronic rejection, akin to the principles applied for antibody therapy or chronic rejection or prevention of immunization in (RhD)-negative women [53].

The investigation of the possible molecular mechanisms that could be in account for the development of long-term transplant acceptance in recipients treated with sMHC-conditioned serum we analyzed alterations in NFκB expression [54, 55]. NF-κB is a key player in the regulation of pro-inflammatory genes in vascular endothelial cells. Moreover, this transcription factor involved into B cell development, differentiation and IgM/IgG immunoglobulin switch. In addition, it had been shown that p50 subunit of NF-κB down-regulates IgM and IgG synthesis in B cells [42]. We have detected decreased expression of NFκB in sMHC-serum treated allografts as compared to those undergoing chronic rejection, and long-term surviving cardiac recipients showed impaired allo-Abs production as well. The inhibition of NFκB following sera transfer in our experiments is consistent with the recent finding that intravenous immunoglobulin (IVIG) inhibits NFκB [56].

In summary, donor-like MHC class I therapy orchestrates the development of protective allo-Abs that can be transferred to a new recipient. Modulated protective alloAbs can induce specific tolerance to MHC mismatching graft in allogeneic transplant. These novel findings demand further investigation of modified class I MHC molecules ability to induce tolerance and inhibit chronic rejection.

REFERENCES

[1] K. Shimomura, M. A. Hardy, S. F. Oluwole, *Transplantation,* 60, 806 (1995)

[2] G. Remuzzi, M. Rossini, O. Imberti, N. Perico, *Lancet* 337, 750, (1991)

[3] N. C. Chowdhury, D.V. Saborio, M. Garrovillo, A. Chandraker, C.C. Magee, A. M. Waaga, et al., *Transplantation,* 66, 1059, (1998)

[4] J. S. Odorico, C. F. Barker, A. M. Posselt, A. Naji, *Surgery,* (1992) 112, 370, (1992)

[5] R. R. Ghobrial, T. Hamashima, M. E. Wang, M. Wang, S. M. Stepkowski, B. D. Kahan, *Transplantation,* 62, 1002, (1996)

[6] T. Hamashima, S. Stepkowski, T. C. Chou, B. Kahan, *Transplant Immunol,* 3, 335, (1995)

[7] H. Shirwan, L. Barwari, N. Sattar-Khan, *Transplantation,* 32, 345, (1998)

[8] H. Shirwan, *Transplantation,* 68, 715, (1999)

[9] N. Semiltova, X. D. Shen, M. C. Fishbein, F. Gao, S. J. Slomowitz, Q. Jiao, et al., *Transplantation,* 75, 550 (2003)

[10] J. W. Fry, P. J. Morris, K. J. Wood, *Gene Therapy*, 9, 22, (2002)

[11] J. C. Madsen, R. A. Superina, K. J. Wood, P. J. Morris, *Nature,* 332, 161, (1988)

[12] R. J. Duquesnoy, L. T. White, J. W. Fierst, M. Vanek, B. F. Banner, Y. Iwaki Y, T. E. Starzl, *Transplantation,* ***50,*** 427, (1990)

[13] A. C. Papassavas, A. Iniotaki-Theodoraki, J. Boletis, P. Douramani, A. Kostakis, *Hum Immunol,* 61, 705, (2000)

[14] T. E. Starzl, M. Eliasziw, D. Gjertson, P. I. Terasaki, J. J. Fung, M. Trucco, et al., *Transplantation* 64, 983, (1997)

[15] N. V. Semiletova, X. D. Shen, B. Baibakov, D. M. Feldman, K. Mukherjee, J. M. Frank, et al., *Transplantation*, 80, 1535, (2005)

[16] D. Liu, X. D. Shen, Z. Fang, F. Gao, N. Semiletova, M. J. Cao, et al., *Transplant Proc,* 37, 1942, (2005)

[17] N. V. Semiletova, X. D. Shen, D. M. Feldman, R. W. Busuttil, J. W. Kupiec-Weglinski, et al., *Transplant Proc,* (2005) 37, 193, (2005)

[18] N. V. Semiletova, X. D. Shen, S. J. Slomowitz, B. Baibakov, D. M. Feldman, R. W. Busuttil, et al., *Transplant Proc* 37, 35, (2005)

[19] N. Semiletova, X. D. Shen, F. Gao, S. J. Slomowitz, Q. Jiao, R. W. Busuttil,et al., *Transplant Proc,* 34, 1402, (2002)

[20] J. S. Singer, A. Mhoyan, M. C. Fishbein, X. D. Shen, F. Gao, D. Zhao, et al., *Transplantation,* 72, 1408 (2001)
[21] S. Hayashi, D. Leu, Y. Yamii, G. Mei, H. Takagi, A. Nakao, *Transplantation*, 80, 494, (2005)
[22] S. M. Stepkowski, M. Wang, J. Langowski, R. Ghobrial, X. Qu, J. Yu,et al., *Transplant Proc,* 29, 1663, (1997)
[23] J. S. Madsen, K. Yamada, J. S. Allan, J. K. Choo, A. E. Erthon, M. R. Pins,et al., *Transplantation,* 65, 304, (1998)
[24] S. C. Chueh, L. Tian, M. Wang, M. E. Wang, S. M. Stepkowski, B. D. Kahan, *Transplantation,* 64, 1407, (1997)
[25] S. Strobel, A. M Mowat, H. E. Drummond, M. G. Pickering, A. Ferguson, *Immunology,* 49, 51, (1983)
[26] T. G. Harriott-Smith, W. J. Halliday, *Clin Exp Immunol,* 71, 144, (1988)
[27] S. Ostman, M. Taube, E. Telemo, Immunology, 116, 464, (2005)
[28] K. L. Elkins, P. W. Stashak, P. J. Baker, *Infection and Immunity,* 55, 3093, (1987)
[29] M. Ghio, P. Contini, C. Mazzei, A. Merlo, G. Filaci, M. Setti, et al., *Transfusion,* 41, 988, (2001)
[30] S. Dzik, M. A. Blajchman, N. Blumberg, S. A. Kirkley, J. M. Heal, K. Wood, *Vox Sang,* 70, 187, (1996)
[31] J. Wang, E. K. Geissler, J. Fechner, W. J. Burlingham, S. Knechtle, *J Surg Res,* 57, 150, (1994)
[32] S. F. Oluwole, K. Tezuka, T. Wasfie, M. D. Stegall, K. Reemtsma, M. A. Hardy, *Transplantation,* 48, 751, (1989)
[33] M. Ferraresso,R. Ghobrial, S. M. Stepkowski, B. D. Khan, *Transplantation,* 55, 888, (1993)
[34] S-C., Chueh, L. Tian, M. Wang, M-Er. Wang, S. M. Stepkowski, B. D. Kahan, *Transplantation,* 64, 1407, (1997)
[35] R. Hausmann, N. Zavazava, J. Steinmann, W. Muller-Ruchholtz, *Clin Exp Immunol,* 91, 183, (1993)
[36] M. H. Sayegh, C. B. Carpenter, *Int Rev Immunol,* 13, 221, (1996).
[37] N. Zavazava, M. Kronke, *Nature Med,* 2, 1005, (1996)
[38] K. Ono, E. S. Lindsey, *J Thorac Cardiovascular Surg,* 57, 225, (1969)
[39] Rattus norvegicus nuclear factor kappa B p105 subunit mRNA, 3' end. ACCESSION #L26267, *http://www.ncbi.nlm.nih.gov/nuccore/425471*
[40] A. L. Kenter, R. Wuerffel, C. Dominguez, A. Shanmugam, H. Zhang, *J Exp Med,* 199, 617, (2004)
[41] N. V. Semiletova, X. D. Shen, D. M. Feldman, F. Gao, A. Mhoyan, D. Liu, et al., *Cell Immunol*, (2007) 248, 48, (2007)
[42] P. J. Morris, *Immunol. Rev,* 48, 93, (1980)
[43] H. D. Kim, Y. Cao, F. K. Kong, K. R. Kampen, T. L. Lewis, Z. Ma, et al., *Vaccine,* 23, 2977, (2005)
[44] B. Heyman, *Annu Rev Immunol,* 18, 709, (2000)
[45] D. Nemazee, A. Gavin, K. Hoebe, B. Beutler, *Nature,* 441, E4, (2006)
[46] C. Henry, N. Jerene, *J. Exp. Med,* 128:133-152, (1968)
[47] P. Coulie, J. Van Snick, *Eur. J. Immunol,* 15, 793, (1985)

[48] S. Applequist, E. J. Dahlström, N. Jiang, H. Molina, B. Heyman, *J. Immunol*, 165, 2398, (2000)
[49] E. J. Wiersma, M. Nose, B. Heyman. *Eur. J. Immunol,* 20, 2585, (1990)
[50] S. Wernersson, M. C. Karlsson, J. Dahlström, R. Mattsson, J. S. Verbeek, B. Heyman, *J. Immunol,* 163, 618, (1999)
[51] *A. Getahun, F. Hjelm, B. Heyman, J. Immunol,* 175, 1473, *(2005)*
[52] Y. Kaneko, F. Nimmerjahn, J. V. Ravetch, *Science,* 313, 670, (2006)
[53] G. D. Wu, E. Gochi, Y-S. Jin, J. Swensson, V. A. Starnes, D. V. Cramer, *Xenotransplantation,* 8, 291, (2001)
[54] A. Lubenko, M. Williams, A. Johnson, J. Pluck, D. Armstrong, S. MacLennan, *Transfusion Medicine,* 9, 331, (1999)
[55] M. A. Read, M. Z. Whitley, A. J. Williams, T. Collins, *J. Exp. Me*, 179, 503, (1994)
[56] T. Ichiyama , Y. Ueno, M. Hasegawa, A. Niimi, T. Matsubara, S. Furukawa, Naunyn Schmiedebergs Arch. *Pharmacol,* 369, 428, (2004).

INDEX

A

acetylation, 93
acid, x, 69, 76, 77, 95
acquired immunity, x, 119, 130
acquired immunodeficiency syndrome, 66
ACs, 3, 4, 5
activation state, 31
acute infection, 152
acute myeloid leukemia, 95, 101, 114
adaptation, 47, 129
adaptive immunity, 19, 123
adenocarcinoma, 102, 116
adhesion, 28, 161, 163
adult T-cell, 12, 13, 14, 15
Adult T-cell leukemia-lymphoma (ATL), vii, 1, 2, 3, 4, 5, 6, 7, 11, 13
adults, 63, 67
adverse effects, 19
age, 2, 45, 46, 59, 60, 64, 65, 101
AIDS, 15, 65, 66, 67, 75, 100, 113, 114, 137, 138
alanine, 74
algorithm, 60
allele, 44, 53, 58, 59, 64, 67, 71, 72, 73, 74, 77, 78, 79, 80, 84, 85, 88, 94, 105, 109, 129, 133, 136, 138, 142, 144
allelic loss, 49
allergic rhinitis, 96, 111
allergy, 93
allograft survival, 154, 161, 162, 165, 169
alters, 52
alveolitis, 2, 14, 15
amino, ix, 69, 72, 74, 76, 77, 79, 80, 81, 89, 120, 121, 122, 123, 140, 154, 158
amino acid(s), ix, 69, 72, 74, 76, 77, 79, 80, 81, 89, 120, 121, 122, 123, 141, 154, 158
amphibia, 51
ancestral haplotype (AH), viii, 23, 40, 56, 57, 60, 61, 65
angiogenesis, 106
antibody, 5, 7, 12, 37, 64, 90, 98, 103, 125, 128, 144, 156, 158, 160, 162, 164, 168, 169, 170
anti-cancer, 103
antigen, vii, viii, x, 2, 4, 7, 9, 10, 11, 12, 13, 14, 17, 18, 19, 20, 21, 22, 25, 26, 27, 28, 29, 32, 33, 34, 35, 36, 37, 38, 39, 40, 41, 44, 45, 47, 48, 50, 51, 53, 61, 70, 76, 77, 81, 87, 91, 92, 97, 102, 104, 105, 106, 107, 108, 112, 113, 115, 116, 117, 119, 120, 123, 124, 125, 130, 131, 132, 133, 134, 136, 140, 141, 144, 145, 146, 147, 148, 149, 150, 151, 154, 156, 170
antigen processing pathway, 22, 76, 77, 81
antigenicity, 139, 143
antigen-presenting cell(s) (APCs), 11, 14, 26, 27, 28, 29, 30, 31, 32, 33, 34, 35, 36, 37, 38, 39, 40, 41, 71, 91, 92, 105, 107, 117, 120, 133, 140, 141, 144, 145, 146, 156
antiretrovirals, 75
antitumor, 18, 20, 22, 23, 103
apoptosis, 36, 90, 91, 106, 113, 124, 125, 133, 134, 151, 154, 156, 162, 169
ARC, 50
arginine, 90, 122
arteries, 126
artery, 93, 97
arthritis, ix, 2, 56
ascites, 102, 116, 128
assessment, 85, 162
asthma, 111, 128, 137
astrocytoma, 129
asymptomatic, 3, 12, 75, 128
ATP, 96, 111
autoimmune disease(s), 3, 70, 93, 103, 120, 125, 133, 134
autoimmunity, x, 14, 35, 36, 64, 87, 88, 120
avian, 48, 54

avian influenza, 48, 54

B

Baars, 52
BAC, 48
bacteria, ix, x, 39, 44, 61, 69, 119, 126
bacterial infection, ix, 45, 56, 138, 140, 155
barriers, 46
beneficial effect, 63, 88
benign, 102, 116
bias, 74
bicarbonate, 158
biochemistry, 76
biodiversity, 48
bioinformatics, x, 69, 75, 78, 140
biological systems, 77
biopsy, 98, 112, 136
biotechnology, 83, 85
bird flu, 148
birth rate, 127
birth weight, 127
blood, xi, 63, 91, 97, 99, 126, 127, 137, 139, 143, 153, 155, 156, 158, 161, 163, 168, 169
blood flow, 97, 127
blood supply, 126
blood transfusion, 155, 156
blood transfusions, 156
blueprint, 84
bonds, 89, 150
bone, 8, 10, 34, 39, 101, 127, 140
bone marrow, 8, 10, 34, 39, 101, 127, 140
bone marrow transplant, 127
breast cancer, 95, 101, 102, 110, 115, 128, 137, 149
breast carcinoma, 102, 115, 128
breeding, 45, 50
bronchial epithelial cells, 98
bronchiolitis, 98

C

Ca^{2+}, 158
cancer, vii, viii, 7, 13, 14, 17, 18, 21, 22, 37, 43, 45, 46, 52, 53, 88, 95, 96, 100, 101, 102, 103, 107, 109, 110, 116, 132, 134, 136, 147, 148, 149
cancer cells, 18
candidates, 72, 149
carbohydrate, 102
carcinoembryonic antigen, 102
carcinoma, 101, 102, 115, 116, 123, 128
cardiac allografts, xi, 153, 154, 155, 156, 157, 158, 161, 162, 164
carnivores, 52
case studies, 45
Caucasian population, 61, 65
Caucasians, 60, 61, 64
CD8+, vii, xi, 1, 3, 4, 5, 6, 7, 8, 9, 10, 12, 13, 18, 23, 27, 28, 30, 31, 32, 33, 36, 37, 39, 40, 79, 82, 83, 90, 91, 92, 100, 101, 106, 124, 125, 129, 132, 133, 134, 135, 137, 139, 140, 142, 144, 147, 148, 152, 156
CD95, 133, 152
cDNA, 160
cell cycle, 128
cell death, 14, 152
cell differentiation, 15, 101
cell line, 13, 20, 22, 46, 94, 95, 96, 99, 100, 110, 113, 128
cell lines, 22, 94, 95, 96, 99, 110, 113, 128
cell surface, viii, 18, 19, 25, 26, 29, 30, 31, 33, 36, 38, 44, 80, 93, 94, 95, 96, 99, 100, 103, 105, 113, 114, 120, 121, 122, 123, 124, 125, 133, 141, 142, 145, 146, 147, 152
cellular immunity, 10, 46, 74
cervical cancer, 102
challenges, 49, 71, 75, 84, 85
chaperones, 141
chemical, 44, 76, 78, 80, 95
chemical properties, 80
chemokine receptor, 27, 38, 91, 107
chemokines, 90, 93
chemotaxis, 91, 107
chemotherapy, vii, 1, 2, 11, 15, 103, 115
chimpanzee, 49, 51
choriocarcinoma, 95, 96, 103, 110
chromosome, ix, 18, 56, 70, 71, 87, 88, 89, 95, 120, 121, 123, 137
chronic lymphocytic leukemia, 101, 114, 115
chronic myelogenous, 136
chronic rejection, xi, 98, 99, 153, 154, 155, 156, 161, 162, 164, 167, 168, 169, 170, 171
chronic venous insufficiency, 60
cirrhosis, 73
classes, ix, 44, 69
classification, 74, 101, 142
cleavage, 76, 77, 80, 84, 97, 126, 143
clinical application, 19, 103, 112
clinical trials, 62, 155
clone, 126, 150, 156
clustering, 149
clusters, 38, 57
CMC, 51
CO2, 143, 158
coding, 57, 72, 88, 105, 130
codon, 88, 89

collagen, 159
colon, 123, 128
colon cancer, 128
colorectal cancer, 22, 101, 102, 116, 132
combination therapy, 22
communication, 26, 29
compatibility, 81
competition, 45
complement, ix, 56, 61, 65, 69, 170
complexity, viii, 25, 133, 142
complications, 62, 67, 127, 131
composition, x, 69, 90
computer, xi, 49, 139, 140, 143, 146
conditioning, 161
conduction, 63
confounders, 62
connectivity, 40
consensus, 15, 83, 88, 95
conservation, 46, 48, 49, 51, 53
conserving, 52
construction, 48, 78, 79, 155
control group, 60, 63, 168, 169
controversies, 108
cooperation, 147
cornea, 30, 36, 93, 108
correlation, 45, 78, 126, 144
correlations, 65, 97
cost, 78
costimulatory molecules, 37, 39
crystal structure, 105, 122
CSF, 15, 20, 94
cultivation, 104, 159
culture, 97, 144
cycles, 97
cyclosporine, 96, 127, 153, 157
cysteine, 89, 123
cytokine production, viii, 55, 56, 62, 97, 125
cytokines, 19, 47, 62, 66, 67, 71, 90, 91, 93, 94, 97, 108, 121, 126, 156
cytomegalovirus, 5, 94, 99, 108, 110, 113, 114, 131, 137
cytometry, 147, 163
cytoplasm, 124, 145, 146
cytoplasmic tail, xi, 88, 89, 90, 104, 114, 123, 153
cytosine, 88
cytotoxic T-lymphocytes (CTLs), vii, 1, 2, 3, 4, 5, 7, 12, 18, 37, 74, 103, 126, 129, 131, 133, 140, 141
cytotoxicity, 90, 91, 106, 107, 122, 123, 125, 126, 127

D

database, 76, 78, 81, 84
deacetylation, 95
deep venous thrombosis, 60
defects, 19, 122, 134
defence, viii, 25, 26
deficiency, ix, 56, 114
degradation, 48, 76, 100, 114
dementia, 63, 67
dendritic cell, x, 7, 26, 28, 36, 37, 38, 39, 40, 41, 71, 87, 91, 98, 107, 112, 134
dephosphorylation, 137
deposits, 162, 164, 170
derivatives, 145
dermatitis, 128
dermatitis herpetiformis, 128
destruction, viii, 17, 44
detectable, 75, 155
detection, 13, 26, 47, 48, 94, 102, 115, 122, 160, 168
detection techniques, 26
deviation, xi, 153
Devil facial tumor disease (DFTD), viii, 43, 45, 46, 47, 48, 50, 52
diabetes, 61, 65, 125, 128
diabetic nephropathy, 62
diabetic neuropathy, 62
dilation, 97
dimerization, 89, 105, 123, 133
dimorphism, 66
discrimination, 44, 135
disease activity, 128
disease progression, 12, 75, 101, 115
diseases, vii, viii, x, 2, 7, 9, 11, 14, 43, 44, 45, 48, 50, 51, 54, 56, 60, 62, 65, 72, 76, 80, 82, 87, 93, 101, 102, 103, 116, 126, 128, 130
disequilibrium, viii, 55, 56, 61, 63, 66, 128
disorder, 127
dissociation, 40, 143
distribution, 77, 80, 82, 88, 97, 105, 144
divergence, 57
diversification, 74
diversity, vii, viii, x, 3, 13, 21, 43, 44, 45, 46, 47, 48, 49, 50, 51, 52, 53, 54, 81, 82, 88, 119, 120, 142
DNA, ix, xi, 23, 51, 56, 57, 90, 93, 95, 105, 106, 119, 137, 160, 162, 164
dogs, 46, 52, 53
donors, 4, 57, 59, 60, 61, 65, 98, 102, 137, 139, 143, 145, 155
down-regulation, 18, 19
drug design, 85
drugs, 103

E

EAE, 125

ECM, 159
ecology, 53, 82
ECs, 159, 161, 163, 165, 166
egg, 45
ELISA, 102, 159, 163
e-mail, 25
encoding, ix, 44, 56, 90, 128
endangered, 48, 50
endangered species, 50
endocrine, 112
endometrial carcinoma, 102
endothelial cells (ECs), 29, 91, 93, 106, 121, 158, 161, 162, 170
endothelium, 170
energy, 78, 79
environment, viii, x, 43, 45, 50, 63, 69, 70, 103
environmental conditions, 32
environmental factors, 93
environmental stimuli, ix, 56
enzyme, 7, 102, 141, 149
enzyme-linked immunosorbent assay, 102
enzymes, 76
epidemic, 142
epidemiology, 14, 65, 75
epigenetic modification, 93
epithelial cells, 30, 32, 35, 40, 99, 112, 113, 123
epithelial ovarian cancer, 115
epitopes, vii, x, xi, 2, 3, 7, 13, 15, 69, 71, 74, 75, 77, 83, 84, 85, 121, 124, 125, 126, 139, 140, 142, 143, 144, 146, 147, 148, 152, 154, 155
Epstein-Barr virus, 5, 94
equilibrium, 143
erythrocytes, 101, 170
erythropoietin, 137
estrogen, 95
ethnic groups, xi, 82, 119, 142
ethnicity, 57
eukaryotic, 44, 126
evidence, xi, 18, 30, 33, 34, 35, 45, 46, 49, 62, 64, 88, 120, 130, 133, 154, 164
evolution, xi, 26, 44, 50, 73, 82, 109, 119
exclusion, 60, 124
exons, 88, 123
experimental autoimmune encephalomyelitis, 125
exposure, 62, 73
extinction, 46, 48, 52, 57

F

families, 54, 57, 65
fertilization, 97, 136
fetus, x, 46, 87, 97, 126, 127
fever, 48
fiber, 159
fibroblasts, 137
filters, 159
fish, 43
fitness, viii, 43, 44, 45, 49
fluctuations, 50
fluid, 26, 60
fluorescence, 9, 105, 158
force, 49, 73
formation, 29, 30, 36, 89, 107, 141
founder effect, 49
fragments, 29, 37, 40, 92
fusion, 127, 142, 145, 146

G

ganglion, 22
gel, 157, 160, 168
gene expression, 19, 47, 63, 95, 96, 100, 109, 110, 111, 167, 168
gene promoter, 95
gene therapy, 19, 22
genes, ix, 18, 19, 21, 22, 43, 44, 48, 51, 54, 56, 57, 60, 61, 65, 66, 67, 69, 70, 71, 72, 73, 88, 90, 93, 104, 109, 120, 121, 132, 142, 170
genetic diversity, viii, 43, 45, 46, 49, 51, 53
genetic drift, 49
genetic factors, 73, 75
genetic marker, 49, 60, 75
genetics, 51, 131
genome, 49, 70, 83, 128, 140, 142, 146, 148, 149
genomics, 51, 52, 76, 82, 148
genotype, 67, 74, 83, 84, 94, 98, 99, 127, 132, 136, 138
genotyping, 46, 59, 65, 73
geometry, 84
gestation, 126, 127, 133
glioblastoma, 128
glioma, 102, 128
glucose, 22
glutamine, 143
glutathione, 63
glycine, 122
glycoproteins, 156
glycosylation, 80
GPS, 85
grants, 104
granules, 6
growth, 47, 127, 136
Guillain-Barre syndrome, 62, 66

H

HAART, 66, 96, 110
habitat, 48
haplotypes, viii, 48, 49, 55, 56, 57, 58, 59, 60, 61, 62, 63, 64, 65, 66, 82, 130
harvesting, 159
HBV infection, 99
healing, 60, 65
health, vii, xi, 48, 49, 52, 73, 104, 120, 132
heart transplantation, xi, 111, 112, 153
heat shock protein, ix, 56
height, 59, 64
hematopoietic stem cells, 140
hemoglobin, 101
hepatitis, vii, 2, 7, 14, 45, 53, 72, 82, 83, 99, 113, 114, 129, 138
hepatocellular carcinoma, 73, 101, 115
herpes, 100, 114
herpes simplex, 100
herpes simplex virus type 1, 100
herpes virus, 100, 114
histocompatibility antigens, 50, 128, 130
histology, 115
histone, 89, 93, 95
histone deacetylase, 95
history, 14, 46, 47, 52
HIV, v, ix, 4, 12, 40, 55, 56, 59, 62, 63, 64, 65, 66, 67, 72, 74, 75, 83, 96, 99, 100, 110, 113, 114, 129, 137, 138, 150
HIV/AIDS, 72
HIV-1, 40, 65, 67, 75, 83, 96, 110, 114, 137, 138
HLA-B27, 82, 150
HM, 84, 110, 114, 150
homeostasis, 140
hormone, 95, 110, 137
host, vii, 1, 2, 3, 4, 11, 21, 31, 39, 44, 45, 46, 47, 48, 49, 52, 62, 73, 83, 93, 99, 113, 127, 136, 147, 154, 161
HTLV, vii, 1, 2, 3, 4, 5, 6, 7, 8, 9, 10, 11, 12, 13, 14, 15
human genome, 70, 72, 82
human immunodeficiency virus, 38, 66, 67, 83, 96, 99, 110
human leukocyte antigen, vii, xi, 2, 3, 18, 36, 39, 71, 82, 83, 87, 97, 107, 109, 111, 113, 114, 115, 116, 117, 130, 131, 132, 137, 139
Human leukocyte antigen-F (HLA-F), x, 104, 119, 120, 122, 123, 124, 127, 128, 129, 130, 133
Human leukocyte antigen-G (HLA-G), v, x, 38, 87, 88, 89, 90, 91, 92, 93, 94, 95, 96, 97, 98, 99, 100, 101, 102, 103, 104, 105, 106, 107, 108, 109, 110, 111, 112, 113, 114, 115, 116, 117, 119, 120, 121, 122, 123, 124, 125, 126, 127, 128, 129, 130, 131, 132, 133, 134, 135, 136, 137, 138
human skin, 108
human T-cell leukemia virus-1 (HTLV-1), vii, 1, 2, 3, 4, 5, 6, 7, 8, 9, 10, 11, 12, 13, 14
hydatidiform mole, 114
hydrogen, 159
hydrogen peroxide, 159
hydrolysis, 145
hypersensitivity, 155
hypertension, 127
hypothesis, 26, 44, 46, 48, 74
hypoxia, 93, 95, 96
hypoxia-inducible factor, 96

I

ICAM, 26, 28, 30, 39
identification, viii, 55, 61, 72, 73, 74, 78, 85, 123, 140, 144, 147, 148, 170
identity, 123
IFN, 3, 6, 7, 8, 9, 10, 19, 22, 23, 47, 52, 79, 91, 93, 94, 97, 106, 109, 110, 121, 124, 125, 126, 159, 161, 163, 165
IL-8, 90
immune modulation, 107
immune reaction, 88, 103
immune regulation, 130
immune response, vii, viii, ix, xi, 1, 4, 7, 9, 11, 13, 18, 19, 20, 22, 25, 26, 32, 33, 34, 39, 40, 56, 69, 70, 71, 72, 73, 74, 75, 76, 80, 81, 88, 90, 91, 99, 106, 108, 119, 122, 123, 126, 132, 136, 139, 140, 144, 146, 147, 154
immune system, vii, viii, x, 2, 17, 18, 21, 25, 26, 35, 36, 44, 48, 52, 67, 71, 76, 80, 93, 119, 123, 128, 129, 131, 136, 140, 147, 155, 169
immunity, vii, 2, 4, 11, 13, 14, 22, 36, 54, 73, 82, 91, 107, 126, 131, 133, 134, 140, 147, 148, 151
immunization, 7, 8, 9, 10, 155, 170
immunodeficiency, 49, 83, 114
immunogen, 7
immunogenetics, 65, 137
immunogenicity, x, 69, 80, 81
immunoglobulin, 26, 38, 66, 89, 90, 123, 125, 141, 159, 161, 162, 163, 164, 168, 169, 170
immunoglobulins, 159, 169, 170
immunoinformatics, x, 69, 75, 76, 78, 80, 81
immunomodulation, 154
immunomodulatory, ix, 56, 133, 156
immunoreactivity, 94, 102
immunosuppression, 48, 121, 123, 156
immunosuppressive agent, 93
immunosuppressive drugs, 156

immunosurveillance, 21, 120, 128, 132
immunotherapeutic strategies, viii, 17, 20
immunotherapy, 7, 13, 18, 19, 20, 21, 22, 23, 96, 103, 107, 111, 117, 130, 148
imprinting, 95, 133
in situ hybridization, 105
in vitro, viii, 2, 3, 8, 10, 22, 25, 27, 30, 31, 32, 34, 61, 62, 63, 75, 76, 81, 89, 92, 95, 97, 99, 100, 107, 108, 110, 117, 136, 137, 155, 159, 165
in vivo, viii, 3, 22, 25, 27, 30, 34, 35, 36, 38, 39, 62, 63, 75, 76, 78, 81, 89, 91, 97, 107, 108, 145, 148, 170
inbreeding, 46, 49
incidence, 30, 48, 60, 62, 64, 112
indirect measure, viii, 43
individuals, viii, xi, 4, 15, 43, 46, 47, 48, 60, 61, 73, 74, 75, 83, 99, 110, 119, 120, 128
induction, vii, 1, 4, 7, 8, 12, 13, 14, 22, 34, 61, 91, 94, 95, 96, 99, 100, 103, 106, 107, 113, 123, 124, 131, 144, 154
industry, 78
INF, 127
infection, vii, viii, ix, x, 1, 2, 4, 11, 12, 14, 25, 36, 38, 66, 69, 72, 73, 74, 75, 81, 83, 87, 99, 100, 108, 113, 125, 128, 129, 134, 137, 138, 155
infectious agents, xi, 121, 129, 139, 140, 147
infectious diseases, vii, viii, x, 2, 7, 9, 11, 43, 44, 45, 51, 54, 82, 87, 93, 103
inflammation, 30, 60, 61, 62, 67, 93, 107
inflammatory bowel disease, ix, 56, 102, 125
inflammatory disease, viii, 2, 55, 62, 64, 88
inflammatory mediators, ix, 56
inflammatory responses, 44, 62
infliximab, 64
influenza, xi, 99, 113, 139, 140, 142, 143, 144, 147, 148, 151, 152
influenza virus, 99, 113, 148
inguinal, 7, 8, 10
inhibition, 19, 26, 28, 63, 90, 91, 107, 122, 169, 171
inhibitor, 66, 95, 107, 131
initiation, 60, 93, 111
injuries, xi, 153, 156
innate immunity, 19
inoculation, 46, 154
insertion, 94, 99, 109
insulin, 65, 133, 141, 149
integration, 30, 81
integrin, 30
integrity, 80, 111
intercellular adhesion molecule, 26, 28
interface, x, 29, 87, 93, 97, 105, 111, 123, 131
interference, 91
interferon, 3, 19, 22, 93, 107, 109, 111, 121, 127, 131, 138
interferon (IFN), 109
interferon gamma, 22
interferon-γ, 127
internalization, 37, 92
intervention, 26, 35, 116
intravenously, 157
intron, 63, 89, 105, 132
introns, 88
invading pathogens, viii, 25, 26, 29
inversion, 92
iron, 96
irradiation, 20, 161, 165, 168, 169
ischemia, 157
islands, 95
isolation, 14
issues, x, 52, 69, 80, 81, 101, 115

K

karyotype, 46
keratinocytes, 93, 108
kidney, 35, 98, 112, 113, 127, 136
kidney transplantation, 35
kill, x, 44, 119, 126, 148
killer cells, 22, 40, 135

L

latency, 2, 100
lead, 19, 20, 52, 90, 93, 122, 142, 147
leishmaniasis, 72
leprosy, 72
lesions, 100, 101, 116
leucine, 109
leucocyte, 99, 113, 115, 116, 117, 132, 136, 148
leukemia, vii, 1, 2, 12, 13, 14, 15, 94, 95, 110, 136
leukocytes, 35, 97, 126, 127, 136
LFA, 26, 30, 38, 39
life expectancy, 62
lifetime, 2
ligand, 4, 20, 29, 31, 36, 38, 78, 84, 89, 90, 105, 130, 133, 134, 135, 137, 156
light, 18, 75, 140
lipids, 40
liposomes, vii, 2, 7, 13, 14
liver, 73, 98, 112, 124, 127, 128, 136
liver cancer, 128
liver disease, 73
liver transplant, 98, 112
localization, ix, 56, 105

loci, ix, 44, 47, 49, 51, 56, 57, 60, 70, 71, 82, 88, 110, 121, 123, 137
locus, 44, 61, 65, 70, 71, 72, 77, 120, 121, 136
low risk, 98, 112
LTA, 57, 61, 66
lumen, 97, 145, 146
lung cancer, 94, 101, 102, 116, 117
Luo, 111, 114
lymph, 7, 8, 10, 40, 101
lymph node, 7, 8, 10, 40
lymphocytes, vii, viii, 1, 2, 6, 14, 17, 18, 36, 37, 39, 44, 71, 74, 77, 92, 100, 121, 124, 133, 140
lymphocytosis, 101, 102
lymphoid, 121, 123, 124, 125
lymphoid organs, 121
lymphoid tissue, 124, 125
lymphoma, vii, 1, 2, 12, 14, 15, 39, 94, 95, 96
lysine, 90
lysis, 19, 97, 121, 122, 123, 125, 150, 160
lysosome, 145, 146, 151

M

mAb, 160
macrophage inflammatory protein, 90
macrophages, 7, 14, 20, 26, 30, 36, 39, 62, 71, 90, 100, 106, 113, 121, 126, 145, 146, 151, 152
major histocompatibility complex (MHC), vii, viii, ix, x, xi, 7, 17, 18, 21, 26, 36, 39, 43, 51, 52, 54, 55, 65, 66, 70, 82, 84, 85, 87, 104, 109, 114, 119, 120, 130, 131, 134, 137, 140, 148, 149, 150, 151, 153
majority, 18, 102, 140, 154
malaria, 45, 52, 72, 75
malignancy, 2, 11, 53, 103
malignant cells, x, 44, 87
malignant melanoma, 19, 22, 102, 128
malignant mesothelioma, 115
malignant tumors, 155
mammal(s), 50, 95
mammalian cells, 18
mapping, 60, 61, 137
masking, 33, 73
mass, 48
materials, 84
mathematics, 76
matrix, 76, 93, 108
measles, 150
media, 159, 165
median, 2
medicine, 53
melanoma, 19, 20, 22, 94, 95, 96, 100, 105, 108, 110, 114, 123, 125, 128, 132, 134, 147, 150
mellitus, 66
membranes, xi, 30, 92, 153
memory, 33, 37, 39, 40, 147, 152
mesenchymal stem cells, 93, 99, 108, 113, 123, 126, 135
messenger ribonucleic acid, 132
metabolic changes, 63
metastasis, 101
metastatic disease, 102
methodology, 78, 80
methylation, 95
Mg^{2+}, 158
MHC class I antigen, vii, 17, 19, 22, 155, 156
MHC class II molecules, 20, 34, 35, 36, 40, 44, 140, 141, 145, 146, 149, 151, 152
mice, vii, 2, 4, 7, 8, 9, 10, 14, 18, 19, 22, 34, 35, 60, 78, 97, 111, 120, 125, 129, 134, 137, 140, 141, 148, 155
microorganism, 146
microorganisms, 145, 146
microparticles, 38
microRNA, 96
microsatellites, 60
migration, 29, 36, 57
MIP, 90
miscarriage, 97, 109
models, 20, 49, 63, 76
modifications, 72, 110
molecular biology, 111
molecular dynamics, x, 69, 78, 85
molecular targeting, 11
monomers, 89
morbidity, 66, 72, 128
morphology, 97, 112
mortality, 46, 66, 72, 148
Moses, 105
motif, 44, 90
MR, 38, 53, 111, 148, 152
mRNA, 63, 88, 89, 94, 95, 96, 104, 105, 109, 123, 124, 132, 136, 168, 172
mRNAs, 96
multiple factors, 93
multiple myeloma, 102, 117, 148
multiple sclerosis, ix, 56, 107, 125, 134
multivariate, 62, 64
multivariate analysis, 62, 64
mutation, 57, 88, 128
mutations, 48, 74
myasthenia gravis, ix, 56
myeloid cells, 123
myocardium, 164
myopathy, 2
myositis, ix, 56

N

nanotube, 30
nasopharyngeal carcinoma, 128, 137
National Academy of Sciences, 50, 51, 52, 53, 156
National Institutes of Health, 17, 147, 156
natural killer (NK) cell(s), vii, x, 17, 36, 39, 40, 87, 106, 111, 117, 121, 131, 132, 133, 137, 138
natural selection, 44
necrosis, ix, 56, 64
nematode, 45, 52
neoplasm, vii, 1
nerve, 63, 67
nerve conduction velocity, 63
neural network(s), 76, 77
neuroblastoma, 102, 117
neurological disease, 13, 66
neuronal cells, 114
neurons, 67, 100
neuropathy, 59, 62, 63, 64, 66, 67
neurotoxicity, 62, 66
neutral, 49
New England, 53
NK cells, 19, 23, 26, 28, 29, 30, 31, 34, 38, 40, 47, 90, 91, 92, 97, 106, 108, 120, 121, 123, 124, 125, 126, 127, 129, 132, 133, 134, 135, 137, 138
NMR, 77
NRT, 62, 63, 64, 67
Nuclear Magnetic Resonance, 77
null, 34, 89, 105

O

oedema, 127
omentum, 7
optimization, 125, 152
oral cavity, 46
organ, viii, xi, 25, 36, 103, 112, 120, 129, 153, 154, 155
organelle, 39
organism, 73
organize, 75
organs, 93
oryx, 49, 52
ovarian cancer, 96, 101, 137
ovarian tumor, 110
overnutrition, 67
oxygen, 96

P

pain, 62, 63
palpation, 157
pancreas, 93
parallel, 72, 141, 159
parasite, 51, 53
parasites, ix, 44, 69
paresis, 15
pathogenesis, ix, 56, 60, 62, 63, 64, 155
pathogens, viii, x, 25, 26, 29, 44, 48, 71, 74, 75, 81, 119, 120, 122, 132
pathology, 52, 103
pathophysiology, 64
pathways, ix, 4, 20, 56, 64, 80, 117, 139, 140, 144, 146, 151
PBMC, 28, 99, 144, 147
PCR, 160, 167, 168
pemphigus, 137
penicillin, 143, 158
peripheral blood, 3, 61, 91, 99, 102, 107, 113, 126, 127, 136, 137, 144
peripheral blood mononuclear cell, 3, 61, 137, 144
peripheral neuropathy, 66
permeability, 63
permission, 57, 58
pH, 31, 78, 80, 159
phagocytic cells, 13
phagocytosis, 70, 151, 152
pharmaceutical, 84
phenotype, ix, 30, 56, 73, 126, 135, 147
phenotypes, viii, 21, 55, 56, 57, 63
phosphate, 8, 158, 159
phosphatidylserine, 30, 38, 41
phosphorylation, 19
physics, 76
physiopathology, 65
placenta, 96, 97, 110, 123, 124, 125, 126, 129
plasma cells, 15
plasma levels, 67
plasma membrane, 29, 30, 33
platelets, 101
platform, 72
playing, 90, 129
pneumonitis, 100
Poland, 148
polycythemia, 128, 137
polycythemia vera, 128, 137
polymerase, xi, 74, 119
polymerase chain reaction, xi, 119
polymerization, 89
polymerization process, 89

polymorphism(s), viii, xi, ix, 44, 45, 47, 49, 51, 53, 54, 55, 56, 60, 63, 65, 67, 75, 88, 94, 96, 98, 99, 104, 109, 111, 113, 119, 120, 124, 125, 127, 128, 130, 132, 133, 136, 137, 150
polyp, 102
polypeptide, 121
population, viii, 5, 10, 43, 44, 45, 46, 47, 48, 49, 50, 51, 52, 53, 56, 57, 58, 60, 61, 64, 65, 66, 73, 74, 75, 81, 83, 98, 105, 113, 120, 142
population group, 57
population structure, 52
portal vein, 168
positive correlation, 63, 99
post-transplant, 155, 157, 168, 169
potential benefits, 19
preeclampsia, 97, 136
pregnancy, x, xi, 87, 97, 103, 106, 111, 112, 119, 120, 121, 123, 124, 126, 127, 130, 131, 135, 136
preparation, iv, 51
preservation, 83
prevention, 170
primary function, 70, 120
primary tumor, 46
priming, 14, 22, 36, 39, 40, 91, 147
principles, 36, 170
probability, 49, 58, 76, 77, 142
probe, 84
progesterone, 93, 94, 95, 109, 128, 135
prognosis, vii, x, xi, 1, 22, 87, 101, 102, 110, 114, 116, 120, 127, 131, 137
programming, 152
pro-inflammatory, ix, 56, 63, 90, 170
proliferation, 2, 3, 33, 91, 92, 97, 99, 111, 115, 123, 125, 128, 147, 155, 158, 162
promoter, 57, 63, 65, 67, 93, 94, 109, 110
prophylactic, vii, 2, 11, 13, 20
prophylaxis, vii, 1, 2, 9, 11
prostate cancer, 22
proteasome, 71, 76, 80, 84, 141, 145, 146, 149, 151
protection, ix, 2, 45, 52, 56, 65, 72, 75, 93, 129, 134, 148, 169
protective role, 74
protein sequence, xi, 76, 78, 139, 140, 143
protein structure, 78
protein synthesis, 96
proteins, vii, ix, xi, 27, 29, 31, 33, 37, 40, 44, 69, 71, 76, 78, 81, 88, 89, 93, 104, 108, 119, 121, 129, 132, 134, 141, 142, 144, 146, 150, 151, 153, 156, 159, 160, 161, 162, 165, 166, 168, 169, 170
proteinuria, 127
proteomics, 76, 82
purification, 157, 160, 168
purity, 157, 168

Q

quality of life, 62

R

rabies virus, 99, 100, 113, 114
radiation, 23, 39
radiotherapy, 20
reactions, 155
reactive arthritis, 126
reactivity, 66, 80, 83, 84, 85, 92, 139, 144, 147, 148
reading, 89
receptors, x, xi, 4, 19, 20, 27, 30, 31, 32, 33, 38, 39, 40, 62, 64, 65, 66, 67, 87, 89, 90, 91, 92, 97, 103, 106, 119, 121, 122, 123, 124, 125, 128, 129, 131, 133, 134, 135, 138
recognition, vii, viii, x, 4, 12, 13, 15, 17, 19, 25, 38, 39, 44, 46, 48, 49, 50, 61, 69, 74, 75, 78, 81, 83, 106, 120, 122, 127, 130, 131, 132, 134, 135, 138, 140, 150, 154
reconstruction, 85
recruiting, 92
recurrence, 101, 155
red blood cells, 120
redistribution, 33
reflexes, 62
Registry, 65
regression, 52, 64
regression model, 64
regulations, 17, 20
rejection, viii, ix, xi, 25, 40, 43, 44, 46, 52, 56, 98, 99, 111, 112, 126, 127, 136, 153, 154, 155, 156, 157, 162, 164, 169, 170
relevance, x, 35, 41, 87, 88, 97, 101, 115, 116, 117, 132, 137
remission, 102, 125
renal cell carcinoma, 101, 110, 116, 117, 128
replication, ix, 56, 62, 83
repression, 95, 96, 110
reproduction, x, 46, 87, 88, 97, 131, 135
requirements, 70, 81, 154
researchers, 73, 76, 102
resection, 115
residues, x, 44, 69, 81, 85, 89, 90, 91, 121, 123, 124, 141, 154, 155
resistance, 43, 45, 53, 54, 61, 114
resolution, x, 69, 73, 134, 136
response, viii, ix, xi, 7, 11, 12, 15, 19, 20, 23, 25, 26, 29, 32, 33, 35, 56, 70, 71, 73, 75, 77, 82, 83, 90, 93, 94, 95, 96, 106, 109, 110, 111, 119, 126, 135, 137, 144, 145, 146, 153, 154, 162, 165, 170

responsiveness, 22
restoration, 65
restrictions, 74
reticulum, 76, 81, 105, 141
retinopathy, 62
retrovirus, 14
reverse transcriptase, 62, 160
rheumatoid arthritis, ix, 56, 57, 60, 64, 65, 96, 111
risk, viii, 2, 3, 48, 49, 55, 56, 62, 63, 64, 66, 67, 111, 127, 128, 136, 138
risk factors, 3, 62, 64, 66
RNA, 48, 74, 75, 99, 100, 103, 159, 160, 165, 166
root, 22, 66
routes, 109, 145
Royal Society, 50, 53

S

saliva, xi, 153
Salmonella, 125, 126, 129, 134, 135
salt concentration, 80
SARS, 54, 142, 149
saturation, 143
schistosomiasis, 72
scope, 71
SDS-PAGE, 157, 160, 168
secrete, 39, 40, 92, 108, 112, 126, 136
secretion, 39, 40, 90, 97, 106, 111, 113, 127
segregation, 38, 144
sensations, 63
sensitivity, 20, 67
septic shock, ix, 56
sequencing, 47, 48
serum, xi, 14, 62, 63, 98, 101, 111, 112, 114, 123, 127, 128, 132, 136, 143, 153, 155, 156, 157, 158, 159, 160, 161, 162, 163, 164, 165, 166, 167, 168, 169, 170
services, iv, 31, 142, 145, 147
severe acute respiratory syndrome, 48
sex, 101
sheep, 45
shellfish, 54
shock, 93, 121
side chain, 79
signal peptide, 122, 124, 127, 131
signal transduction, 19, 107, 121
signaling pathway, 90, 92, 106, 107
signals, 19, 44, 92, 125, 134
signs, 127, 164
simulation, 49, 51, 85
simulations, 84
smallpox, 139, 143
smoking, 67
smooth muscle, 93, 95, 109
smooth muscle cells, 93, 95, 109
SNP, 57, 58, 59, 60, 61, 63, 64, 65
sodium, 95
software, 79, 160
solid tumors, x, 87, 100, 101, 123
solution, 80, 158
somatic cell, 18
South America, 2
spastic, 2, 12, 13, 15
species, viii, 43, 44, 45, 48, 49, 53, 112, 126, 170
sperm, 97
spin, 157, 168
spleen, 7, 8, 35, 124, 150, 158, 166
spontaneous abortion, 97, 127, 155
squamous cell, 101, 102, 116
squamous cell carcinoma, 101, 102, 116
stability, x, 31, 34, 69, 78, 80, 94, 109
stabilization, 125
state, xi, 3, 15, 27, 31, 70, 85, 124, 126, 153, 155
stimulation, 8, 10, 32, 33, 35, 38, 61, 75, 80, 91, 92, 94, 126, 166
stimulus, 32, 33, 99
stress, 48, 49, 93, 96, 112, 121, 130
stressors, 93
stromal cells, 93, 108
structure, viii, 44, 46, 49, 52, 55, 57, 65, 72, 76, 77, 78, 79, 82, 88, 89, 90, 91, 104, 105, 122
subcutaneous injection, 40
substitution, 74, 85, 122
substitutions, 74
Sun, 117, 134, 149, 152
suppression, 32, 63, 88, 90, 96, 103, 107, 135, 155, 166, 170
surveillance, vii, ix, 17, 18, 28, 53, 69, 71, 140, 151
survival, vii, xi, 1, 2, 17, 19, 49, 53, 101, 102, 125, 126, 127, 153, 154, 156, 157, 161, 168, 169, 170
survival rate, 101
susceptibility, viii, 55, 56, 57, 60, 61, 64, 65, 66, 70, 72, 115, 128, 137
symptoms, 46
synapse, 29, 30, 32, 33, 36, 37, 39, 40, 81, 107, 134
syndrome, 2, 12, 14, 15, 60, 98, 100, 114
synthesis, 141, 159, 165, 168, 171
systemic lupus erythematosus, ix, 56, 128

T

T cell receptor (TCR), 4, 27, 36, 38, 90, 133, 140, 154
T cells, vii, viii, x, 1, 3, 4, 5, 7, 9, 10, 12, 13, 18, 19, 23, 25, 26, 27, 28, 29, 30, 31, 32, 33, 34, 36, 37, 38, 39, 40, 41, 44, 47, 48, 87, 91, 92, 99, 100,

101, 103, 107, 108, 113, 116, 119, 120, 121, 123, 124, 125, 126, 127, 128, 129, 130, 131, 132, 133, 134, 135, 136, 137, 138, 139, 140, 141, 143, 144, 147, 148, 150, 151, 152, 154, 156, 158, 165, 166, 170
T lymphocytes, vii, ix, 6, 12, 13, 15, 17, 37, 38, 40, 46, 69, 70, 83, 90, 100, 107, 114, 121, 130, 132, 137, 140, 150, 152, 154
T regulatory cells, 107
tactics, vii, 17
tamoxifen, 128
TAP, 71, 76, 80, 84, 121, 124, 132, 133, 141, 143, 145, 146, 151
target, vii, x, 1, 2, 7, 8, 10, 28, 29, 30, 34, 36, 37, 38, 40, 43, 73, 75, 80, 87, 92, 93, 103, 106, 117, 125, 148, 158, 161, 163
T-cell receptor, 141, 155
technology, 140, 142, 145
temperature, 78
testing, 97
testis, 149
Th cells, 170
therapeutic agents, 96
therapeutic effects, 18
therapy, x, 2, 7, 11, 14, 62, 87, 96, 100, 103, 107, 111, 114, 147, 148, 156, 161, 162, 163, 164, 170, 171
thermodynamics, 135
thymus, 32, 34, 93, 124, 125, 126, 134, 150, 154
tissue, 48, 88, 93, 100, 104, 108, 136, 158, 160, 162, 167, 168
TLR4, 7, 9
TNF, v, viii, 6, 20, 22, 55, 56, 57, 59, 60, 61, 62, 63, 64, 65, 66, 67, 90
TNF block haplotypes, viii, 55, 56, 57, 60, 61, 63, 64, 65, 66
TNF-alpha, 20, 65, 66, 67
TNF-α, ix, 6, 56, 62
topology, 77, 79, 80
toxicity, 62
transcription, 67, 93, 95, 96, 109, 131, 132, 168, 170
transcription factors, 67, 168
transcripts, 48, 88, 89, 93, 96, 104, 127, 132
transduction, 19
transfection, 121
transferrin, 33
transformation, 14, 21, 114, 128
transforming growth factor, 91
transfusion, 156
transitional cell carcinoma, 116, 128
transmembrane region, 89, 141
transmissible cancer, viii, 43, 53
transmission, 2, 40, 48, 52, 53, 76
transplant, ix, x, xi, 56, 87, 96, 98, 103, 111, 112, 113, 127, 136, 153, 154, 156, 167, 168, 170, 171
transplant recipients, 96, 98, 112, 168
transplantation, vii, viii, x, xi, 11, 12, 25, 29, 34, 35, 36, 43, 81, 87, 88, 98, 103, 112, 113, 120, 129, 136, 137, 153, 154, 155, 157, 161, 162, 165, 168, 169
transport, 34, 39, 76, 80, 151
transportation, 81, 142
treatment, vii, 1, 2, 11, 14, 46, 64, 65, 74, 94, 95, 96, 100, 110, 112, 114, 127, 128, 136, 137, 147, 155, 157, 161, 164, 170
trichostatin A, 95
triggers, 19, 92, 133
tuberculosis, ix, xi, 56, 72, 126, 134, 135, 139, 140, 142, 143, 144, 145, 147, 148
tumo(u)r(s), v, vii, viii, x, 1, 2, 4, 7, 9, 11, 12, 13, 17, 18, 19, 20, 21, 22, 23, 40, 41, 43, 45, 46, 47, 48, 51, 52, 53, 55, 65, 66, 67, 87, 88, 90, 91, 92, 93, 100, 101, 103, 107, 110, 111, 115, 116, 120, 125, 128, 130, 131, 132, 134, 136, 140, 142, 156
tumor cells, viii, 18, 19, 20, 22, 23, 43, 46, 47, 48, 92, 93, 103, 111, 132, 140
tumor development, vii, 17, 18
tumor escape, viii, 4, 17, 21, 107, 136
tumor growth, 47, 100, 134
tumor necrosis factor, viii, 55, 65, 66, 67, 90, 93
tumour necrosis factor (TNF), v, viii, 6, 20, 22, 55, 56, 57, 59, 60, 61, 62, 63, 64, 65, 66, 67, 90
tunneling, 40
Turkey, 99
turnover, 88, 159, 166
type 1 diabetes, 66, 67, 131
Type 1 Diabetes Mellitus (T1DM), ix, 56, 60, 61, 62, 63
type 2 diabetes, 67
typhoid, 135
tyrosine, 90, 92

U

ulcer, 65
underlying mechanisms, 64, 169
unique features, 90
urine, xi, 153
uveitis, 2

V

vaccine, vii, x, 2, 7, 9, 15, 41, 46, 69, 75, 81, 83, 135, 142, 149
validation, 149

variations, ix, 56, 57, 62, 64, 120, 122, 128
vascularization, 97
vasculitis, 128
velocity, 63
venous insufficiency, 60
venules, 134
vertebrate classes, 43
vertebrates, 43, 51
viral infection, viii, ix, 4, 21, 25, 69, 72, 74, 81, 88, 99, 100, 103, 114
virology, 83, 84
virus infection, 45, 53, 83, 99, 113, 114
viruses, ix, x, 54, 69, 71, 74, 81, 99, 119, 125, 148
vision, 84
visualization, 76, 82
vulnerability, 53

W

water, 85
wells, 159, 165
Western blot, 124, 160
whales, 53
wild animals, 48
wild type, 34, 154
wildlife, vii, viii, 43, 45, 48, 49
wildlife conservation, viii, 43, 45
World Health Organization (WHO), 88
worldwide, 2, 81, 142

X

xenotransplantation, 131